EMERGENCY MEDICINE

DIAGNOSIS AND MANAGEMENT

Seventh edition

Anthony F. T. Brown

MB ChB, FRCP, FRCS(Ed), FRCEM, FACEM
Professor
Discipline of Anaesthesiology and Critical Care
School of Medicine MD Program
University of Queensland, Brisbane.
Senior Staff Specialist (Pre-eminent)
Department of Emergency Medicine
Royal Brisbane and Women's Hospital
Brisbane.
Past Editor-in-Chief
Emergency Medicine Australasia.
Senior Court of Examiners
Australasian College for Emergency Medicine (ACEM).
Inaugural ACEM Teaching Excellence Award 2001.

Mike D. Cadogan

MA(Oxon), MB ChB (Ed), FACEM
Staff Specialist in Emergency Medicine
Department of Emergency Medicine
Sir Charles Gairdner Hospital
Perth.
Chief Medical Editor and Co-Founder
Lifeinthefastlane.com
Winner, Gold Medal/Buchanan Prize
ACEM Fellowship Exam 2003.

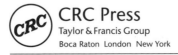
CRC Press
Taylor & Francis Group
Boca Raton London New York

CRC Press is an imprint of the
Taylor & Francis Group, an **informa** business

CRC Press
Taylor & Francis Group
6000 Broken Sound Parkway NW, Suite 300
Boca Raton, FL 33487-2742

© 2016 by Taylor & Francis Group, LLC
CRC Press is an imprint of Taylor & Francis Group, an Informa business

No claim to original U.S. Government works

Printed on acid-free paper
Version Date: 20151207

Printed and bound in India by Replika Press Pvt. Ltd.

International Standard Book Number-13: 978-1-4987-1427-3 (Paperback)

Visit the Taylor & Francis Web site at
http://www.taylorandfrancis.com

and the CRC Press Web site at
http://www.crcpress.com

DEDICATION

To Edward, with love, admiration and my highest regard from a proud father. I hope this book inspires your fascination and respect for medicine as much as it does mine.

A.F.T.B.

To the most important people in my life, William, Hamish and Olivia, this book is for you. Your strength, love, support, and pure extraordinariness leave a legacy beyond the imagining.

M.D.C.

CONTENTS

Section III ACID–BASE, ELECTROLYTE AND RENAL EMERGENCIES

Section IV INFECTIOUS DISEASE AND FOREIGN TRAVEL EMERGENCIES

Section V SURGICAL EMERGENCIES

Section VI ORTHOPAEDIC EMERGENCIES

Section VII MUSCULOSKELETAL AND SOFT-TISSUE EMERGENCIES

Section XI ENT EMERGENCIES

Section XII MAXILLOFACIAL AND DENTAL EMERGENCIES

Section XIII PSYCHIATRIC EMERGENCIES

Section XIV TOXICOLOGY

Section XVII ADMINISTRATIVE AND LEGAL ISSUES

Section XVIII PRACTICAL PROCEDURES

PREFACE TO THE 7TH EDITION OF
EMERGENCY MEDICINE

Updates, changes and new additions have been made throughout this 7th edition, which incorporates the very latest ideas and evidence base underpinning best practice emergency medicine care. The whole text has been updated to include the latest 2015 international consensus guidelines on Cardiopulmonary Resuscitation and Emergency Cardiovascular Care, through to new 2014 case definitions for HIV. The sections on General Medical Emergencies, Surgical Emergencies, Paediatric Emergencies and Infectious Disease and Foreign Travel Emergencies in particular have been expanded with new topics, tables and practical tips.

A standardized approach to each and every condition has been retained with the text consistently formatted to maximize ease of use and the practical delivery of care. This edition is as much aimed at the bedside as it is for studying.

The text is again supported by a wealth of additional online material at **http://lifeinthefastlane.com/**. This includes high-resolution clinical images, videos, case-based questions, examination material and links to online references, all available for *free*.

The emergency department is rightly regarded as the 'front door' to the hospital. No matter how busy or time-pressured you may be, or how much inpatient beds are at a premium, each new patient deserves quality care from the moment he or she arrives. We hope this new edition helps you deliver on this promise.

Anthony F T Brown
Mike Cadogan
November 2015

ACKNOWLEDGEMENTS

Special thanks in particular to Dr Kate Edgworth and Dr Jamie Thomas for their invaluable expert contributions on Paediatrics, and to Dr Peter Logan on the Major Incident and Dr Tor Ercleve for his fine illustrations.

In addition, our special thanks to Stephen Clausard, Editor, CRC Press, Taylor & Francis Group for his outstanding and professional assistance, advice and ongoing responsibility that made this new edition possible. Also to Alice Oven, Senior Editor in the UK, and particularly to Linda Van Pelt, Senior Project Manager – Medical in the US for her truly amazing ability to make the production stages so smooth. We could not have asked to work in a more responsive or encouraging partnership.

Tony Brown and Mike Cadogan
November 2015

Section I

CRITICAL CARE EMERGENCIES

CARDIOPULMONARY RESUSCITATION

INITIAL APPROACH

DIAGNOSIS

1   Cardiopulmonary resuscitation (CPR) is required if a collapsed person is unresponsive, not breathing, and has no palpable pulse in a large artery such as the carotid or femoral.
    (i)   The following may also be seen:
          (a) occasional, ineffectual (agonal) gasps
          (b) pallor or cyanosis
          (c) dilated pupils
          (d) brief tonic grand mal seizure.

2   Sudden cardiac arrest still causes over 60% of deaths from coronary heart disease in adults.

MANAGEMENT

1   This is based on the International Liaison Committee on Resuscitation (ILCOR) 2015 International Consensus on CPR and ECC Science with Treatment Recommendations (CoSTR).
    (i)   The first person calls for help to arrange arrival of additional people and equipment, then assists with the resuscitation.
    (ii) The second person on the scene stays with the patient, checks for danger and commences resuscitation, making a note of the time.

2   **Immediate actions**
    The aim is to maintain oxygenation of the brain and myocardium until a stable cardiac output is achieved.
    (i)   Lay the patient flat on a hard surface such as a trolley. If the patient is on the floor and enough people are available, lift the patient onto a trolley to facilitate the resuscitation procedure.
    (ii) Rapidly give a single, sharp precordial thump within the first few seconds of the onset of a witnessed or monitored arrest, where the rhythm is pulseless ventricular tachycardia (pVT) or ventricular fibrillation (VF), and a defibrillator is not immediately to hand.
    (iii) Check the victim for a response, and then open the airway by tilting the head and lifting the chin if there is no response ('head tilt, chin lift'):
          (a) this prevents the tongue from occluding the larynx
          (b) look, listen and feel for breathing for no more than 10 s, while keeping the airway open.
    (iv) If breathing is not normal or absent, check for signs of a circulation:
          (a) assess a large pulse such as the carotid or femoral, or look for signs of life for no more than 10 s.

    (v)   Start CPR immediately if there are no signs of life:
       (a) commence external cardiac massage
       (b) commence assisted ventilation.

3   External cardiac massage

    (i)   Place the heel of one hand in the centre of the patient's chest. Place the heel of the other hand on top, interlocking the fingers.

    (ii)   Keeping the arms straight and applying a vertical compression force, depress the sternum 5–6 cm at a rate of at least 100 compressions/min (but not exceeding 120/min):
       (a) release all the pressure on the chest without losing contact with the sternum after each compression
       (b) do not apply pressure over the upper abdomen, lower end of sternum or the ribs, and take equal time for compression and for release.

    (iii) Perform 30 compressions, which should create a palpable femoral pulse.

    (iv) Use a one- or two-hand technique to compress the lower half of the sternum in small children by approximately one-third of its depth, at a rate of at least 100 compressions/min but not greater than 120/min:
       (a) use a two-handed encircling technique in infants, also at a rate of at least 100/min (see p. 290).

Warning: avoid using excessive or malpositioned force causing rib fractures, flail chest, liver lacerations, etc.

4   Assisted ventilation

    (i)   Open the airway again using head tilt and chin lift.

    (ii)   Start mouth-to-mouth/nose or mouth-to-mask respiration without delay if breathing is absent, using a pocket mask such as the Laerdal.

    (iii) Deliver two effective rescue breaths that should be completed within 5 s total time, and immediately resume compressions.

    (iv) Use a bag-valve mask setup such as an Ambu or Laerdal bag with oxygen reservoir attached and face mask instead, if trained in the technique
       (a) quickly look in the mouth and remove any obstruction with forceps or suction. Leave well-fitting dentures in place
       (b) or try inserting an oropharyngeal (Guedel) airway if necessary
       (c) check for leaks around the mask or convert to a two-person technique if the chest fails to inflate
       (d) consider possible obstruction of the upper airway, if ventilation is still ineffective (see p. 13).

> **Warning:** adequate oxygenation is achieved by the above measures. Endotracheal intubation should *only* be attempted by those who are trained, competent and experienced.

5 **Basic life support: external cardiac massage with assisted ventilation**

    (i)   Continue with chest compressions and rescue breaths in a ratio of 30:2.

    (ii)   Change the person providing chest compressions every 2 min, but ensure minimum interruption to compressions during the changeover.

6 **Defibrillation**

    (i)   As soon as the defibrillator arrives, apply self-adhesive pads or paddles to the patient whilst continuing chest compressions

       (a) rapidly shave excessive male chest hair, without delay

       (b) place one self-adhesive defibrillation pad or conventional paddle to the right of the sternum below the clavicle, and the other adhesive pad or paddle in the mid-axillary line level with the V6 electrocardiogram (ECG) electrode or female breast

       (c) avoid positioning self-adhesive pads or paddles over an ECG electrode, medication patch, or implanted device, e.g. pacemaker or automatic cardioverter defibrillator.

    (ii)   Analyse the rhythm with a brief pause, and charge the defibrillator if the rhythm is VF or pulseless VT. Continue chest compressions until fully charged.

    (iii) Quickly ensure that all rescuers are clear, then give the patient an immediate 150–200 J direct current (DC) shock using a biphasic waveform defibrillator (all modern defibrillators are now biphasic)

       (a) minimize the delay in delivering the shock, which should take less than 5 s

       (b) ensure good electrical contact is made when applying manual paddles by using gel pads or electrode jelly, and apply firm pressure of 8 kg force in adults.

    (iv) Immediately resume chest compressions without reassessing the rhythm or feeling for a pulse.

    (v)   The *only* exception is when VF is witnessed in a patient already connected to a manual defibrillator, or during cardiac catheterization, and/or early post-cardiac surgery

       (a) use a stacked, three-shock strategy rapidly delivering three shocks in a row *before* starting chest compressions.

    (vi) Continue external chest compressions and assisted ventilation for 2 min, then pause briefly to assess the rhythm again.

7 Observe one of four possible traces (see Fig. 1.1 for a rapid overview of treatment):

   (i) Shockable rhythms such as VF (see p. 7) or pulseless VT (see p. 7).

   (ii) Non-shockable rhythms such as asystole (see p. 8) and pulseless electrical activity (PEA) (see p. 8).

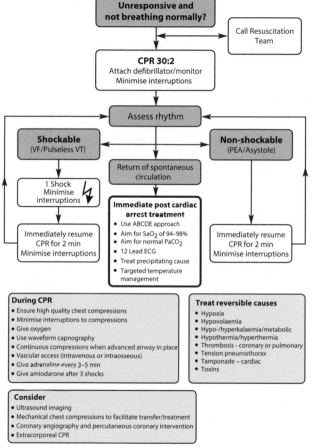

Figure 1.1 **Adult advanced life support algorithm**. ABCDE, Airway, Breathing, Circulation, Disability, Exposure; CPR, cardiopulmonary resuscitation; ECG, electrocardiogram; $PaCO_2$, partial pressure carbon dioxide in arterial blood; PEA, pulseless electrical activity; SaO_2, oxygen saturation; VF/Pulseless VT, ventricular fibrillation/pulseless ventricular tachycardia.

Reproduced with kind permission from European Resuscitation Council (2015) European Resuscitation Council Guidelines for Resuscitation 2015. Section 1. Executive summary. *Resuscitation* **95**: 1–80.

8   Establish an initial i.v. line in the antecubital fossa.

    (i)   Give at least 20 mL of normal saline to flush any drugs administered, that are given after the third DC shock.

    (ii)   Elevate the limb for 10–20 s to facilitate drug delivery to the central circulation.

    (iii)   Establish a second i.v. line unless the cardiac resuscitation is rapidly successful

        (a)   ideally this line should be inserted into a central vein, either the external or internal jugular or the subclavian

        (b)   a central line should *only* be inserted by a skilled doctor, as inadvertent arterial puncture, haemothorax or pneumothorax may invalidate further resuscitation attempts

        (c)   also, the central venous route poses additional serious hazards should thrombolytic therapy be indicated

        (d)   all drugs are then given via this central line.

9   **Endotracheal intubation**

A skilled doctor with airway training may insert a cuffed endotracheal tube (see p. 466). This maintains airway patency, prevents regurgitation with inhalation of vomit or blood from the mouth or stomach, and allows lung ventilation without interrupting chest compressions.

    (i)   Confirm correct endotracheal tube placement by seeing the tube pass between the vocal cords, and by observing bilateral chest expansion, and auscultating the lung fields and over the epigastrium.

    (ii)   Immediately connect an exhaled carbon dioxide detection device such as a waveform capnograph, and look for a tracing, as the signs above are not completely reliable.

    (iii)   Never delay CPR to intubate the airway except for a brief pause in chest compressions of not more than 10 s, as the tube is passed between the vocal cords.

    (iv)   Once the airway has been secured, continue cardiac compressions uninterrupted at a rate of at least 100/min, and ventilate the lungs at 10 breaths/min (without any need now to pause for the chest compressions)

        (a)   take care not to hyperventilate the patient at too fast a rate.

10   Subsequent management depends on the cardiac rhythm and the patient's condition. Keep the ECG monitor attached to the patient at all times.

DEFINITIVE CARE

DIAGNOSIS

The ECG trace will show shockable rhythms such as VF or pulseless VT, or non-shockable rhythms such as asystole or PEA (see Fig. 1.1).

MANAGEMENT

1   Ventricular fibrillation or pulseless ventricular tachycardia

VF is asynchronous, chaotic ventricular depolarization and repolarization producing no cardiac output. Pulseless VT is a wide-complex, regular tachycardia associated with no clinically detectable cardiac output.

   (i)   Give a DC shock once VF/pVT is confirmed on the monitor:
         (a) deliver 150–200 J using a biphasic defibrillator
         (b) deliver this shock with less than 5 s delay to cardiac compressions.

   (ii) Immediately resume CPR, continuing with chest compressions to ventilations at a ratio of 30:2, if the airway has not yet been secured
         (a) do **not** delay CPR by reassessing the rhythm or feeling for a pulse
         (b) perform compressions at 100/min and ventilations at 10/min without interruption if the airway has been secured by now.

   (iii) Continue CPR for 2 min, then briefly pause to reassess the rhythm on the monitor
         (a) if there is still VF/VT, give a second DC shock of 150–360 J biphasic
         (b) immediately resume CPR after this shock.

   (iv) Briefly pause after another 2 min of CPR to check the monitor:
         (a) give by a third shock of 150–360 J biphasic and resume CPR.

   (v)   Continue compressions and give:
         (a) 10 mL of 1 in 10 000 adrenaline (epinephrine) (1 mg) i.v.
         (b) a bolus of amiodarone 300 mg i.v. diluted in 5% dextrose to a volume of 20 mL if VF/pVT persist.

2   Irrespective of the arrest rhythm, give additional 1 in 10 000 adrenaline (epinephrine) 1 mg (10 mL) every 3–5 min until return of spontaneous circulation (ROSC).

   (i)   This will be once every two cycles of the algorithm (see Fig. 1.1).

   (ii) Meanwhile continue providing CPR and make sure to change the person performing cardiac compressions every 2 min, to preserve optimum efficacy.

3   Continue the drug–shock–CPR–rhythm check sequence.

   (i)   Analyse the rhythm again after another 2 min of CPR:
         (a) immediately deliver a fourth shock if still in VF/pVT.

4   Look for signs of life suggesting ROSC, or palpate for a pulse once a non-shockable rhythm is present with regular or narrow complexes.

   (i)   Resume CPR if the pulse is absent or difficult to feel.

   (ii) Begin post-resuscitation care when a strong pulse is felt, or the patient shows signs of life suggesting ROSC. See page 11.

5   During this period of CPR:
    (i)   If not already done:
          (a) check the defibrillator pad or paddle position and contact
          (b) attempt/verify the endotracheal tube position, and successful
              i.v. access
          (c) review all potentially reversible causes. See the '*4 Hs*' and the
              '*4 Ts*' on next page (point 7).

Tip: if venous access is impossible, insert an intraosseous cannula,
particularly in children (see p. 291).

    (ii) Consider the following drugs even though there are no data in
          support of their increasing survival to hospital discharge:
          (a) *amiodarone* – give initial bolus of 300 mg i.v. after the third
              shock, repeated once at a dose of 150 mg for recurrent or
              refractory VF/VT. Follow with an infusion of 900 mg over 24 h
          (b) *lignocaine (lidocaine)* – give initial bolus of 1 mg/kg i.v.
              if amiodarone is unavailable, followed by 0.5 mg/kg if
              necessary. Omit if amiodarone has been given
          (c) *magnesium* – give 2 g (8 mmol or 4 mL) of 49.3% magnesium
              sulphate i.v., particularly in torsades de pointes, or for
              suspected hypomagnesaemia such as a patient on a
              potassium-losing diuretic, and for digoxin toxicity. Repeat
              the dose after 10–15 min if ineffective.
    (iii) Consider buffering agent:
          (a) *8.4% sodium bicarbonate* – particular indications are for
              life-threatening hyperkalaemia or tricyclic antidepressant
              overdose (see p. 134 and p. 401)
          (b) give 50 mmol (50 mL) i.v., then as guided by arterial blood
              gases (ABGs).

6   **Asystole or pulseless electrical activity**
    These are non-shockable rhythms. See Figure 1.1 for a rapid overview of
    treatment.
    (i)   Asystole is absence of any cardiac electrical activity
          (a) make sure the ECG leads are not disconnected or broken
              by observing the cardiac compressions artefact on the ECG
              screen during CPR
          (b) check appropriate ECG lead selection and gain setting,
              without stopping chest compressions or ventilation
          (c) do *not* rely on a gel pad–manual paddle combination to
              diagnose asystole, but use independent ECG electrodes
          (d) continue chest compressions and ventilation if there is
              difficulty in differentiating from fine VF, in an attempt to
              'coarsen' unsuspected VF.

(ii) Pulseless electrical activity (PEA) was formerly known as electromechanical dissociation. It is the presence of a coordinated electrical rhythm *without* detectable cardiac output

    (a) survival is unlikely unless a reversible cause can be found and treated. See the '*4 Hs*' and the '*4 Ts*' below.

(iii) Asystole and PEA have a poor prognosis because defibrillation is of no use

    (a) continue CPR at a compression/ventilation (C/V) ratio of 30:2, unless the airway has been secured, in which case give compressions at a rate of 100/min and ventilations at a rate of 10/min

    (b) give 1 in 10 000 adrenaline (epinephrine) 1 mg (10 mL) i.v.

    (c) recheck the rhythm after 2 min of CPR. If organized with a palpable pulse, begin post-resuscitation care

    (d) resume CPR immediately if asystole or PEA persist

    (e) give repeated 1 in 10 000 adrenaline (epinephrine) 1 mg (10 mL) every 3–5 min, i.e. every second cycle of the algorithm (see Fig. 1.1)

    (f) continue CPR unless the rhythm changes to VF/VT. If VF is identified midway through a 2-min cycle, complete that cycle of CPR before shock delivery.

7 Potentially reversible causes: the *4 Hs* and the *4 Ts*.

Always look out for the following conditions, which may precipitate cardio-respiratory arrest and/or decrease the chances of a successful resuscitation (see Fig. 1.1).

(i) *Hypoxaemia*

    (a) make sure maximal up to 100% oxygen is being delivered at 15 L/min

    (b) confirm ventilation at 500–600 mL tidal volume (6–7 mL/kg) is creating a visible rise and fall of both sides of the chest.

(ii) *Hypovolaemia*

    (a) major blood loss following trauma, gastrointestinal haemorrhage, ruptured aortic aneurysm or ruptured ectopic pregnancy may cause cardiac arrest

    (b) alternatively severe vasodilation from anaphylaxis or sepsis may be responsible

    (c) consider these in any case of unexplained cardiovascular collapse

    (d) get senior emergency department (ED) help, and search for a source of bleeding, such as by abdominal ultrasound

    (e) give warmed fluid replacement and call the surgical, vascular, or obstetrics and gynaecology team as appropriate.

(iii) *Hyper/hypokalaemia, hypocalcaemia, acidaemia and other metabolic disorders*

    (a) rapidly check the potassium and calcium initially as suggested by the medical history, e.g. in renal failure (see p. 143)

       (b) give 10% calcium chloride 10 mL i.v. for hyperkalaemia, hypocalcaemia or calcium-channel blocking drug overdose

       (c) give a bolus of potassium 5 mmol i.v. for hypokalaemia.

(iv) *Hypothermia*

       (a) check the core temperature particularly in any drowning or exposure incident (see p. 435)

       (b) moderate (29–32°C) or severe (under 29°C) hypothermia will require heroic measures such as active core re-warming with warmed pleural, peritoneal or gastric lavage, or even extracorporeal re-warming, when a patient is in cardiac arrest (see p. 434)

       (c) get a senior ED doctor's help. Do not cease CPR until the temperature is at least 33°C, or the team leader determines futility.

(v) *Tension pneumothorax*

       (a) tension usually follows a traumatic rather than a spontaneous pneumothorax, particularly if positive-pressure ventilation is used

       (b) it results in extreme respiratory distress and circulatory collapse. It may follow attempts at central venous cannulation

       (c) the patient becomes increasingly breathless and cyanosed, and develops a tachycardia with hypotension
  - there is decreased chest expansion on the affected side, a hyper-resonant percussion note, and absent or diminished breath sounds
  - the trachea is displaced towards the other side, and the neck veins are usually distended

       (d) this is a life-threatening situation requiring immediate relief, **without** waiting for a chest radiograph (CXR)

       (e) insert a wide-bore needle or cannula through the second intercostal space in the mid-clavicular line. This will be followed by a rush of air outwards (see p. 471)

       (f) insert an intercostal drain (see p. 473).

(vi) *Tamponade*

       (a) cardiac tamponade may follow trauma, usually penetrating, myocardial infarction, dissecting aneurysm or pericarditis

       (b) there is hypotension, tachycardia, pulsus paradoxus and engorged neck veins that rise on inspiration (Kussmaul's sign). The heart sounds are quiet, the apex beat is impalpable and PEA may ensue

       (c) arrange an immediate focused ultrasound to demonstrate pericardial fluid

       (d) perform pericardiocentesis if the patient is *in extremis*. Insert a cardiac needle between the angle of the xiphisternum and the left costal margin at 45° to the horizontal, aiming for the left shoulder (see p. 475)

(d) sometimes aspirating as little as 50 mL restores the cardiac output, although immediate resuscitative thoracotomy is usually indicated in cases resulting from trauma (see p. 187).

(vii) *Toxins/poisons/drugs*

(a) many substances cause cardiorespiratory arrest following accidental or deliberate ingestion, such as poisoning with tricyclic antidepressants (see p. 401), calcium-channel blocking drugs (see p. 410) or β-blockers (see p. 409), and hydrofluoric acid burns (see p. 417)

(b) consider these based on the history, recognize early, and treat supportively or with antidotes where available.

(viii) *Thromboembolism with mechanical circulatory obstruction*

(a) perform external cardiac massage, which may break up a massive pulmonary embolus (PE), and give a fluid load of 20 mL/kg

(b) give thrombolysis such as alteplase (recombinant tissue plasminogen activator [rt-PA]) 100 mg i.v. if clinical suspicion is high and there are no absolute contraindications

(c) consider performing CPR for at least another 60–90 min before termination of the resuscitation.

8 The prognosis is usually hopeless if a patient is still in asystole. However, consider pacing if P waves or any other electrical activity, such as a severe bradycardia, are present with poor perfusion:

(i) Use an external (transcutaneous) pacemaker to maintain the cardiac output until a transvenous wire is inserted.

(ii) A temporary transvenous pacemaker wire should ideally be passed under X-ray guidance, but may be inserted blind via a central vein.

9 **Post-resuscitation care**

It is important to continue effective CPR until the heartbeat is strong enough to produce a peripheral pulse, and/or there are signs of life.

(i) Titrate oxygen delivery to maintain oxygen saturation 94–98%. Avoid hyperoxaemia.

(ii) Check the ABG to exclude hypocarbia from over-ventilation, which causes cerebral vasoconstriction with decreased cerebral blood flow

(a) adjust ventilation to aim for normocarbia with a $PaCO_2$ from 35 to 45 mmHg (4.5 to 6 kPa).

(iii) Insert a gastric tube to decompress the stomach.

(iv) Contact the cardiology service *urgently* after cardiac arrest in a suspected acute coronary syndrome, such as a cardiac arrest following chest pain

(a) immediate percutaneous coronary intervention (PCI) may be possible

(b) do not rely on any particular early ECG abnormality, or necessarily expect to see ST elevation.

(v) Give 1 in 10 000 adrenaline (epinephrine) 50 µg (0.5 mL) i.v. if there is persistent hypotension, and other treatable causes such as hypoxia, hypovolaemia, tension pneumothorax, hyperkalaemia or hypokalaemia have been excluded.

    (a) repeat the adrenaline (epinephrine) to maintain a blood pressure similar to the patient's usual blood pressure, or a systolic blood pressure greater than 100 mmHg, aiming for an adequate urine output of 1 mL/kg/h

    (b) give the adrenaline (epinephrine) and other vasoactive drugs as soon as possible via a dedicated central venous line, which should be inserted under ultrasound control if not already sited.

(vi) Control seizures with midazolam 0.05–0.1 mg/kg up to 10 mg i.v., diazepam 0.1–0.2 mg/kg up to 20 mg i.v. or lorazepam 0.07 mg/kg up to 4 mg i.v.

    (a) follow this with phenytoin 15–18 mg/kg i.v. no faster than 50 mg/min by slow bolus, or preferably as an infusion in 250 mL normal saline (never in dextrose) over 30 min under ECG monitoring.

(vii) Maintain blood glucose at ≤10 mmol/L, but avoid hypoglycaemia.

(viii) Commence targeted temperature management to maintain a constant temperature between 32–36°C, according to local policy:

    (a) initiate temperature management particularly following out-of-hospital VF arrest, and consider in post asystole/PEA patients

    (b) when cooling is adopted, infuse 30 mL/kg cold 4°C normal saline or Hartmann's

    (c) place ice packs to the groin and axillae, and use a cooling blanket if available.

(ix) Transfer the patient to the ICU, catheter laboratory or coronary care unit (CCU). Perform the following investigations but do not delay the transfer:

    (a) serum sodium, potassium, glucose and ABG, if not already done

    (b) 12-lead ECG

    (c) CXR to look for correct positioning of the endotracheal tube, nasogastric tube and central line – exclude a pneumothorax, pulmonary collapse and pulmonary oedema

    (d) CT brain scan and/or chest, if a neurological or respiratory cause is suspected with headache, seizures, neurological deficit or shortness of breath respectively immediately pre-collapse.

(x) Transfer the patient with a trained nurse and doctor in attendance. A minimum of a portable cardiac monitor, defibrillator, oxygen and suction should be available on the trolley.

10 When to stop

The decision to cease further attempts at resuscitation is difficult. Only the senior ED doctor should take this. Survival from out-of-hospital cardiac arrest is greatest when:

   (i)   The event is witnessed and help is called early.
   (ii) A bystander starts resuscitation, even if only chest compressions (doubles or triples survival rate).
   (iii) The heart arrests in VF or VT (20% or higher survival).
   (iv) Defibrillation is carried out at an early stage, with successful cardioversion achieved within 3–5 min (50–75% survival), and not more than 8 min:
        (a) each minute of delay before defibrillation reduces survival to discharge by 10–12%
        (b) survival after more than 12 min of VF in adults without ROSC is less than 5%.

Tip: make special considerations in near-drowning, hypothermia and acute poisoning (especially with tricyclic antidepressants). Full recovery has followed in apparently hopeless cases (fixed dilated pupils, non-shockable rhythm) with resuscitation prolonged for several hours.

ACUTE UPPER AIRWAY OBSTRUCTION

DIAGNOSIS

1 Acute upper airway obstruction may be due to choking on an inhaled foreign body, epiglottitis, croup, facial burns and/or steam inhalation, angioedema, trauma, carcinoma or retropharyngeal abscess.

2 There may be sudden wheeze, coughing, hoarseness or complete aphonia, with severe distress, ineffective respiratory efforts, stridor and cyanosis, followed by unconsciousness.

3 Attach a cardiac monitor and pulse oximeter to the patient.

MANAGEMENT

This depends on the suspected cause.

1 Sit the patient up and give 100% oxygen via a face mask. Aim for an oxygen saturation above 94%.

2 **Inhalation of a foreign body**
      (i) Perform up to five back blows between the shoulder blades, using the heel of your hand with the victim leaning well forwards or lying on the side.

(ii) Perform up to five abdominal thrusts if back blows fail (Heimlich's manoeuvre) in adults and children over 1 year:
- (a) stand behind the patient, place your arms around the upper abdomen with your hands clasped between the umbilicus and xiphisternum
- (b) give thrusts sharply inwards and upwards to expel the obstruction.

(iii) Continue alternating five back blows with five abdominal thrusts if the obstruction is still not relieved.

(iv) Hold babies and infants up to 1 year head-down, and deliver up to five back blows with the heel of the free hand.

(v) Perform up to five chest thrusts if this fails, using the same landmark as for cardiac compression, to dislodge foreign material in the airway.

(vi) Attempt removal under direct vision if the foreign body is still present, using a laryngoscope and a pair of long-handled Magill forceps.

(vii) *Cricothyrotomy*

Perform a cricothyrotomy if the patient is *in extremis*, and all else has failed (see p. 469):
- (a) make an incision through the cricothyroid membrane with a scalpel blade, and insert a 4–6 mm endotracheal tube (or small tracheostomy tube) over a bougie, and connect this tube to an Ambu or Laerdal bag and oxygen supply
- (b) alternatively, achieve rapid access by inserting a large-bore 14-gauge i.v. cannula through the cricothyroid membrane and connect to wall oxygen at 15 L/min.

3   Epiglottitis (see p. 301)

Inflammation of the epiglottis presents with sudden onset of fever, difficulty in breathing, soft inspiratory stridor, dysphagia and drooling. The child looks pale, toxic and unwell.

(i) Do *not* examine further, i.e. no temperature, blood pressure, or X-ray. Do *not* attempt to visualize the throat.

(ii) Leave the parent holding the child upright with an oxygen mask held near the child's face.

(iii) Call for senior ED, paediatric, anaesthetic and ENT assistance immediately.

4   Croup (see p. 299)

A child with croup will have a barking cough, harsh stridor and hoarseness, and will be frightened and miserable but not systemically ill.

(i) Give dexamethasone 0.15–0.3 mg/kg orally or i.m., nebulized budesonide 2 mg or prednisolone 1 mg/kg orally.

(ii) Refer to the paediatric team.

5 Facial burns and/or steam inhalation (see p. 199)

    (i) Send blood for ABGs and a carboxyhaemoglobin level.

    (ii) Give 100% oxygen and nebulized salbutamol 5 mg, and refer to intensive care or specialist burns unit if there is an associated respiratory burn.

    (iii) Be prepared to intubate if laryngeal oedema occurs.

6 Angioedema with laryngeal oedema (see p. 112)

    (i) Give high-dose oxygen and 1 in 1000 adrenaline (epinephrine) 0.3–0.5 mg (0.3–0.5 mL) i.m. into the upper outer thigh, repeated every 5–10 min as necessary.

    (ii) Change to adrenaline (epinephrine) 0.75–1.5 µg/kg i.v. if circulatory collapse occurs, i.e. 50–100 µg or 0.5–1.0 mL of 1 in 10 000 adrenaline (epinephrine), or 5–10 mL of 1 in 100 000 adrenaline (epinephrine) for a 70 kg patient, given slowly.

    (iii) Endotracheal intubation may still be required, performed by a skilled doctor with airway training, or even a cricothyrotomy.

SHOCKED PATIENT

GENERAL APPROACH

DIAGNOSIS

1 'Shock' is defined as acute circulatory failure leading to inadequate end-organ tissue perfusion with oxygen and nutrients. It is a clinical diagnosis with a high mortality that depends on the underlying cause, its duration and response to treatment.

    (i) Shock progresses from an initial insult to compensated (reversible), decompensated (progressive) then finally refractory (irreversible) shock.

    (ii) *Compensated shock*
Physiological mechanisms initially compensate to combat the circulatory failure. These include hyperventilation as a result of acidosis, sympathetic mediated tachycardia and vasoconstriction, and the diversion of blood from the gastrointestinal and renal tracts to the brain, heart and lungs.

    (iii) *Decompensated shock*
Inadequate tissue perfusion results in increasing anaerobic glycolysis and metabolic acidosis, cellular injury with fluid and protein leakage, and deteriorating cardiac output from vascular dilatation and myocardial depression.

    (iv) *Irreversible shock*
This ensues when vital organs fail and cell death occurs. Severe and progressive shock states cause multi-organ failure (MOF) or end

in cardiac arrest with pulseless electrical activity. Once shock deteriorates to this degree, it is difficult or impossible to reverse.

2   Aim to identify abnormal tissue perfusion early, ideally **before** the systolic blood pressure (SBP) drops, treat aggressively and avoid the irreversible phase. Investigation and treatment are concurrent – get senior help early.

     (i)   A normal blood pressure does not exclude the diagnosis of shock.

     (ii)   The absolute value of the SBP associated with poor perfusion varies greatly, but an SBP <90 mmHg is usually insufficient to maintain adequate vital organ perfusion.

3   Consider causes in four broad categories (see Fig. 1.2). Often more than one mechanism is present:

     (i)   Hypovolaemic shock (*'insufficient circulatory volume'*) (see p. 19):

         (a)   haemorrhagic – traumatic or non-traumatic; external (revealed) or internal (concealed)

         (b)   non-haemorrhagic fluid losses – external (revealed), internal (concealed).

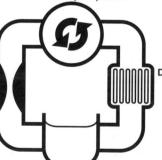

Cardiogenic shock
Depressed contractility
     Acute coronary syndrome
     Myocarditis
     Cardiomyopathy
     Drug toxicity
Acute valvular dysfunction
Arrhythmia
     Bradyarrhythmia
     Tachyarrhythmia

Obstructive shock
Pulmonary embolism
Tension pneumothorax
     Traumatic
     Non-traumatic
Cardiac tamponade
     Traumatic
     Non-traumatic
Dynamic hyperinflation

Distributive shock
Anaphylaxis
Sepsis
Neurogenic
Drug related
Acute adrenal
     insufficiency

Hypovolaemic shock (most common)
Haemorrhage
     Traumatic
         External (revealed)
         Internal (concealed)
     Non-traumatic
         External (revealed)
         Internal (concealed)
Non-haemorrhagic
     External fluid loss

Figure 1.2 Different types of shock.

(ii) Cardiogenic shock (*'pump failure'*):

    (a) decreased contractility – acute coronary syndrome, myocarditis, myocardial contusion, end-stage cardiomyopathy, drug toxicity, severe acidaemia

    (b) acute valvular dysfunction – acute valve leak (papillary muscle/chordae tendinae rupture, infective endocarditis), severe aortic stenosis

    (c) arrhythmia – tachycardia such as SVT, AF or VT, bradycardia including heart block.

(iii) Distributive shock (*'circulation unable to be filled'*):

    (a) sepsis (see p. 21)

    (b) anaphylaxis

    (c) neurogenic – spinal cord trauma, epidural

    (d) drug-related – nitrates, vasodilators

    (e) adrenal insufficiency – inadequate steroid replacement, Addison's.

(iv) Obstructive shock (*'obstructed circulation'*):

    (a) pulmonary embolism – thrombotic, air, fat, amniotic fluid

    (b) tension pneumothorax – traumatic, non-traumatic

    (c) cardiac tamponade – traumatic; non-traumatic such as uraemia, pericarditis, malignancy

    (d) dynamic hyperinflation – over-ventilated asthma, or COPD.

4 Ask about the onset whether sudden or gradual, associated symptoms such as chest pain, abdominal or back pain, and the past medical history, drugs taken including illicit drugs, allergies, recent travel abroad, alcohol use or immunosuppression and prior cardiorespiratory status.

5 Assess for features of circulatory shock including abnormal vital signs.

(i) Tachycardia occasionally bradycardia, tachypnoea, hypotension, hypothermia (or hyperthermia in sepsis), reduced oxygen saturation and a reduced conscious level (Glasgow Coma Scale [GCS] score) occur

    (a) check for a postural change in blood pressure, if the SBP is normal

      – increase in heart rate of >20 beats/min, a fall in SBP of >20 mmHg, or a fall in DBP of >10 mmHg indicates postural hypotension and suggests hypovolaemia

      – make certain the orthostatic readings are taken after at least 2 min sitting or standing up.

(ii) Look at the skin for sweating, pallor or mottling and feel whether it is cold or clammy

    (a) check the capillary refill time (CRT) by pressing on a nailbed (held at the level of the heart) for 5 s. Observe the time taken to refill the blanched area with blood

    (b) over 2 s is prolonged and suggests hypoperfused or cool peripheries.

6 Estimate preload volume status to help determine the cause, and to monitor treatment effect.
  (i) Low preload with non-visible jugular venous pressure (JVP) occurs in hypovolaemic and distributive shock states.
  (ii) High preload with raised JVP occurs in cardiogenic and obstructive shock.

7 Establish venous access with two large-bore (14- or 16-gauge) cannulae into the antecubital veins and attach a cardiac monitor and pulse oximeter to the patient.

8 Send blood for full blood count (FBC), coagulation profile, electrolyte and liver function tests (ELFTs), lipase, cardiac troponin I (cTnI) or troponin T (cTnT), lactate, paired blood cultures from two sites and a group and save (G&S) or cross-match blood according to the suspected cause.
  (i) Check a venous or arterial blood gas.

9 Perform an ECG, and arrange immediate review by a senior ED doctor.
  (i) Look for acute changes suggesting an acute coronary syndrome, or for an arrhythmia
    (a) acute changes may be the cause or the effect of the shock state.
  (ii) A normal ECG effectively rules out cardiogenic shock.

10 Request a CXR to look for cardiomegaly, pneumothorax, consolidation, pulmonary oedema and atelectasis.

11 Insert a urethral catheter to measure the urine output, and check a urinalysis for blood, protein, nitrites and sugar. Send for microscopy and culture if positive.
  (i) Oliguria suggests ongoing renal hypoperfusion.
  (ii) Check a urinary β-human chorionic gonadotrophin (hCG) pregnancy test in pre-menopausal females.

12 Organize a rapid bedside ultrasound to look for a ruptured abdominal aortic aneurysm (AAA), ectopic pregnancy, cardiac tamponade or free fluid in the peritoneal cavity.

MANAGEMENT

1 Commence high-dose oxygen via a face mask. Maintain the oxygen saturation above 94%.

2 Begin immediate fluid replacement:
  (i) Give 20 mL/kg normal saline i.v. rapidly and repeat until JVP is 3–5 cm above sternal angle
    (a) omit fluids if JVP is already raised, and/or the patient has pulmonary oedema
    (b) aim for a urine output of 0.5–1 mL/kg per h.

    (ii)   Give cross-matched blood when it is available, if the patient is shocked due to blood loss:

        (a) use O-negative blood if the situation is desperate. Aim for haemoglobin 70–100 g/L, or haematocrit >30%.

3   Optimize afterload:

    (i)   Give a vasopressor such as adrenaline if vasodilated from anaphylaxis (see p. 27) or sepsis (see p. 21).

4   Treat sepsis:

    (i)   Give broad-spectrum antibiotics early if septic shock is suspected, after taking a minimum of two sets of blood cultures from different sites (see p. 21).

5   Admit the patient to ICU, HDU, theatre or coronary care depending on the underlying cause, and response to treatment.

HYPOVOLAEMIC SHOCK

DIAGNOSIS

1   This follows haemorrhage or non-haemorrhagic fluid loss that results in a reduced circulatory volume with inadequate end-organ tissue perfusion.

2   Causes of haemorrhagic shock include (see also p. 16):

    (i)   Trauma with external bleeding:

        (a) arterial laceration, compound fracture, limb avulsion, massive scalping injury.

    (ii)   Trauma with internal (concealed) bleeding:

        (a) haemothorax, haemoperitoneum from liver, spleen or mesenteric injury, retroperitoneal from aortic, pelvic or renal injury, closed long-bone or pelvic fracture.

    (iii) Non-traumatic, external bleeding:

        (a) epistaxis, massive haemoptysis, haematemesis either fresh or coffee-grounds, rectal bleeding either melaena or fresh red, vaginal bleeding either pregnancy-related or non-pregnant, or gross haematuria.

    (iv) Non-traumatic, internal (concealed) bleeding:

        (a) haemothorax, haemoperitoneum including ruptured AAA or ectopic pregnancy, retroperitoneal bleeding including ruptured AAA or spontaneous from warfarin, NOAC or bleeding diathesis.

3   Causes of non-haemorrhagic shock from fluid loss include:

    (i)   External:

        (a) vomiting, diarrhoea, polyuria from renal disease, diabetes insipidus or diabetes mellitus, burns, extensive skin disease including erythroderma, hyperthermia, fistulae.

    (ii)   Internal:

        (a) pancreatitis 'third spacing', bowel obstruction.

4 Ask about external bleeding, previous episodes of bleeding, chest, abdominal or back pain, drugs taken including non-steroidal anti-inflammatory drugs (NSAIDs) or warfarin/NOAC, allergies, alcohol use and travel abroad.

   (i) Enquire about non-specific symptoms of lethargy, breathlessness, light-headedness, syncope and altered mental status such as confusion, particularly in the elderly.

5 Check the vital signs and include a postural blood pressure if SBP is normal.

6 Look for signs of anaemia with pale skin creases and conjunctivae, and for signs of dehydration such as dry mucous membranes, reduced tissue turgor or sunken eyes.

   (i) Assess the JVP which should be low.

7 Examine for specific causes according to the history. Include a per rectal exam for unrecognized gastrointestinal bleeding.

8 Establish venous access with two large-bore (14- or 16-gauge) cannulae into the antecubital veins and attach a cardiac monitor and pulse oximeter to the patient.

9 Send blood for FBC, coagulation profile, ELFTs, lipase, lactate and cross-match blood according to the suspected cause.

   (i) Check a venous or arterial blood gas.

10 Perform an ECG and request a CXR.

11 Insert a urethral catheter to measure the urine output.

   (i)   Oliguria suggests ongoing renal hypoperfusion.
   (ii) Check a urinary β-hCG pregnancy test in pre-menopausal females.

12 Organize a rapid bedside ultrasound to look for a ruptured AAA, ectopic pregnancy or free fluid in the peritoneal cavity.

MANAGEMENT

1 Commence high-dose oxygen via a face mask. Maintain the oxygen saturation above 94%.

2 Compress or pack any external haemorrhage such as epistaxis (see p. 368) or wound bleeding (see p. 170).

3 Begin immediate fluid replacement:

   (i) Give 20 mL/kg normal saline i.v. rapidly and repeat, aiming for a urine output of 0.5–1 mL/kg per h

        (a) then gradually correct any dehydration (rehydration), and include daily maintenance amounts.

   (ii) Give cross-matched blood when it is available, if the patient is shocked due to blood loss

        (a) remember that in healthy adults the only signs associated with loss of up to 30% of the circulatory blood volume (i.e. 1500 mL) may be a tachycardia and a narrowed pulse pressure

(b) thus, a consistent fall in SBP indicates that at least 30% of the blood volume has *already* been lost

(c) full cross-match takes 45 min, a type-specific cross-match takes 10 min, and O rhesus-negative blood is available immediately

(d) use a blood warmer and macropore blood filter for multiple transfusions
   - give fresh frozen plasma 8–10 units and platelets after transfusing 8–10 units of blood or more, i.e. in a 1:1 ratio for a 'massive blood transfusion'

(e) aim for haemoglobin 70–100 g/L, or haematocrit >30%.

4 Consult the surgical, vascular or gynaecological team immediately if there is suspected rapid blood loss causing shock (e.g. ruptured spleen, AAA or ectopic pregnancy).

5 Admit the patient to theatre, intensive care unit (ICU) or a high-dependency unit (HDU) depending on the underlying cause, and response to treatment.

SEPTIC SHOCK

DIAGNOSIS

1 Sepsis is a heterogeneous systemic host response defined by a variety of general, inflammatory, haemodynamic and organ dysfunction variables in response to a presumed infectious aetiology, which is most usually bacterial, or fungal, viral or parasitic.

(i) More than 85% of the causes originate from the chest, abdominal or genitourinary systems, skin and vascular access.

(ii) Worldwide sepsis is one of the most common reasons for admission to an ICU, and up to 20–50% of patients with sepsis die.

2 Updated sepsis definitions include:

(i) *Sepsis*

The presence (probable or documented) of infection together with systemic manifestations such as

(a) *general*: fever >38.3°C or <36°C, heart rate >90/min, tachypnoea >20/min or hyperventilation with $PaCO_2$ <32 mmHg (4.2 kPa), confusion

(b) *inflammatory*: WBC $>12 \times 10^9/L$, $<4 \times 10^9/L$ or >10% immature band forms; raised CRP or procalcitonin

(c) *haemodynamic*: SBP <90 mmHg or MAP <70 mmHg

(d) *organ dysfunction*: hypoxia, oliguria, coagulopathy, thrombocytopaenia, hyperbilirubinaemia, ileus

(e) *tissue hypoperfusion*: raised lactate >1 mmol/L, decreased capillary refill, or skin mottling.

    (ii) *Severe sepsis*
Sepsis plus either sepsis-induced organ dysfunction, or tissue hypoperfusion. These may cause
    (a) hypoxia, hypotension, oliguria, confusion and a raised lactate (see above).

    (iii) *Septic shock*
Sepsis-induced hypotension persisting despite adequate fluid resuscitation (at least 30 mL/kg of crystalloid).

3   Initial symptoms are non-specific and include malaise, fever or rigors, myalgia, nausea or vomiting and lethargy.

    (i)   Ask specifically about focal features such as headache, neck pain, sore throat, ear ache, cough, breathlessness, abdominal pain, frequency, dysuria, joint or skin changes.

    (ii)   Enquire about previous illnesses, use of antibiotics, allergies, immunosuppression including diabetes, chemotherapy, steroids or HIV, alcohol use or travel abroad.

4   Assess for features of circulatory shock including abnormal vital signs.

    (i)   Early signs are non-specific such as tachypnoea, tachycardia, temperature change (high or low), and altered mental status.

    (ii)   Some patients will be hot and flushed with a bounding pulse, but many others are normo- or hypothermic with a tachypnoea and metabolic acidosis.

5   Examine for potential source areas such as the ears, throat, chest, heart, abdomen, back, limbs and skin including between the toes (tinea), skin folds (intertrigo), perineum and axillae (abscess).

    (i)   Look for a rash, particularly petechial.

6   Establish venous access with two large-bore (14- or 16-gauge) cannulae into the antecubital veins and attach a cardiac monitor and pulse oximeter to the patient.

7   Send blood for FBC, coagulation profile, ELFTs, CRP, lactate and two sets of blood cultures from different sites.

    (i)   Check a venous or arterial blood gas.

    (ii)   Swab any infected areas.

8   Perform an ECG and request a CXR.

9   Insert a urethral catheter to measure the urine output, and check a urinalysis for blood, protein, nitrites and sugar. Send for microscopy and culture if positive.

    (i)   Oliguria suggests ongoing renal hypoperfusion.

    (ii)   Check a urinary β-hCG pregnancy test in pre-menopausal females.

10 Arrange an ultrasound, CT scan and/or lumbar puncture (LP) according to the suspected source of infection, but these should **never** delay antibiotic therapy.

MANAGEMENT

1 Commence high-dose oxygen via a face mask. Maintain the oxygen saturation above 94%.

2 Begin aggressive fluid replacement:
- (i) Give 30 mL/kg normal saline i.v. rapidly over the first 30 min and then reassess. Multiple boluses may be required
  - (a) intravascular fluid resuscitation often requires large volumes up to 50–100 mL/kg before volume replacement is adequate
  - (b) ensure haemoglobin is maintained between 70–90 g/L.

3 Administer appropriate antibiotics early. Mortality is reduced if antibiotics are given within 1 h of onset of hypotension. Each additional hour of delay adds 7% to the mortality in septic shock. Get senior advice early and consult local antibiotic guidelines:
- (i) Give flucloxacillin 2 g i.v. 4-hourly plus gentamicin 4–7 mg/kg once daily if no source is apparent in the immunocompetent patient.
- (ii) Add vancomycin 1.5 g i.v. 12-hourly for possible MRSA including community-associated (CA-MRSA), suspected line sepsis and instead of flucloxacillin for immediate hypersensitivity.
- (iii) Give neutropenic patients piperacillin 4 g with tazobactam 0.5 g i.v. 8-hourly, plus gentamicin 4–7 mg/kg stat when no source is apparent, and add vancomycin 1.5 g i.v. 12-hourly for possible line sepsis.
- (iv) Otherwise give antibiotics to cover likely pathogens depending on a known focus, and/or once culture and sensitivities are known.

4 Start vasopressor support for continuing hypotension despite fluid resuscitation.
- (i) Give noradrenaline or adrenaline i.v. by infusion to maintain mean arterial pressure (MAP) $\geq$65 mmHg (see p. 35 for dose and dilution).
- (ii) Inotropic support with dobutamine i.v. by infusion may also be required, particularly in the presence of myocardial dysfunction (see p. 35 for dose and dilution).
- (iii) Give hydrocortisone 50 mg i.v. q.d.s. only if poorly or unresponsive to adequate fluid and vasopressor therapy.

5 Refer the patient urgently to the surgical team if a local cause requires source control or drainage such as wound debridement for necrotising fasciitis, laparotomy for perforation or gangrene, percutaneous drainage for urinary obstruction, etc. Contact theatre and the anaesthetist.

6 Meanwhile arrange admission to ICU for all patients.

Tip: beware patients who are neutropenic from chemotherapy, malnourished, elderly, diabetic, have HIV or are otherwise immunosuppressed, as they have few signs of sepsis. Fever may be minimal, focal features few, and only a non-specific inflammatory response is found in the laboratory tests. Immediate blood cultures and empirical antibiotics are *essential*.

UNCONSCIOUS PATIENT

The aim is to resuscitate the patient and treat urgent precipitating conditions while a picture of the situation is built up. The definitive diagnosis may not be made in the ED.

MANAGEMENT

1 Manage the patient in a monitored resuscitation area, and call the senior ED doctor immediately.

    (i) Clear obstructing material using a tongue depressor or laryngoscope blade if the patient is unconscious with a noisy airway, and remove broken dentures, vomit or blood with a Yankauer sucker.

    (ii) Improve airway opening using a head tilt, chin lift and/or jaw thrust

        (a) open the airway with the jaw thrust alone in trauma cases, avoiding any movement of the neck.

    (iii) Insert an oropharyngeal airway and give high-dose oxygen via a face mask. Attach a cardiac monitor and pulse oximeter to the patient and aim for an oxygen saturation above 94%.

2 Commence cardiopulmonary resuscitation if no pulse is felt (see p. 2).

3 An airway-skilled doctor should now insert an endotracheal tube if there is a reduced or absent gag reflex and an unprotected airway, using a rapid sequence induction technique (see p. 467).

Warning: *never* attempt rapid sequence induction (RSI) unless you have been trained. Use a bag-valve mask technique instead, while waiting for help.

4 Otherwise:

    (i) Apply a semi-rigid collar if there is any suggestion of face, head or neck trauma, before moving the patient.

    (ii) Remove all the clothing, but keep the patient covered and avoid heat loss.

5 Insert an i.v. cannula and take blood for FBC, coagulation profile, blood sugar, ELFTs, blood culture and drug screen for salicylate and paracetamol if not already done.

 (i) Perform ABGs, recording the amount of oxygen being delivered (FiO_2).

 (ii) Give 50% dextrose 50 mL i.v. if the blood glucose test strip is low

 (a) remember dextrose i.v. can precipitate Wernicke's encephalopathy in alcoholic or malnourished patients, who require thiamine 250 mg i.v. immediately.

6 Record the temperature (if 35°C, repeat with a low-reading thermometer to exclude hypothermia), pulse, blood pressure, and the pupil size and reaction.

 (i) Consider naloxone 0.4–2 mg i.v. slowly if there are pinpoint pupils with hypoventilation to reverse narcotic poisoning, but beware of precipitating an acute withdrawal reaction.

7 Consider other critical conditions requiring immediate action:

 (i) *Tension pneumothorax*

 (a) this usually follows trauma, especially if positive-pressure ventilation is being given

 (b) insert a large-bore cannula or intercostal drain without waiting for an X-ray (see p. 471).

 (ii) *Cardiac arrhythmia*

 (a) treat as necessary after recording a formal 12-lead ECG (see p. 60).

 (iii) *Exsanguination*

 (a) bleeding may be external and obvious, or internal and concealed from the gastrointestinal tract, a ruptured AAA or ectopic pregnancy

 (b) cross-match blood, give i.v. fluids, arrange an ultrasound and refer the patient for an urgent surgical opinion.

 (iv) *Anaphylaxis*

 (a) this may follow drug therapy, food ingestion, or an insect sting

 (b) give 1 in 1000 adrenaline (epinephrine) 0.3–0.5 mg (0.3–0.5 mL) i.m. repeated as necessary every 5–10 min

 (c) give 1 in 10 000 or 1 in 100 000 adrenaline (epinephrine) 0.75–1.5 µg/kg i.v. if there is circulatory collapse, i.e. 50–100 µg or 0.5–1.0 mL of 1 in 10 000, 5–10 mL of 1 in 100 000 adrenaline (epinephrine), slowly i.v. for a 70 kg patient (see p. 27).

 (v) *Extradural haemorrhage*

 (a) this may follow even trivial trauma; look for a local bruise on the scalp, for instance in the temporoparietal area over the middle meningeal artery territory

    (b) watch out for deterioration in the level of consciousness, ultimately with the development of Cheyne–Stokes breathing and a unilateral fixed, dilated pupil

    (c) call an airway-skilled doctor to pass a cuffed endotracheal tube if one is not already in place

    (d) arrange an urgent head CT scan, and refer the patient immediately to the neurosurgical team, before critical mass lesion signs develop.

DIAGNOSIS

1 The patient's cardiorespiratory status should have been stabilized by this stage, bloods sent, a blood sugar level checked, an indwelling catheter and a nasogastric tube placed, and an ECG and CXR performed.

2 Now focus on the underlying cause.

The most common causes of an unconscious patient are:

    (i)   Poisoning (accidental or deliberate, including alcohol, carbon monoxide).

    (ii) Hypoglycaemia.

    (iii) Post-ictal state.

    (iv) Stroke.

    (v)   Head injury.

    (vi) Subarachnoid haemorrhage.

    (vii) Respiratory failure.

    (viii) Hypotension (shock – see p. 15).

3 Less common causes of an unconscious patient are:

    (i)   Meningitis or encephalitis.

    (ii) Hepatic or renal failure.

    (iii) Septicaemia.

    (iv) Subdural haematoma.

    (v)   Hyperglycaemia (diabetic ketoacidosis [DKA] or hyperosmolar, hyperglycaemic state [HHS]).

    (vi) Hypothermia or hyperthermia.

4 Rare causes of an unconscious patient are:

    (i)   Cerebral space-occupying lesion.

    (ii) Hyponatraemia or hypercalcaemia.

    (iii) Myxoedema.

    (iv) Addison's disease.

    (v)   Hypertensive encephalopathy.

5 Finally, in those who have recently been abroad, consider:

    (i)   Cerebral malaria.

    (ii) Typhus, yellow fever, trypanosomiasis and typhoid.

    (iii) Rabies, Japanese B encephalitis.

    (iv) Severe acute respiratory syndrome (SARS), viral haemorrhagic fever.

6 These four lists may seem daunting, but aim to build up a picture of the events as follows.

History:

    (i) Any clues from relatives, passers-by or ambulance crew?

    (ii) Witnessed fit, trauma, alcohol or drug ingestion?

    (iii) Prior medical or surgical conditions?

    (iv) Known drug therapy or abuse?

    (v) Recent travel abroad?

7 Further examination:

    (i) Search the clothing for a diabetic card, steroid card or outpatient card.

    (ii) Look particularly for signs of trauma, needle puncture marks, or petechiae on the skin.

    (iii) Repeat the vital signs, including the temperature.

    (iv) Reassess the neurological state, including the level of consciousness using the GCS score (see Table 1.1, p. 30), the pupil responses, eye movements and fundi. Assess the muscle power, tone and reflexes including the plantar responses. Exclude any neck stiffness

        (a) consider head injury, stroke, subdural haematoma or space-occupying lesion in coma with focal neurological signs

        (b) consider meningitis or encephalitis, or subarachnoid haemorrhage in coma with meningeal irritation, usually without focal signs.

    (v) Examine the front of the chest, feel the abdomen and examine the back, inspect the perineum and perform a rectal examination.

8 Arrange:

    (i) CXR and pelvic X-ray in trauma (see p. 172).

    (ii) Head computed tomography (CT) scan, with cervical spine in trauma, if intracranial pathology is suspected or cannot be excluded, which is frequently the case.

9 Refer the patient to the medical (or surgical) team, or ICU if they are not already involved, having stabilized the cardiorespiratory status, treated any urgent conditions and built up a list of the likely causes of unconsciousness.

ANAPHYLAXIS

DIAGNOSIS

1 IgE-mediated allergic anaphylaxis is an immunological, multi-system reaction that may rapidly follow drug ingestion, particularly parenteral penicillin, a bee or wasp sting, or food such as nuts and seafood.

    (i) Non-IgE-mediated, non-allergic anaphylaxis (previously termed an anaphylactoid reaction) is a clinically identical reaction most commonly seen following radio-contrast media or aspirin or NSAID exposure, but which is not triggered by IgE antibodies.

2 Respiratory manifestations:
- (i) Dyspnoea, laryngeal oedema, hoarseness and stridor.
- (ii) Cough, wheeze (bronchospasm), cyanosis.
- (iii) Rhinitis and conjunctivitis.

3 Cardiovascular manifestations:
- (i) Tachycardia, occasionally bradycardia.
- (ii) Hypotension, with massive vasodilation.
- (iii) Light-headedness, confusion, collapse with loss of consciousness.

4 Other manifestations:
- (i) Gastrointestinal:
  - (a) odynophagia (difficult or painful swallowing)
  - (b) abdominal cramps or pain
  - (c) vomiting and diarrhoea.
- (ii) Cutaneous:
  - (a) erythema
  - (b) local or widespread urticaria
  - (c) pruritus
  - (d) angioedema.
- (iii) Miscellaneous:
  - (a) premonitory aura, anxiety, feeling of impending doom
  - (b) back pain, pelvic cramps.

5 Attach a cardiac monitor and pulse oximeter to the patient.

MANAGEMENT

1 Give high-dose oxygen via a face mask aiming for an oxygen saturation above 94%, and place the patient supine or elevate the legs. Stop the delivery of potential causative agent and call for help.

2 **Laryngeal oedema and wheeze**
- (i) Give 1 in 1000 adrenaline (epinephrine) 0.3–0.5 mg (0.3–0.5 mL) i.m. immediately into the upper outer thigh.
- (ii) If rapid deterioration occurs, change to 1 in 10 000 or 1 in 100 000 adrenaline (epinephrine) 0.75–1.5 µg/kg i.v.; i.e. 50–100 µg or 0.5–1.0 mL of 1 in 10 000, or 5–10 mL of 1 in 100 000 adrenaline (epinephrine) given over 5 min i.v. The ECG *must* be monitored.
- (iii) Give 1 in 1000 adrenaline (epinephrine) 2–4 mg (2–4 mL) nebulized in oxygen while preparing the i.v. adrenaline (epinephrine).
- (iv) Give hydrocortisone 200 mg i.v. particularly for bronchospasm.

3 **Shock and circulatory collapse**
- (i) Give 1 in 1000 adrenaline (epinephrine) 0.3–0.5 mg (0.3–0.5 mL) i.m. immediately into the upper outer thigh, repeated every 5–10 min until improvement occurs.

   (ii)   Lie the patient flat and/or elevate the legs.
   (iii) Give a bolus of normal saline 20–40 mL/kg i.v.
   (iv)   If rapid deterioration occurs, change to 1 in 10 000 or
          1 in 100 000 adrenaline (epinephrine) 0.75–1.5 μg/kg i.v.;
          i.e. 50–100 μg or 0.5–1.0 mL of 1 in 10 000, or 5–10 mL of 1 in
          100 000 adrenaline (epinephrine) given over 5 min i.v. The ECG
          must be monitored.

4   Second-line measures only used *after* achieving cardiorespiratory stability.
   (i)   Cetirizine 10 mg orally or fexofenadine 180 mg orally, or
          chlorphenamine 10–20 mg slowly i.v., plus ranitidine 50 mg i.v.
   (ii)   Hydrocortisone 200 mg i.v. (if not given already).
   (iii) Glucagon 1–2 mg i.v. repeated as necessary, for patients on
          β-blockers resistant to the above treatment.

5   Admit any patient receiving adrenaline (epinephrine) for 6–8 h observation
       as late deterioration may occur in up to 5%, known as biphasic anaphylaxis.

6   Then discharge home on prednisolone 50 mg once daily, cetirizine 10 mg or
       fexofenadine 180 mg once daily plus ranitidine 150 mg b.d., all orally for 3 days.
   (i)   Inform the GP by fax or letter.
   (ii)   Refer all significant or recurrent attacks to the allergy clinic,
          especially if the cause is unavoidable or unknown.
   (iii) Prescribe an EpiPen or Anapen 300 μg in adults as part of an
          Anaphylaxis Management Plan.

SEVERE HEAD INJURY

DIAGNOSIS

1   The head injury may be obvious from the history or on immediate examination.

2   The possibility of a head injury must also be considered in every instance of
       coma or abnormal behaviour, in at-risk groups such as alcohol intoxication
       and epileptics, non-accidental injury in children, and in falls in the elderly.

3   Confirm a history from the ambulance crew, police or any witnesses as to the
       circumstances and nature of the injury, period of loss of consciousness or
       subsequent seizures.

4   Obtain other medical details, if a relative or friend is available, of current
       medical or surgical conditions, drug therapy, allergies and any previous
       head injury or epilepsy.

5   Check the temperature, pulse, blood pressure, respiratory rate, and attach an
       ECG monitor and pulse oximeter to the patient. Record the level of
       consciousness using the GCS score (Table 1.1).

   (i)   A patient in coma has a score of 8 or less.

   (ii) A decrease in score of 2 or more points indicates a significant deterioration.

   (iii) Repeat neurological examinations, including the GCS, are essential for detecting and managing secondary brain damage.

6   Insert a large-bore i.v. cannula and send blood for FBC, U&Es, coagulation profile, blood sugar, and G&S, and save serum for a drug screen in case alcohol or drug intoxication is subsequently suspected.

7   Send ABGs, recording the percentage of inspired oxygen administered at the time the sample was drawn.

8   Perform a neurological examination, including:

   (i)   Conscious level: regularly record the GCS and look for any deterioration (decrease in score).

   (ii) Pupil size and reactions: look in particular for an unequal or dilating pupil, indicating a focal mass lesion and/or rising intracranial pressure.

Table 1.1 The Glasgow Coma Scale (GCS) score

		Score
Eye opening	Spontaneously	4
	To speech	3
	To pain	2
	None	1
Verbal response	Oriented	5
	Confused	4
	Inappropriate	3
	Incomprehensible	2
	None	1
Motor response	Obeys commands	6
	Localizes pain	5
	Withdraws (pain)	4
	Flexion (pain)	3
	Extension (pain)	2
	None	1

The maximum score is 15. Any reduction in score indicates deterioration in the level of consciousness.

     (iii) Eye movements and fundoscopy:
        (a) intact eye movements are one indicator of brainstem function
        (b) fundoscopy may reveal papilloedema, subhyaloid haemorrhage or retinal detachment.
     (iv) Other cranial nerves: include examination of the corneal reflex, facial movements and the cough and gag reflexes.
     (v) Limb movements:
        (a) assess for abnormal tone, weakness or loss of movement, or an asymmetrical response to pain if the patient is unconscious
        (b) check the limb reflexes, including the plantar responses.

9   Examine the scalp for bruising, lacerations and haematomas, and palpate for a deformity indicating a depressed skull fracture.

10   Examine the face and mouth for signs of facial fracture or basal skull fracture. A basal skull fracture is indicated by:
     (i) Periorbital and subconjunctival haemorrhage.
     (ii) Haemotympanum, external bleeding, or cerebrospinal fluid (CSF) leak from the ear.
     (iii) Haemorrhage or CSF leakage from the nose.
     (iv) Nasopharyngeal haemorrhage, which may be profuse.
     (v) Mastoid bruising (Battle's sign), which may not appear for many hours.

11   Perform a head-to-toe assessment for other injuries to the neck, chest, abdomen and perineum including a rectal examination (loss of anal tone may indicate spinal cord damage), back and limbs.

12   Request radiological examinations:
     (i) CXR and pelvic X-ray in all multiply injured patients.
     (ii) CT head scan with cervical spine scan.
        The airway **must** be protected first, before a head CT is performed. Indications for CT head scan include:
        (a) GCS <13 on initial assessment
        (b) GCS 14 or less 2 h post injury
        (c) focal neurological deficit including hemiparesis, diplopia
        (d) neurological deterioration, i.e. 2 points or more on the GCS
        (e) post-traumatic seizure
        (f) coagulopathy (history of bleeding, clotting disorder, or patient on warfarin or NOAC)
        (g) fracture known or suspected, including base of skull
        (h) penetrating injury, known or suspected.
     (iii) Skull X-rays are of no value in the early management of a major head injury, when there is ready access to CT scanning
        (a) **only** consider if CT scanning is not available. They may demonstrate a radio-opaque foreign body or depressed skull fracture, but cannot exclude serious injury if normal.

MANAGEMENT

1 Clear the airway by sucking out any secretions, remove loose or broken dentures, and insert an oropharyngeal airway. Give 100% oxygen by tight-fitting mask with reservoir bag. Aim for an oxygen saturation above 94%.
   (i) Position head-up at 20–30 degree elevation.

2 Immobilize the cervical spine by applying a semi-rigid collar, as up to 10% of patients with blunt head trauma have a concomitant neck injury. Use sandbags in addition on either side of the head taped to the forehead, unless the patient is excessively restless.

3 The patient must be intubated to protect and maintain the airway, prevent aspiration and guarantee oxygenation and ventilation, if the gag reflex is reduced or absent. Take great care to minimize neck movements by an assistant providing in-line manual immobilization of the neck throughout.
   (i) Call the senior ED doctor immediately.
   (ii) Prepare for an RSI intubation (see p. 467).

4 Regularly repeat the temperature, pulse, blood pressure and respiratory rate.

5 Consider whether a tension pneumothorax (see p. 170), open pneumothorax (see p. 170), massive haemothorax (see p. 182) or flail chest (see p. 182) is responsible if the respiratory rate is rapid or ineffective.

6 Commence i.v. fluid to maintain normotension. Use a crystalloid such as normal saline or Hartmann's.
   (i) Aim for a MAP of >90 mmHg, to ensure adequate cerebral perfusion pressure.
   (ii) Avoid excessive fluid administration if the patient is normotensive, as this may contribute to cerebral oedema.

7 Search for associated injuries including chest, abdominal or pelvic bleeding, long-bone fracture and cardiac tamponade if the patient is hypotensive. Note shock is rarely ever due to an isolated head injury:
   (i) Occasionally, brisk scalp bleeding alone is found to be responsible, usually in children.
   (ii) Alternatively, a cervical or high thoracic spinal cord injury with loss of sympathetic vascular tone may be the cause.

8 Treat the following complications immediately, as they worsen the existing primary cerebral injury and may lead to secondary brain damage.
   (i) *Hypoglycaemia*
      (a) perform a bedside glucose test; if it is low, send a formal blood glucose to the laboratory and give 50% dextrose 50 mL i.v.
      (b) remember this especially if the patient has been drinking alcohol.
   (ii) *Hypoxia*
      (a) PaO_2 <70 mmHg (9 kPa) breathing air or 100 mmHg (13 kPa) on supplemental oxygen and hypercarbia with $PaCO_2$ over

45 mmHg (6 kPa) in the spontaneously breathing patient requires active intervention

(b) call for urgent senior ED doctor help and prepare for endotracheal intubation using an RSI technique (see p. 467) to protect the airway, if not already performed.

(iii) *Seizures*

    (a) give midazolam 0.05–0.1 mg/kg up to 10 mg i.v., diazepam 0.1–0.2 mg/kg up to 20 mg i.v. or lorazepam 0.07 mg/kg up to 4 mg i.v.

    (b) follow with phenytoin 15–18 mg/kg i.v. (see p. 93).

(iv) *Pinpoint pupils*

    (a) give naloxone 0.8–2 mg i.v.

    (b) no response may indicate pontine or cerebellar damage.

(v) *Restless or aggressive behaviour*

Check if any of the following are present:

    (a) hypoxia: make sure the airway is still patent and high-flow oxygen is being delivered

    (b) hypotension: repeat the blood pressure

    (c) pain: catheterize the bladder, splint fractures and exclude a constricting bandage or tight cast.

(vi) *Gastric distension*

    (a) pass a large-bore nasogastric tube

    (b) use an orogastric tube if a basal skull or mid-face fracture is present.

9 Look out for signs of increasing intracranial pressure and uncal transtentorial herniation ('coning') causing a deteriorating level of consciousness, bradycardia, hypertension and focal neurological signs, e.g. a dilated pupil:

(i) Call for a skilled doctor to perform an RSI intubation, if an endotracheal tube is not already positioned.

(ii) Mildly hyperventilate the patient to maintain $PaCO_2$ at 30–35 mmHg (4.0–4.7 kPa).

(iii) Give 20% mannitol 0.5–1 g/kg (2.5–5 mL/kg) as an osmotic diuretic, provided adequate circulatory volume resuscitation has occurred.

(iv) Arrange immediate neurosurgical intervention.

10 Give flucloxacillin 1 g i.v. or cephazolin 2 g i.v. if a penetrating or compound skull fracture or intracranial air is found, and tetanus prophylaxis.

11 **Criteria for neurosurgical consultation**:

Refer all the following patients to the neurosurgery team:

(i) Coma continues after resuscitation (GCS <9).

(ii) Deterioration in neurological status, e.g. worsening in conscious state (2 points or more decrease in GCS), seizures, increasing headache, focal neurological signs.

(iii) Skull fracture:
   (a) compound depressed fracture
   (b) basal skull fracture (see p. 31)
   (c) any skull fracture with confusion, decreased level of consciousness or focal neurological signs.
(iv) Penetrating head injury.
(v) Confusion or other neurological disturbance (GCS 9–13) for more than 2 h with no defined skull fracture.
(vi) Radiological abnormality on CT head scan.

12 Stabilize the patient's condition **first** including airway protection, and make sure any associated injuries have been dealt with before transferring the patient, if transfer is necessary.
   (i) The transport team must be trained and suitably experienced and carry appropriate monitoring equipment (see p. 455).

13 Refer all other patients for admission under the care of the surgical team.

CRITICAL CARE AREAS DRUG INFUSION GUIDELINES

These infusion guidelines were developed for use in critical care areas only. Most require close monitoring with titration to response, and are thus **inappropriate** for general ward areas. All calculations assume an adult weight of 70–80 kg.

Paediatric resuscitation drug doses are available in Table 8.4 (p. 292) in Section VIII, Paediatric Emergencies.

Other paediatric doses are available in any paediatric formulary.

Readers are strongly advised to **re-check all doses** with another medical person before commencing therapy.

Drug	Loading dose	Paediatric infusion range (< 30 kg)	Dilution			Adult dose (70–80 kg)		
			Infusion pump (IP)	Syringe driver	Concentration	Dose per hour	Volume per hour	
Adrenaline (epinephrine)	According to condition 1–100 µg/kg	0.05–1 0 µg/kg/min	6 mg in 100 mL DS	3 mg in 50 mL DS	60 µg/mL	2–20 µg/min	2–20 mL/h	
Amiodarone [b]*Standard*	2–5 mg/kg in 100 mL DW over 30 min by IP	5–15 µg/kg/min	600 mg in 500 mL DW glass bottle. Discard at 12 h	—	1.2 mg/mL	20–60 mg/h (max. 15 mg/kg/24h)	17–52 mL/h	
[a]*Transport*	2–5 mg/kg in 100 mL DW over 30 min by IP	5–15 µg/kg/min	300 mg in 100 mL DW	150 mg in 50 mL DW	3 mg/mL	20–60 mg/h (max. 15 mg/kg/24h)	7.5–22 mL/h	
Clonazepam	1.0–2.0 mg	5–10 µg/kg/h	10 mg in 100 mL DS	5 mg in 50 mL DS	0.1 mg/mL	0.35–0.7 mg/h	3.5–7.0 mL/h	
Dobutamine	—	2–30 µg/kg/min	250 mg in 100 mL DS	125 mg in 50 mL DS	2.5 mg/mL	2–30 µg/kg/min	2–30 mL/n	
Dopamine	—	Renal: 0.5–2.5 µg/kg/min Inotrope: 5–20 µg/kg/min	200 mg in 100 mL DS	100 mg in 50 mL DS	2 mg/mL	Renal: 0.5–2.5 µg/kg/min Inotrope: 5–20 µg/kg/min	Renal: 1–5 mL/h Inotrope: 10–40 mL/h	
Fentanyl	1–5 µg/kg	1–10 µg/kg/h	1000 µg in 100 mL DS	500 µg in 50 mL DS	10 µg/mL	50–200 µg/h	5–20 mL/h	

[a,b] See key, page 40. Abbreviations see key, page 40.

Drug	Loading dose	Paediatric infusion range (<30 kg)	Dilution		Concentration	Adult dose (70–80 kg)	
			Infusion pump (IP)	Syringe driver		Dose per hour	Volume per hour
Glyceryl trinitrate (GTN) [b]*Standard*	—	1–10 µg/kg/min	200 mg in 500 mL DW. Use glass bottle/low-absorption set	—	400 µg/mL	0.4–8 mg/h	1–20 mL/h
[a]*Transport*	—	1–10 µg/kg/min	50 mg in 100 mL DW	25 mg in 50 mL DW	500 µg/mL	0.5–10 mg/h	1–20 mL/h
Insulin (short-acting)	2–20 units	0.03–0.3 units/kg/h	100 units in 100 mL NS	50 units in 50 mL NS	1 unit/mL	2–20 units/h	2–20 mL/h
Isoprenaline *Low dose*	50–100 µg increments	0.5–7.5 µg/min	1 mg in 100 mL DS	0.5 mg in 50 mL DS	10 µg/mL	0.5–7.5 µg/min	2–30 mL/h
High dose	—	0.05–1.0 µg/kg/min	6 mg in 100 mL DS	3 mg in 50 mL DS	60 µg/mL	2–20 µg/min	2–20 mL/h
Ketamine	IV: 1–2 mg/kg IM: 5–10 mg/kg	5–20 µg/kg/min	1000 mg in 100 mL DS	500 mg in 50 mL DS	10 mg/mL	0.3–1.2 mg/kg/h	2–10 mL/h
Lignocaine (lidocaine) [b]*Standard*	1–2 mg/kg	15–50 µg/kg/min	Pre-mixed: 2 g in 500 mL DW	Pre-mixed: 2 g in 500 mL DW	4 mg/mL	*8 mg/min **4 mg/min ***2 mg/min	*120 mL/h for 20 min **60 mL/h for 60 min ***30 mL/h for 24 h
[a]*Transport*	1–2 mg/kg	15–50 µg/kg/min	2 g in 100 mL DW	1 g in	20 mg/mL	8 mg/min	24 mL/h

Continued

Drug	Loading dose	Paediatric infusion range (<30 kg)	Dilution		Concentration	Adult dose (70–80 kg)	
			Infusion pump (IP)	Syringe driver		Dose per hour	Volume per hour
				50 mL DW		**4 mg/min ***2 mg/min	for 20 min **12 mL/h for 60 min ***6 mL/h for 24 h
Magnesium sulphate *49.3% solution in 5 mL = 10 mmol = 2.47 g*	0.15–0.3 mmol/kg = 10–20 mmol (adult) Dilute in 50 mL DS Infuse: 2 min (VT) to 20 min (pre-eclampsia)	0.05–0.1 mmol/kg/h	40 mmol in 100 mL DS	20 mmol in 50 mL DS	0.4 mmol/mL or 0.1 g/mL	2–8 mmol/h 0.5–2.0 g/h	5–20 mL/h
Midazolam	0.05–0.1 mg/kg in 1–2.5 mg increments	10–100 µg/kg/h	50 mg in 100 mL DS	25 mg in 50 mL DS	0.5 mg/mL	2.5–10 mg/h	5–20 mL/h
Morphine	2.5–15 mg in 2.5 mg increments	10–50 µg/kg/h	100 mg in 100 mL DS	50 mg in 50 mL DS	1 mg/mL	2–10 mg/h	2–10 mL/h
Naloxone	0.4–2.0 mg (max. 10 mg)	10 µg/kg/r	4 mg in 100 mL DS	2 mg in 50 mL DS	40 µg/mL	0.5–1.0 mg/h	12.5–25 mL/h
Nimodipine	—	6–30 µg/kg/h	10 mg in 50 mL dispensed	10 mg in 50 mL dispensed	0.2 mg/mL	0.4–2.0 mg/h. Titrate to maintain MAP	Start 2 mL/h Increase 2 mL/h every hour to max. of 10 mL/h
Noradrenaline (norepinephrine)	—	0.05–1.0 µg/kg/min	6 mg in 100 mL DS	3 mg in 50 mL DS	60 µg/mL	2–20 µg/min	2–20 mL/h

a, b See key, page 40. Abbreviations see key, page 40.

Drug	Loading dose	Paediatric infusion range (<30 kg)	Dilution		Concentration	Adult dose (70–80 kg)		
			Infusion pump (IP)	Syringe driver		Dose per hour	Volume per hour	
Octreotide	50–200 µg	3–5 µg/kg/h	1000 µg in 100 mL DS	500 µg in 50 mL DS	10 µg/mL	25–100 µg/h	2.5–10 mL/h	
Phenobarbitone (phenobarbital)	15–25 mg/kg in 100 mL DS over 20–30 min (max. 50 mg/min) by IP	—	—	—	—	—	—	
Phenytoin	15–18 mg/kg in 100 mL NS over 20–30 min (max. 50 mg/min) by IP	—	—	—	—	—	—	
Procainamide	10 mg/kg (max. 1000 mg) in 100 mL DW over 30 min by IP	20–80 µg/kg/min	1000 mg in 100 mL DW	500 mg in 50 mg DW	10 mg/mL	2–6 mg/min	12–36 mL/h	
Propofol	Sedation: 0.5–1.0 mg/kg Induction: 2–3 mg/kg	1–10 mg/kg/h	—	500 mg in 50 mL (dispensed as 20-mL and 50-mL amps, both with 10 mg/mL)	10 mg/mL	Sedation 1–2 mg/kg/h Anaesthesia 5–10 mg/kg/h	Sedation 7–15 mL/h Anaesthesia 35–70 mL/h	

Continued

Drug	Loading dose	Paediatric infusion range (<30 kg)	Dilution		Concentration	Adult dose (70–80 kg)	
			Infusion pump (IP)	Syringe driver		Dose per hour	Volume per hour
rt-PA (alteplase)	15-mg bolus (15 ml)	—	100 mg in 100 ml water BP	—	1 mg/ml	(a) 15-mg bolus (b) 0.75 mg/kg (max 50 mg) over 30 min (c) 0.5 mg/kg (max 35 mg) over 60 min	
r-PA (reteplase)	10-U bolus in 2 min. After 30 min, second 10-U bolus in 2 min	—	—	2 vials/prefilled syringes/ reconstitution devices and needles			
Salbutamol (asthma)	5–10 µg/kg in 100 ml DS over 10 min	1.0–5.0 µg/kg/min	6 mg in 100 mL DS	3 mg in 50 ml DS	60 µg/ml	5–50 µg/min	5–50 ml/h
Salbutamol (asthma)	5–10 µg/kg in 100 ml DS over 10 min	0.2–1.0 µg/kg/min	6 mg in 100 ml DS	3 mg in 50 ml DS	60 µg/ml	10–50 µg/min	10–50 ml/h
Sodium nitroprusside	—	0.05–10 µg/kg/min	100 mg in 500 mL DW in glass bottle Protect from light Discard at 24 h	—	Min 200 µg/mL Max 800 µg/min	0.05–10 µg/kg/min (max. 1.5 mg/kg/24h)	1–210 mL/h 500 mL/24h
Streptokinase *AMI*	1.5 million units in 100 mL NS over 45 min by IP	—	—	—	15 000 units/mL	2.5 mL/min	150 mL/h
PE, DVT, etc.	250 000 units in 100 mL NS over 30 min by IP	1500–2000 units/kg/h	500 000 units in 100 mL NS	—	5000 units/mL	100 000 units/h	20 mL/h

a, b See key, page 40. Abbreviations see key, page 40.

| Drug | Loading dose | Paediatric infusion range (<30 kg) | Dilution | | Concentration | Adult dose (70–80 kg) | |
			Infusion pump (IP)	Syringe driver		Dose per hour	Volume per hour
Thiopentone (thiopental)	3–6 mg/kg (0.5 mg/kg in shock)	1–5 mg/kg/h	2500 mg in 100 mL water BP Protect from light	1250 mg in 50 mL water BP Protect from light	25 mg/mL	75–350 mg/h	3–15 mL/h
Vecuronium	0.1 mg/kg	0.05–0.1 mg/kg/h	100 mg in 100 mL. Reconstitute in water BP Dilute in DS	50 mg in 50 mL. Reconstitute in water BP Dilute in DS	1.0 mg/mL	4–8 mg/h	4–8 mL/h

AMI, acute myocardial infarct; DS, dextrose saline, or any isotonic crystalloid; DVT, deep vein thrombosis; DW, 5% dextrose in water; IM, intramuscular; IP, infusion pump; IV, intravenous; MAP, mean arterial pressure; NS, normal saline; PE, pulmonary embolus; VT, ventricular tachycardia; water BP, water for injection.

ᵇStandard: use in Emergency department.

ᵃTransport: use for retrievals/interhospital transfers.

Reproduced by kind permission of Associate Professor CT Myers, Director and Head, Department of Emergency Medicine, The Prince Charles Hospital, Brisbane.

Allergy UK. http://www.allergyuk.org/ (anaphylaxis).

American Heart Association. https://eccguidelines.heart.org/index.php/circulation/cpr-ecc-guidelines-2/ (2015 CPR and ECC guidelines).

American Heart Association (2015) Part 1: Executive Summary: 2015 American Heart Association guidelines update for cardiopulmonary resuscitation and emergency cardiovascular care. *Circulation* **132**: S315–S367.

American Heart Association (2015) Part 7: Adult advanced cardiovascular life support: 2015 American Heart Association guidelines update for cardiopulmonary resuscitation and emergency cardiovascular care. *Circulation* **132**: S444–S464.

Australian Resuscitation Council. http://www.resus.org.au/ (resuscitation guidelines 2015).

Australasian Society of Clinical Immunology and Allergy. http://www.allergy.org.au/ (anaphylaxis).

Dellinger R, Levy M, Rhodes A *et al.* (2013) Surviving Sepsis Campaign: International Guidelines for Management of Severe Sepsis and Septic Shock: 2012. *Critical Care Medicine* **41**: 580–637.

European Resuscitation Council. http://cprguidelines.eu/ (ERC Guidelines 2015).

European Resuscitation Council (2015) European Resuscitation Council Guidelines for Resuscitation 2015 Section 1. Executive summary. *Resuscitation* **95**: 1–80.

European Resuscitation Council (2015) European Resuscitation Council Guidelines for Resuscitation 2015 Section 3. Adult advanced life support. *Resuscitation* **95**: 100–147.

Lieberman P, Nicklas R, Oppenheimer J *et al.* (2010) The diagnosis and management of anaphylaxis practice parameter: 2010 Update. *Journal of Allergy and Clinical Immunology* **126**: 480.e1–41.

National Health and Medical Research Council (Australia). http://www.nhmrc.gov.au/guidelines/search

National Institute for Health and Care Excellence, NHS UK. http://www.nice.org.uk/guidance/published

Scottish Intercollegiate Guidelines Network. http://www.sign.ac.uk/

Trauma.org http://trauma.org/ (severe head injury).

GENERAL MEDICAL EMERGENCIES

DIFFERENTIAL DIAGNOSIS

Always consider the life-threatening diagnoses first:

- Acute coronary syndrome (ACS), such as myocardial infarction or unstable angina.
- Pulmonary embolus.
- Aortic dissection.

Warning: patients with these can present with few physical signs and/or a non-diagnostic chest radiograph (CXR) and electrocardiogram (ECG), so may have to initially be managed on clinical suspicion alone. Attach a cardiac monitor and pulse oximeter to the patient, establish venous access and give 35% oxygen.

Other causes to consider include:

- Pericarditis.
- Pleurisy.
- Pneumonia.
- Pneumothorax.
- Abdominal – oesophagitis, oesophageal rupture, gall bladder disease, etc.
- Musculoskeletal and chest wall pain.

ACUTE CORONARY SYNDROME

The term acute coronary syndrome (ACS) encompasses the spectrum of patients presenting with chest pain or other symptoms due to myocardial ischaemia that ranges from ST elevation myocardial infarction (STEMI), non-ST elevation myocardial infarction (NSTEMI) to unstable angina pectoris (UA), with the latter two often referred to as NSTEAC (non-ST elevation acute coronary syndrome).

The common pathophysiology of ACS is rupture or erosion of an atherosclerotic plaque.

ST ELEVATION MYOCARDIAL INFARCTION (STEMI)

DIAGNOSIS

1   Predisposing factors include cigarette smoking, hypertension, diabetes, hyper-cholesterolaemia, male sex, increasing age and a positive family history.

2   There may be a prior history of angina, myocardial infarction or heart failure, or alternatively the condition may arise *de novo*.

3   'Typical' pain is central, heavy, burning, crushing or tight retrosternal, usually lasting for several minutes or longer, unrelieved by sublingual nitrates, and is associated with anxiety, dyspnoea, nausea and vomiting.

4   The pain may radiate to the neck, jaw, one or both arms, the back and occasionally the epigastrium, or may present at these sites alone.

    (i)   Atypical symptoms occur more frequently in people with diabetes, the elderly and in females.

5   The patient may be clammy, sweaty, breathless and pale or the patient may appear deceptively well.

6   Alternatively, the patient may present with a complication such as a cardiac arrhythmia (fast or slow), heart failure, severe hypotension with cardiogenic shock, ventricular septal rupture or papillary muscle rupture, systemic embolism or pericarditis.

7   Establish venous access with an i.v. cannula and attach a cardiac monitor and pulse oximeter to the patient.

8   Send blood for full blood count (FBC), coagulation profile, electrolyte and liver function tests (ELFTs), cardiac biomarker assay such as cardiac troponin I (cTnI) or troponin T (cTnT) and lipid profile.
    (i)   Do not delay definitive management while awaiting a result.
    (ii)   Cardiac biomarkers can be normal early on.
    (iii) Higher elevated troponin levels identify an increase in adverse outcome risk.

9   Electrocardiogram (ECG). Perform this within 10 min of patient arrival, and arrange for immediate review by a senior emergency department (ED) doctor.
    (i)   Look for ST elevation in two or more contiguous leads.
    (ii)   The greater the number of leads affected and the higher the ST segments, the higher the mortality.
    (iii) Inferior myocardial infarction causes changes in leads II, III and aVF.
    (iv)   Anterior myocardial infarction causes changes in I, aVL and V1–V3 (anteroseptal) or V4–V6 (anterolateral).
    (v)   True posterior myocardial infarction causes mirror-image changes of tall R waves and ST depression in leads V1–V4.
    (vi)   Repeat the ECG after 5–10 min in symptomatic patients with an initial non-diagnostic ECG.

10 Perform a CXR to look for pulmonary oedema, cardiomegaly and atelectasis. Request a portable X-ray in the ED, provided this does not delay definitive management.

MANAGEMENT

1   Give high-dose 40–60% oxygen only in patients with hypoxia (oxygen saturation <93%), or for those with shock. If there is a prior history of obstructive airways disease, give 28% oxygen.

2   Give aspirin 150–300 mg orally unless contraindicated by known hyper-sensitivity.
    (i)   Also give clopidogrel 300 mg oral loading dose if followed by thrombolysis, or 600 mg if PCI will follow.
    (ii)   Alternatively give prasugrel 60 mg orally if undergoing PCI (see below), or ticagrelor 180 mg orally, according to cardiologist preference.

3 Maximize pain relief:
  (i) Give glyceryl trinitrate (GTN) 300–600 µg sublingually, maintaining systolic blood pressure (BP) above 100 mmHg and avoiding excessive hypotension.
  (ii) Add morphine 2.5–5 mg i.v. with an antiemetic, e.g. metoclopramide 10 mg i.v., if pain persists.

4 *Reperfusion therapy*
Consider reperfusion therapy in consultation with the senior ED doctor. Aim to either commence thrombolysis within a maximum of 30 min of the patient's arrival in hospital, without delay by transferring to the CCU, or arrange for percutaneous coronary intervention (PCI) if this is available in under 60–90 min.

5 *Thrombolysis*
This is indicated within 12 h (ideally 6 h) of the onset of myocardial ischaemic pain in patients with a STEMI, e.g. ECG evidence of ST elevation MI, with ST elevation of at least 1 mm in two contiguous limb leads or 2 mm in two contiguous precordial chest leads, and for presumed new left bundle branch block (LBBB).
  (i) *Absolute contraindications* to thrombolysis:
      (a) intracerebral or subarachnoid haemorrhage ever, intracranial malignancy
      (b) thrombotic stroke in previous 3 months
      (c) known bleeding diathesis or active bleeding (excluding menses)
      (d) significant head or facial trauma in previous 3 months
      (e) aortic dissection (see p. 57).
  (ii) *Relative contraindications* (thrombolysis may still be considered in those at highest risk of death, or with greatest net clinical benefit, such as a large anterior infarction presenting within 3 h of symptom onset):
      (a) oral anticoagulant therapy
      (b) pregnancy or within 1 week post partum
      (c) major surgery in last 3 weeks
      (d) non-compressible arterial puncture or central line
      (e) refractory hypertension (systolic BP over 180 mmHg, diastolic BP over 110 mmHg)
      (f) history of severe or poorly controlled hypertension
      (g) prolonged CPR over 10 min
      (h) severe hepatic or renal disease.
  (iii) Administer tenecteplase (TNK) as the lytic agent of choice:
      (a) give tenecteplase 30 mg (weight <60 kg), 35 mg (weight ≥60 to <70 kg), 40 mg (≥70 to <80 kg), 45 mg (≥80 to <90 kg) and 50 mg (weight ≥90 kg) as a single bolus over 10 s
      (b) tenecteplase is easiest to administer, safe given weight-based, has greater fibrin specificity and efficacy up to 12 h
      (c) continue ECG monitoring for reperfusion arrhythmias.

(iv) Start unfractionated heparin by i.v. bolus 60 units/kg (maximum 4000 units), then i.v. infusion at 12 units/kg/h (maximum 1000 units/h) adjusted according to APTT

    (a) alternatively, give low-molecular-weight (LMW) heparin such as enoxaparin 30 mg i.v. immediately, then after 15 min 1 mg/kg up to 100 mg subcutaneously (s.c.) 12-hourly

    (b) omit i.v. bolus if age over 75 yr and give enoxaparin 0.75 mg up to 75 mg s.c. 12-hourly.

(v) Other fibrin-specific lytic agents to consider if tenecteplase is unavailable include:

    (a) reteplase 10 units as a bolus over no more than 2 min, followed after 30 min by a further 10 units bolus i.v.

    (b) alteplase (rt-PA) 15 mg (15 mL) bolus, followed by an infusion of 0.75 mg/kg over 30 min (to maximum 50 mg), then 0.5 mg/kg over 60 min (to maximum 35 mg).

(vi) Give streptokinase (SK) 1.5 million units over 45–60 min in 100 mL normal saline only if none of the above fibrin-specific agents are available. The early infarct-related artery vessel patency rate is less than with those agents

    (a) avoid SK if it has been given between 3 days and 12 months previously, or immediately after a severe streptococcal infection

    (b) slow or stop the infusion if hypotension or rash occurs. Restart the infusion as soon as they have resolved

    (c) occasionally, severe hypotension and anaphylaxis may occur, requiring oxygen, adrenaline (epinephrine) and fluids, etc. (see p. 27).

6   *Percutaneous coronary intervention (PCI)*

Organize primary percutaneous coronary intervention in preference to thrombolysis, when it is available locally in less than 90 min of patient arrival, or in less than 60 min if the chest pain onset was within the last hour.

(i) It is superior to thrombolysis, particularly in a high-volume centre preferably with cardiac surgery capability.

(ii) It is preferred in cardiogenic shock, and if thrombolysis is contraindicated.

(iii) Give thrombolysis with tenecteplase if the PCI will take longer than the 60–90 min to organize.

**7   **Transfer the patient to the CCU following thrombolysis, or to the catheter lab for PCI, with a doctor and nurse escort, and resuscitation equipment and drugs available.

NON-ST ELEVATION MYOCARDIAL INFARCTION (NSTEMI) AND UNSTABLE ANGINA

DIAGNOSIS

1   The predisposing factors and pathophysiology are the same as for STEMI (see p. 44).

2   It is not possible from the character of the chest pain alone to accurately exclude ACS, **unless** a clear alternative cause for the pain is apparent (see Table 2.1).
    (i)   Older patients, females, diabetics and chronic renal failure patients may present with atypical ACS pain.
    (ii) Unstable angina (UA) includes increasing severity or frequency of angina, angina at rest and new-onset angina that markedly limits physical activity or following a recent myocardial infarction.

3   As NSTEMI and UA take time to differentiate, they are often referred to collectively as NSTEAC (non-ST elevation acute coronary syndrome).

4   Establish venous access with an i.v. cannula, and attach a cardiac monitor and pulse oximeter to the patient.

5   Send blood for FBC, coagulation profile, ELFTs, cardiac biomarker assay such as cardiac troponin I (cTnI) or troponin T (cTnT) and lipid profile, exactly as for STEMI.

6   Perform an ECG within 10 min of patient arrival, with immediate review by a senior ED doctor.
    (i)   This may show ST depression, T wave inversion or flattening, non-specific or transient changes, or
    (ii) The ECG may be normal.

MANAGEMENT

1   Give aspirin 150–300 mg orally unless contraindicated by known hypersensitivity.
    (i)   Give clopidogrel 300 mg oral loading dose, then 75 mg once daily if aspirin-intolerant, or in addition if this is local policy.

2   Give GTN 300–600 µg sublingually, and add morphine 2.5–5 mg i.v. with an antiemetic, e.g. metoclopramide 10 mg i.v., if pain persists.

3   Commence heparin for all patients with a suspected NSTEMI or UA, without necessarily awaiting the first cardiac biomarker results particularly with new ECG changes.
    (i)   Give LMW heparin such as enoxaparin 1 mg/kg s.c. or dalteparin 120 units/kg s.c. both 12-hourly, or
    (ii) Give unfractionated (UF) heparin i.v. bolus 60–70 units/kg (maximum 5000 units), followed by an infusion at 12–15 units/kg/h (maximum 1000 units/h)
        (a) UF heparin may be preferred in hospitals likely to offer coronary angioplasty (PCI) within 24–36 h of symptom onset

Table 2.1 Differential diagnosis of chest pain in patients presenting with possible acute coronary syndrome (ACS)

Diagnosis	Classic history	Physical examination	Diagnostic testing
Acute coronary syndrome (see p. 44)	Band-like, tight, or pressure pain with radiation to neck and arms, sweating, dyspnoea, cardiac risk factors	May be normal, or may have evidence of heart failure, hypotension	Cardiac biomarkers, ECG, possibly stress testing
Pulmonary embolus (see p. 51)	Sudden onset, pleuritic pain, dyspnoea, risks for venous thrombo-embolism	Tachycardia, tachypnoea, pleural rub, low-grade fever	CXR, V/Q scan, CTPA
Aortic dissection (see p. 57)	Sudden, sharp, tearing pain radiating to back, neurologic symptoms	Unequal pulses or BP, new murmur, bruits	CXR, echocardiogram, CT angiogram
Pericarditis (see p. 58)	Pleuritic, positional ache, worse lying down	Fever, pericardial rub, tachycardia	ECG, CXR, echocardiogram
Pneumonia (see p. 68)	Cough, fever, dyspnoea, pleuritic pain, malaise	Fever, hypoxia, tachypnoea, tachycardia, abnormal breath sounds	CXR, WCC
Pneumothorax (see p. 73)	Pleuritic pain, dyspnoea	Reduced breath sounds over hemithorax	CXR
Oesophageal rupture (Boerhaave's syndrome) (see p. 186)	Constant, severe retrosternal pain, dysphagia	Subcutaneous emphysema	CXR, CT chest
Gastrointestinal causes (see p. 59)	Burning, nocturnal pain, gastrointestinal symptoms	Abdominal tenderness, rebound or guarding	Lipase, AXR, ultrasound
Musculoskeletal causes (see p. 60)	Pain increased with movement or muscular activity	Chest-wall tenderness to palpation (may occur in ACS!)	Normal

ACS, acute coronary syndrome; AXR, abdominal X-ray; BP, blood pressure; CT, computerized tomography; CTPA, computerized tomography pulmonary angiogram; CXR, chest X-ray; ECG, electrocardiograph; V/Q, ventilation perfusion; WCC, white cell count.

      (b) titrate the UF heparin infusion to an activated partial thromboplastin time (aPTT) of 50–70 s by 6 h post infusion

      (c) alternatively give bivalirudin 0.1 mg/kg i.v. bolus followed by 0.25 mg/kg/h if PCI is planned, so check your local policy.

4 Admit **all** patients.

The final diagnosis of NSTEMI (rise in cardiac troponin biomarker), UA (no rise in troponin or cardiac biomarker) or non-cardiac chest pain (normal cardiac biomarkers, normal ECGs, normal non-invasive test) takes time to establish.

    (i) Admit patients with '**high-risk**' features directly to the coronary care unit (CCU). These include any one or more of:

      (a) elevated troponin on arrival blood test, repetitive or prolonged chest pain over 10 min, diabetic patient or chronic kidney disease patient with estimated glomerular filtration rate of <60 mL/min and typical symptoms of ACS, associated syncope, symptoms or signs of heart failure (see p. 75), signs of new mitral incompetence (pansystolic murmur), PCI in the last 6 months or prior revascularization (coronary artery bypass graft [CABG]), haemodynamic instability or ECG changes.

    (ii) Admit patients with '**intermediate-risk**' features under the medical team, possibly to a shared chest pain assessment unit (CPAU). These include any one or more of:

      (a) chest pain or discomfort within the past 48 h occurring at rest, or that was repetitive or prolonged (but currently resolved), age over 65 years, two or more risk factors of hypertension, family history, active smoking or hyperlipidaemia, and diabetic patient or chronic kidney disease patient with estimated glomerular filtration rate of <60 mL/min and atypical symptoms of ACS

      (b) lack of CCU beds may necessitate that all diabetic or chronic renal impairment patients are treated as intermediate-risk and are admitted to a general ward (rather than to CCU as high-risk if they have typical symptoms of ACS)

      (c) repeat the ECG and troponin by 6–8 h post arrival in the ED, or earlier than this according to local policy

      (d) admit the patient to CCU if chest pain recurs, the ECG changes, or the repeat cardiac troponin is elevated, as they have now become a high-risk patient.

    (iii) Meanwhile, arrange a non-invasive test such as an ECG exercise stress test (EST) if the repeat ECG and cardiac biomarkers remain normal and the pain does not recur:

      (a) ideally this non-invasive test is performed as an inpatient

      (b) only if this test is normal has ACS finally now been excluded and the patient can go home

(c) local policy may instead be to arrange an outpatient non-invasive test preferably within 72 h of discharge as determined by local availability, such as EST, stress echo, myocardial perfusion scan or CT coronary angiography (CTCA)

(d) make sure the general practitioner (GP) is kept informed.

> **Warning:** never discharge any chest pain patient after a single normal troponin test as a second paired test plus repeat ECG by 6–8 h post-arrival is mandatory, followed by some form of non-invasive test to definitely rule out ACS.

NON-CARDIAC CHEST PAIN

DIAGNOSIS

1 A stabbing, pleuritic, positional or palpation-induced pain is less characteristic of ACS, but can **not** absolutely exclude it.

2 Thus non-cardiac chest pain is a diagnosis of exclusion, unless there are clear positive features that indicate its origin such as immediate rib pain following a fall or blow, or a sudden onset related to a sneeze or deep cough.

3 Non-cardiac chest pain is diagnosed by finding definite features of an alternative diagnosis such as a PE, aortic dissection, pericarditis, pleurisy, pneumothorax, etc. (see Table 2.1).

    (i) Otherwise perform serial ECGs and troponins, and arrange a non-invasive test to rule out ACS.

MANAGEMENT

1 Give every patient in whom the diagnosis is not immediately clear aspirin 150–300 mg orally unless contraindicated by known hypersensitivity.

2 Management will depend on which cause is suspected or found (see above or following pages).

PULMONARY EMBOLUS

DIAGNOSIS

1 Venous thromboembolism (VTE) includes PE and deep venous thrombosis (DVT).

2 Predisposing risk factors for VTE are best divided into acute provoking and chronic predisposing, and apply to both PE and DVT (see Table 2.2).

3 A small PE causes sudden dyspnoea, cough, pleuritic pain and possibly haemoptysis, with few physical signs. Look for a low-grade pyrexia (37.5°C), tachypnoea over 20/min, tachycardia, crepitations and a pleural rub.

4 A major PE causes dyspnoea, chest pain and light-headedness or syncope. Look for cyanosis, tachycardia, hypotension, a parasternal heave, raised jugular venous pressure (JVP) and a loud delayed pulmonary second sound.

Table 2.2 Predisposing risk factors for venous thromboembolism (VTE)

Acute provoking factors
Hospitalization, i.e. reduced mobility
Surgery, particularly abdominal, pelvic, leg
Trauma or fracture of lower limbs or pelvis
Immobilization (includes plaster cast)
Long haul travel – over 3000 miles or 5000 km
Recently commenced oestrogen therapy (e.g. within previous 2 weeks)
Intravascular device (e.g. venous catheter)

Chronic predisposing factors		
Inherited	**Acquired**	**Inherited or acquired**
Natural anticoagulant deficiency such as protein C, protein S, antithrombin III deficiency	Increasing age	High plasma homocysteine
Factor V Leiden	Obesity	High plasma coagulation factors VIII, IX, XI
Prothrombin G20210A mutation	Cancer (chemotherapy)	Antiphospholipid syndrome (anticardiolipin antibodies and lupus anticoagulant)
	Leg paralysis	
	Oestrogen therapy	
	Pregnancy or puerperium	
	Major medical illness[a]	
	Previous venous thromboembolism (DVT/PE)	

[a] Chronic cardiorespiratory disease, inflammatory bowel disease, nephritic syndrome, myeloproliferative disorders.
DVT, deep vein thrombosis; PE, pulmonary embolus.
Modified from Ho WK, Hankey GJ (2005) Venous thromboembolism: diagnosis and management of deep venous thrombosis. *Med J Aust* **182**:476–81.

5   Establish venous access with an i.v. cannula, send blood for FBC, coagulation profile and ELFTs, and attach a cardiac monitor and pulse oximeter to the patient.

   (i)   Only request a D-dimer test after assessing the clinical pre-test probability as low and one or more PE rule-out criteria (PERC) are positive. See points 9 to 11 below.

6   Consider a blood gas that may reflect hypocapnia from hyperventilation, and less commonly hypoxia, but will be normal in over 20% patients with PE.

    (i)   Do **not** perform an arterial blood gas (ABG) routinely, unless there is an unexplained low pulse oximeter reading on room air. ABGs rarely help.

7   Perform an ECG, mainly to exclude other diagnoses such as ACS or pericarditis.

    (i)   It may show a tachycardia alone or possibly right axis deviation, right heart strain, right bundle branch block (RBBB) or atrial fibrillation (AF) in PE.

    (ii)   The well-known 'S1Q3T3' pattern is neither sensitive nor specific for PE.

8   Request a CXR, again mainly to exclude other diagnoses such as pneumonia or a pneumothorax.

    (i)   It may be normal in PE, or show a blunted costophrenic angle, raised hemidiaphragm, an area of linear atelectasis or infarction, or an area of oligaemia.

9   Determine the clinical pre-test probability now **before** requesting any further diagnostic imaging (see Table 2.3).

    (i)   A low pre-test probability on Wells' criteria with a score of <2 has up to 3.6% probability of PE.

    (ii)   A moderate pre-test probability with a Wells' criteria score of 2–6 has a 20.5% probability of PE.

Table 2.3 Estimation of the clinical pre-test probability for suspected pulmonary embolus (PE)

Feature	Score
Clinical signs and symptoms of DVT (minimum of leg swelling and pain with palpation of the deep veins. See p. 55)	3
Alternative diagnosis less likely than PE	3
Heart rate >100 beats/min	1.5
Immobilization or surgery in previous 4 weeks	1.5
Previous DVT or PE	1.5
Haemoptysis	1
Cancer	1

Low pre-test probability = score <2. **Moderate** pre-test probability = score 2–6.
High pre-test probability = score >6.
DVT, deep venous thrombosis; PE, pulmonary embolus.
Modified from Wells PS, Anderson DR, Rodger M *et al.* (2001) Excluding pulmonary embolism at the bedside without diagnostic imaging: management of patients with suspected pulmonary embolism presenting to the emergency department by using a simple clinical model and D-dimer. *Ann Intern Med* **135**:98–107.

(iii) A high pre-test probability with a Wells' criteria score of >6 has a 66.7% probability of PE.

10 Patients under 50 years old *and* with a low pre-test probability:

(i) Check if the PERC rule score is negative (see Table 2.4) and if all criteria are fulfilled, no further testing is required and a PE is ruled out.

11 Send a D-dimer test only in patients ≥50 years with a low pre-test probability, or in any patient under 50 with a low pre-test probability but with one or more PERC criteria positive (see Table 2.4).

(i) Check with the laboratory which D-dimer test they use and their test's reference ranges, in particular their normal cut-off range.

(ii) Arrange imaging if the D-dimer test comes back positive (see below).

(iii) Discharge the patient if this D-dimer test is negative, i.e. there is no PE.

12 Perform a multislice, helical computed tomography pulmonary angiogram (CTPA) if available, in all patients with a moderate or high pre-test probability, and in those low pre-test probability patients with a positive D-dimer.

(i) Follow this if negative in a high pre-test probability patient, with a lower-limb venous Doppler ultrasound to rule out an embolic source.

13 Alternatively, start with a ventilation–perfusion isotope lung scan, the V/Q scan.

(i) A V/Q scan is preferred when the patient is allergic to contrast dye, has renal failure or is younger than 40 years, particularly in females.

(ii) In addition the CXR should be normal with no history of chronic lung disease.

Table 2.4 Pulmonary embolism rule-out criteria (PERC) rule in the low pre-test probability patient

Age <50 years
Pulse <100 beats/min
Pulse oximetry >94%
No unilateral leg swelling
No haemoptysis
No recent trauma or surgery
No prior pulmonary embolism or deep vein thrombosis
No oral hormone use

When all eight factors are fulfilled (negative), no further testing is required.
Modified from Kline JA, Mitchell AM, Kabrhel C *et al.* (2004) Clinical criteria to prevent unnecessary diagnostic testing in ED patients with suspected pulmonary embolism. *Journal of Thrombosis and Haemostasis* **2:** 1247–55.

(iii) Unfortunately, over half the V/Q results will not help, i.e. are low or intermediate probability results, and *must* still be followed by further testing, such as CTPA or lower-limb venous Doppler ultrasound.

MANAGEMENT

1 Give high-dose oxygen through a face mask. Aim for an oxygen saturation above 94%.

2 Relieve pain if it is severe with morphine 5 mg i.v. and give an antiemetic such as metoclopramide 10 mg i.v.

3 Commence heparin in intermediate or high pre-test probability patients, unless a diagnostic imaging test is imminently available, and contraindications such as active bleeding, thrombocytopenia, recent trauma or cerebral haemorrhage are absent:

    (i) Give LMW heparin such as enoxaparin 1 mg/kg s.c. or dalteparin s.c. according to body weight, both 12-hourly.

    (ii) Alternatively, give UF heparin 80 units/kg i.v. bolus, followed by 18 units/kg/h infusion

        (a) this is preferred with a major PE, as a first dose bolus or according to local policy.

4 Admit all patients with a confirmed PE under the medical team, or if the test results remain indeterminate.

    (i) Arrange sequential testing with a V/Q scan then a CTPA or vice versa, plus or minus a lower-limb venous Doppler ultrasound to finally rule in or out the diagnosis.

    (ii) Commence heparin once a positive result is confirmed, if not already started.

5 Get help from a senior ED doctor for any apparent major, life-threatening PE patient:

    (i) Arrange a bedside echocardiograph to look for RV dilatation and hypokinesis, and involve the intensive care team early.

    (ii) Reserve thrombolysis with recombinant tissue plasminogen activator (rt-PA) 10 mg i.v. over 1–2 min, then 90 mg over 2 h (or 1.5 mg/kg maximum if under 65 kg) for patients with a massive PE in shock, with acute right heart failure and systolic hypotension.

VENOUS THROMBOEMBOLISM WITH DEEP VEIN THROMBOSIS

DIAGNOSIS

1 Predisposing risk factors are as for venous thromboembolism. Up to two-thirds of patients have acute provoking factors (see Table 2.2).

2 Typical symptoms include leg pain, swelling, tenderness and redness or discoloration.

3   Examination may reveal unilateral oedema, warmth, superficial venous dilatation, increased limb girth or tenderness along the deep venous system.

    (i)   Unfortunately, a similar picture is seen in cellulitis, lymphoedema, musculoskeletal injury and varicose vein insufficiency.

    (ii)   Homan's sign of pain on forced ankle dorsiflexion is unreliable, unhelpful and not recommended.

4   Ask about any associated features of a concomitant PE (see p. 51), particularly in suspected proximal DVT above the knee.

5   Exactly as with PE, determine the clinical pre-test probability of a DVT now **before** requesting diagnostic testing (see Table 2.5).

    (i)   A low pre-test probability on Wells' criteria with a score ≤0 has up to a 5% probability of DVT.

    (ii)   A moderate pre-test probability with a Wells' score 1–2 has a 17% probability of DVT, and a high pre-test probability with a Wells' score ≥3 has up to a 53% probability of DVT.

6   Send blood for D-dimer only when the pre-test probability is low.

    (i)   Discharge the patient if this D-dimer is negative, that is no DVT, provided alternative diagnoses do not require further care.

Table 2.5 Estimation of the clinical pre-test probability for suspected deep venous thrombosis (DVT)

Clinical feature	Score
Active cancer (treatment ongoing or within 6 months or palliative)	1
Paralysis, paresis or recent plaster immobilization of the lower extremities	1
Recently bedridden for ≥3 days, or major surgery within the previous 12 weeks	1
Localized tenderness along the distribution of the deep venous system	1
Entire leg swollen	1
Calf swelling >3 cm when compared with the asymptomatic leg (at 10 cm below the tibial tuberosity)	1
Pitting oedema: confined to the symptomatic leg	1
Collateral superficial veins (non-varicose)	1
Previously documented deep venous thrombosis	1
Alternative diagnosis as likely or greater than that of deep venous thrombosis	−2

In patients with symptoms in both legs, the more symptomatic leg is scored.
Low pre-test probability = score ≤0.
Moderate pre-test probability = score 1–2.
High pre-test probability = score ≥3.
From Wells PS, Owen C, Doucette S et al. (2006) Does this patient have deep vein thrombosis? *J Amer Med Assoc* **295**:199–207.

7   Perform Doppler ultrasound on all moderate and high pre-test probability patients, and when the D-dimer test is positive.

MANAGEMENT

1   Give the patient analgesia such as paracetamol 500 mg with codeine 8 mg two tablets orally q.d.s. or an anti-inflammatory such as ibuprofen 200–400 mg orally t.d.s. or naproxen 250 mg orally t.d.s.

2   Commence heparin if the diagnosis is confirmed.
    (i)   Give LMW heparin such as enoxaparin 1 mg/kg s.c. 12-hourly or dalteparin according to body weight s.c. 12-hourly.
    (ii) Alternatively, give UF heparin 80 units/kg i.v. bolus followed by 18 units/kg/h infusion particularly for a large or extensive DVT, according to local policy.

3   Refer all patients to the medical team if the diagnosis is confirmed.
    (i)   Some patients may be discharged for outpatient LMW heparin, or NOAC rivaroxaban 15 mg orally b.d. for 3 weeks then 20 mg once daily, providing the creatinine clearance is >30 mL/min. Check your local policy.
    (ii) Other patients may even be sent home without any treatment at all if the DVT is confined below the knee
        (a) organize a repeat US scan within 5–7 days in those not treated to exclude more proximal extension of the thrombosis.

4   Get senior ED doctor advice if the diagnosis is still indeterminate.

AORTIC DISSECTION

DIAGNOSIS

1   Predisposed to by hypertension typically in males 60–80 years old. Other risk factors include Marfan's syndrome, bicuspid aortic valve, coarctation, cocaine use, iatrogenic trauma or prior cardiovascular surgery.

2   The onset is abrupt with sudden pain that is sharp or tearing, retrosternal, interscapular or lower in the back or migratory, and may be severe and resistant to opiates.

3   Look for unequal or absent pulses, a difference of blood pressure in the arms >20 mmHg, or the following complications of the dissection:
    (i)   Aortic incompetence, myocardial ischaemia and haemopericardium with pericardial rub or cardiac tamponade (see p. 10).
    (ii) Dyspnoea, pleural rub or effusion.
    (iii) Agitation, altered consciousness, syncope, hemiplegia or paraplegia.
    (iv) Intestinal ischaemia or bowel infarction with abdominal pain and bloody diarrhoea.
    (v)   Oliguria and haematuria.

4 Establish venous access with a large-bore (14- or 16-gauge) i.v. cannula, and send blood for FBC, ELFTs, cardiac enzymes and group and cross-match. Attach a cardiac monitor and pulse oximeter to the patient.

5 Perform an ECG, which may look remarkably normal despite the severity of the pain, with left ventricular hypertrophy and non-specific changes.

6 Request a CXR that may show a widened mediastinum, blurred aortic knob and a left pleural effusion, but can be normal.

MANAGEMENT

1 Give high-dose oxygen via a face mask. Aim for an oxygen saturation above 94%.

2 Relieve the pain with morphine 5–10 mg i.v. and give an antiemetic.

3 Reduce the systolic BP to below 110 mmHg using a labetalol infusion or sodium nitroprusside plus propranolol i.v. in consultation with the senior ED doctor or intensive care team, when dissection is diagnosed or highly likely.

4 Organize an urgent helical CT angiogram, transoesophageal echocardiogram or aortogram to confirm the diagnosis.

5 Contact the cardiothoracic surgeons and arrange transfer without delay. Involve the intensive care team early.

PERICARDITIS

DIAGNOSIS

1 This may be post-viral such as Coxsackie or follow a myocardial infarction either early within 24 h or later at 2–3 weeks (Dressler's syndrome), pericardiotomy, connective tissue disorder, uraemia, trauma, tuberculosis or a neoplasm.

2 The pain is sharp, pleuritic, retrosternal and positional, relieved by sitting forward.

3 Listen for a pericardial friction rub, best heard along the left sternal edge with the patient sitting forward, which may be transient or intermittent.

4 Send blood for FBC, ELFTs, cardiac biomarkers and viral serology. Attach a cardiac monitor and pulse oximeter to the patient.

5 Perform an ECG that may show sinus tachycardia alone or AF, widespread concave ST elevation, followed by T wave flattening then inversion.

6 Request a CXR, which is usually normal, even if a pericardial effusion is present.

MANAGEMENT

1 Give high-dose oxygen via a face mask. Aim for an oxygen saturation above 94%.

2 Give the patient a non-steroidal anti-inflammatory analgesic such as ibuprofen 200–400 mg orally t.d.s. or naproxen 250 mg orally t.d.s.

    (i) Use colchicine 500 μg orally b.d. (halve dose if diarrhoea occurs) or prednisone 50 mg orally, when intolerant to NSAIDs.

3 Refer the patient to the medical team for bed rest and cardiac monitoring if there are widespread ECG changes or raised cardiac enzymes.

4 Arrange urgent echocardiography and pericardiocentesis for signs of cardiac tamponade such as tachycardia, hypotension, pulsus paradoxus and a raised JVP that rises on inspiration, known as Kussmaul's sign (see p. 10).

PLEURISY

DIAGNOSIS

1 Pleurisy or pleuritic pain occurs in association with pneumonia, pulmonary infarction from a PE, neoplasia, tuberculosis, connective tissue disorders, uraemia, or following trauma.

2 It may also be due to viruses, especially enteroviruses, and may be mimicked by a pneumothorax or epidemic myalgia (Bornholm's disease).

3 The pain is sharp, knife-like, localized and exacerbated by moving, coughing or breathing, which tends to be shallow. Radiation to the shoulder or abdomen occurs with diaphragmatic involvement.

4 Listen for a pleural rub, although this may be inaudible if pain limits deep breathing, and disappears as an effusion develops.

5 Send ABGs if there are significant signs of pulmonary parenchymal disease. Perform an ECG, which should be normal.

6 Request a CXR that may reveal the underlying cause or may be quite normal.

MANAGEMENT

1 Give the patient oxygen and a non-steroidal anti-inflammatory analgesic such as ibuprofen 200–400 mg orally t.d.s. or naproxen 250 mg orally t.d.s.

2 Rule out a PE if there was sudden dyspnoea, tachypnoea and risk factors for thromboembolism. A PE is possible even with a normal CXR and ECG (see p. 51).

3 Refer the patient to the medical team for treatment of the underlying cause, or discuss with the senior ED doctor before discharging.

ABDOMINAL CAUSES OF CHEST PAIN

DIAGNOSIS AND MANAGEMENT

1 *Oesophagitis*
    (i) This is suggested by burning retrosternal or epigastric pain, worse on stooping or recumbency, exacerbated by alcohol, hot drinks or food, and relieved by antacids.
    (ii) It may mimic cardiac pain and may even be relieved by sublingual GTN, so consult the senior ED doctor
        (a) admit the patient to rule out ACS with serial ECGs and troponins, if there is any doubt at all about the diagnosis.
    (iii) Otherwise give an antacid or proton-pump inhibitor orally.

2 *Oesophageal rupture.* See page 186.

3 *Acute cholecystitis, pancreatitis* and *peptic ulceration* may cause chest pain, but other diagnostic features should be present.

MUSCULOSKELETAL AND CHEST WALL PAIN

DIAGNOSIS AND MANAGEMENT

1 Musculoskeletal disorders cause pain that is worse with movement and breathing. There may have been preceding strenuous exercise, a bout of coughing, or a history of minor trauma.

2 Pain is localized on palpation and the ECG is normal. A CXR may show a fractured rib but is otherwise normal.

3 Give the patient a non-steroidal anti-inflammatory analgesic such as ibuprofen 200–400 mg orally t.d.s., or naproxen 250 mg orally t.d.s. Refer back to the GP.

4 Two specific causes are:

   (i) *Shingles*

      This causes pain localized to a dermatome, unaffected by breathing, associated with an area of hyperaesthesia preceding the characteristic blistering rash

      (a) give the patient (usually elderly) with severe pain a narcotic analgesic and famciclovir 250 mg orally t.d.s, valaciclovir 1 g orally t.d.s, or aciclovir 800 mg orally five times a day all for 7 days, if seen within 72 h of vesicle eruption

      (b) admit to a suitable isolation area if unable to be nursed at home.

   (ii) *Costochondritis (Tietze's syndrome)*

      This causes localized pain, swelling and tenderness typically around the second costochondral junction, related to physical strain or minor injury.

      (a) prescribe ibuprofen 200–400 mg orally t.d.s., or naproxen 250 mg orally t.d.s. Refer the patient back to the GP.

CARDIAC ARRHYTHMIAS

DIAGNOSIS

1 Cardiac rhythm disturbances include atrial, nodal and ventricular tachycardias, atrial flutter and fibrillation, the bradycardias and the various degrees of heart block.

2 Exclude myocardial ischaemia from ACS as a priority (see p. 44).

3 Consider other underlying precipitating factors for the arrhythmia such as hypoxia from any cause, hypovolaemia from blood or fluid loss, electrolyte disturbances particularly hyperkalaemia, thyroid disease, drug, alcohol or noxious gas toxicity whether inadvertent or deliberate, septicaemia, hypothermia, electrocution, or simple pain and fear.

4 Ask the patient about palpitations, 'missed beats', breathlessness, chest pain, light-headedness and fatigue.

5 Measure the temperature and vital signs and attach a cardiac monitor and pulse oximeter to the patient.

    (i) Abnormal vital signs including hypotension, confusion or associated features such as chest pain and breathlessness necessitate urgent management.

6 Send blood for FBC, ELFTs, cardiac biomarkers, coagulation profile, thyroid function and toxicology screen as indicated. Measure the ABGs if in respiratory distress.

7 Perform an ECG. Look systematically at the following:

    (i) Rate: fast or slow; paroxysmal or continuous?
    (ii) Rhythm: regular, regularly irregular or irregularly irregular?
    (iii) P waves: present, absent and relationship to QRS complexes?
    (iv) PR interval: shortened <120 ms or prolonged over 200 ms?
    (v) QRS complexes: narrow or widened >120 ms?
    (vi) QTc interval (corrected for rate): normal or longer than 450 ms (470 ms in females)?
    (vii) ST segment and T waves: elevated, depressed or inverted?

8 Request a CXR and look for cardiomegaly or evidence of acute pulmonary oedema. See page 75.

 Tip: call the senior ED doctor immediately if the patient is hypotensive with a systolic BP <90 mmHg, is breathless, confused or has chest pain.

MANAGEMENT

This depends on the arrhythmia, cardiovascular stability and the presence of associated chest pain, breathlessness or confusion.

1 Give high-dose 40–60% oxygen unless there is a prior history of obstructive airways disease, in which case give 28% oxygen. Aim for an oxygen saturation over 94%.

2 Give aspirin 150–300 mg orally if there is possible or probable ACS, unless contraindicated by known hypersensitivity.

3 Provide pain relief if needed with GTN 300–600 µg sublingually for coronary ischaemic pain, or morphine 2.5–5 mg i.v. with an antiemetic, e.g. metoclopramide 10 mg i.v., for more severe pain, including non-ischaemic.

4 Correct any electrolyte abnormality. See page 134.

5   *Tachycardia*

This may be sinus with normal preceding P waves, narrow-complex or broad-complex.

   (i)   Look urgently for and treat underlying causes such as hypoxia, hypovolaemia, fever, thyrotoxicosis, sympathomimetic drug, anaemia, pain, etc. if it is a sinus tachycardia.

   (ii)   Otherwise give a synchronized DC shock, if the patient is unstable with hypotension and a systolic BP <90 mmHg, is confused, has chest pain or heart failure (see p. 75)

       (a) start with 120–150 J biphasic and repeat up to three times, with stepwise increases in joules

       (b) a senior doctor with airway experience must first give a short-acting general anaesthetic or i.v. midazolam in the conscious patient

       (c) give amiodarone 300 mg i.v. over 10–20 min if three attempts at synchronized DC cardioversion failed, then repeat the DC shock and follow by an infusion of amiodarone 900 mg over 24 h.

   (iii) *Broad-complex tachycardia*

When regular this may be due to ventricular tachycardia (VT) or supraventricular tachycardia with aberrant conduction (block):

       (a) give amiodarone 5 mg/kg i.v. over 20–60 min if the patient is stable, followed by an infusion of amiodarone 900 mg over 24 h

       (b) consider AF with bundle branch block if the rhythm is irregular, or AF with ventricular pre-excitation as in Wolff–Parkinson–White syndrome:

         – seek expert help if not already involved

         – give flecainide 2 mg/kg over 10 min, or amiodarone 5 mg/kg i.v. followed by an infusion

         – **avoid** adenosine, verapamil, digoxin and diltiazem, as they block the atrioventricular (AV) node and may worsen pre-excited AF leading to VT or even ventricular fibrillation (VF).

Tip: frequent ventricular ectopic beats (VEBs) do not require treatment other than reducing caffeine or alcohol, unless they are multi-focal, in runs or arrive on the T wave of the preceding complex.

   (iv) *Narrow-complex supraventricular tachycardia (SVT)*

When regular this may be one of the re-entry tachycardias or atrial flutter with regular AV conduction (usually 2 to 1 block if the rate is about 150/min)

       (a) proceed directly to synchronized DC cardioversion if the patient is shocked, unstable or deteriorating, starting at 70–120 J biphasic, after a senior doctor with airway experience has given a short-acting anaesthetic

(b) use a vagal stimulus such as carotid sinus massage (CSM)
if patient is stable and young with no carotid bruit, or prior
transient ischaemic attack (TIA) or cerebrovascular accident
(CVA)
- press firmly at the upper border of the thyroid
cartilage against the vertebral process with a circular
motion
- or get the patient to perform Valsalva's manoeuvre supine
for 15 s to a pressure of 40 mmHg
(c) give adenosine 6 mg rapidly over 2–5 s i.v. if CSM fails,
followed by 12 mg i.v. rapidly after 1–2 min, then a further
12 mg i.v. rapidly once more if still no response
- make sure to warn the patient to expect transient facial
flushing, headache, dyspnoea, chest discomfort and nausea
from the adenosine
(d) alternatively, give verapamil 5 mg i.v. as a bolus over 30 s to
2 min. Verapamil may cause hypotension and bradycardia,
particularly in elderly patients, who should be pre-treated
with calcium gluconate 10 mL given slowly i.v. to prevent
these
(e) **never** use verapamil after a β-blocker, when digitalis
toxicity is suspected, or if the patient has a wide complex
tachycardia.
(v) *Irregular narrow-complex tachycardia or AF*
Irregularly irregular narrow-complex tachycardia is usually AF or
less frequently atrial flutter with variable AV block
(a) proceed directly to synchronized DC cardioversion starting
at 120–150 J biphasic, if the patient is shocked, unstable or
deteriorating
- in patients on digoxin therapy, temporary transcutaneous
pacing may be required as asystole may follow DC
reversion
(b) otherwise attempt rhythm control, if the patient has been in
the AF for less than 48 h, with amiodarone 5 mg/kg i.v. over
20–60 min, followed by an infusion of amiodarone 900 mg
over 24 h
(c) however, when the patient has been in AF for over
48 h, or the time duration is unclear, rhythm control
with drugs or elective DC reversion is contraindicated
prior to full anticoagulation, due to the risk of clot
embolization:
- attempt rate control only using an oral or i.v. β-blocker,
digoxin, diltiazem or magnesium. Seek senior ED doctor
advice

- commence heparinization with LMW heparin such as enoxaparin 1 mg/kg s.c. or unfractionated UF heparin 5000 units i.v. as a bolus, followed by an infusion
- consider longer term oral anticoagulation with warfarin, or with a NOAC for nonvalvular AF such as dabigatran 150 mg b.d. (110 mg if over 75 yr), or rivaroxaban 20 mg once daily according to the stroke risk given by the CHADS$_2$ score (see Table 2.6).

(vi) Admit all patients who required active treatment to a monitored CCU bed.

6 Bradycardia

This may be sinus, junctional (nodal) or due to atrioventricular block.

(i) Give a bolus of atropine 0.5–0.6 mg i.v.

(ii) Repeat the atropine for sinus or junctional bradycardia if it persists, to a maximum of 3 mg i.v. total.

(iii) Consider insertion of a temporary transvenous pacemaker wire by an expert, if the bradycardia persists with symptomatic second- or third-degree (complete) AV block, or the patient is unstable, or

(a) use an external (transcutaneous) pacemaker until X-ray guidance and expert help are available

(b) small doses of a sedative such as midazolam 0.05 mg/kg and/or morphine 0.05 mg/kg are needed as external pacing is uncomfortable.

(iv) Avoid excessive atropine or using an isoprenaline infusion immediately following an acute myocardial infarction, as these may provoke VF.

(v) Admit all patients who required active treatment to a monitored CCU bed.

Table 2.6 CHADS$_2$ score to estimate thromboembolic risk in nonvalvular atrial fibrillation, with treatment recommendations

		Points
C	Congestive cardiac failure	1
H	Hypertension	1
A	Age ≥75 yr	1
D	Diabetes	1
S$_2$	Previous stroke or TIA	2

Low risk = score 0. No therapy or aspirin.
Moderate risk = score 1. Oral anticoagulant or aspirin.
High risk = score ≥2. Oral anticoagulant, as annual stroke rate is 4% (score 2) up to 18% (score 6).

DIFFERENTIAL DIAGNOSIS

Consider the following, some of which were covered in the preceding section on chest pain:

- Acute asthma
- Community-acquired pneumonia (CAP)
- Chronic obstructive pulmonary disease (COPD)
- Pneumothorax
- Pulmonary embolus (see p. 51)
- Pulmonary oedema
- Acute upper airway obstruction – see page 13
- Metabolic acidosis, such as diabetic ketoacidosis or lactic acidosis - see page 79
- Respiratory muscle weakness from myasthenia gravis or Guillain–Barré syndrome
- Miscellaneous including anaemia, anaphylaxis, interstitial lung disease, obesity, poisoning such as salicylate or carbon monoxide, pain and anxiety

ACUTE ASTHMA

DIAGNOSIS

1 Ascertain the precipitating factors in the present attack, its duration, additional treatment given particularly steroids and the response to treatment.

2 Ask about regular medication such as inhalers, previous attacks, hospital admissions and ventilation in an ICU.

3 Risk factors for a severe or fatal attack are:
  (i) Previous ICU admission.
  (ii) A recent acute attack within the last month, especially if the patient required steroids.
  (iii) ≥3 ED visits, or ≥2 hospitalizations in the previous 1 year.
  (iv) Difficulty perceiving asthma severity, and/or lack of a written Asthma Action Plan.
  (v) Drug or alcohol abuse, mental illness, low socioeconomic status and non-compliance 'denial'.
  (vi) Comorbidities such as food allergy, obesity, chronic lung disease, cardiovascular disease.

4 Assess the severity of the present attack rapidly before any nebulizer therapy is given.
  (i) **Severe** attack is indicated by any one of the following:
    (a) inability to complete sentences in one breath
    (b) respiratory rate of ≥25 breaths/min
    (c) tachycardia of ≥110 beats/min

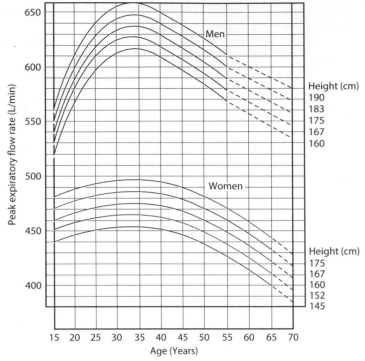

Figure 2.1 Predicted normal peak expiratory flow rates in adult men and women. Reproduced by kind permission of Clement Clark International Ltd.

     (d) peak expiratory flow (PEF) rate or forced expiratory volume in 1 s (FEV_1) 33–50% or less of predicted or known best (see Fig. 2.1).

(ii) **Life-threatening** attack is indicated by any one of the following:

     (a) silent chest, cyanosis or feeble respiratory effort

     (b) bradycardia, dysrhythmia or hypotension

     (c) exhaustion, confusion or coma

     (d) PEF under 33% of predicted or best

     (e) oxygen saturation (SaO_2) <92%, PaO_2 <60 mmHg (below 8 kPa), normal $PaCO_2$ 34–45 mmHg (4.6–6.0 kPa), or worse a raised $PaCO_2$ (imminently fatal).

MANAGEMENT

1 Commence high-dose 40–60% oxygen via a face mask. Maintain the oxygen saturation above 94%.

2 Give salbutamol 5 mg via an oxygen-driven nebulizer, diluted with 3 mL normal saline.

3 Add ipratropium (Atrovent™) 500 µg to a second dose of salbutamol 5 mg via the nebulizer if there is no response, or there is a severe attack.

4 Involve the senior ED doctor if the patient is still wheezy, and perform the following:

    (i) Give prednisolone 50 mg orally or hydrocortisone 200 mg i.v. if unable to swallow.

    (ii) Repeat the salbutamol 5 mg via the nebulizer every 20 min for the first hour, or even by continuous nebulization if not improving.

    (iii) Send blood for white cell count (WCC), urea and electrolytes (U&Es) and blood sugar. Commence an i.v. infusion of normal saline for dehydration, with added potassium if low.

5 Perform a CXR **only** when a pneumothorax, pneumomediastinum or an infection with consolidation is suspected, or the patient is not improving.

6 Take an ABG **only** if the patient is deteriorating, never routinely. ABG markers of a life-threatening attack are:

    (i) Normal 34–45 mmHg (4.6–6 kPa), or high $PaCO_2$ (imminently fatal).

    (ii) Severe hypoxia with PaO_2 under 60 mmHg (8 kPa).

    (iii) Low pH (or high hydrogen ion concentration).

    (iv) Also check potassium, which may be low.

7 Call the ICU and/or the anaesthetist if the patient remains severe or has any life-threatening features.

    (i) Give magnesium 2 g (8 mmol) i.v. over 20 min.

    (ii) Commence an i.v. bronchodilator under ECG control.

        (a) give salbutamol 3–6 µg/kg i.v. over 5 min, followed by an infusion of 5 mg salbutamol in 500 mL of 5% dextrose, i.e. 10 µg/mL at 10 µg/min (60 mL/h or 1.0 mL/min) initially. Titrate to response up to 40–60 µg/min (240–360 mL/h)

        (b) i.v. salbutamol increases risk of hypokalaemia, arrhythmias and lactic acidosis.

    (iii) Arrange immediate ICU or high-dependency unit (HDU) admission.

8 Meanwhile, admit under the medical team the initially severe patient who stabilizes with a PEF maintained over 50%.

9 Alternatively, in the patient with a mild (PEF over 75% predicted) or a moderate (PEF 50–75% predicted) initial attack who improves with prednisolone and nebulizers to a PEF over 75% for at least 1–2 h off treatment:

    (i) Discharge if the GP can provide follow-up within 2 days and the patient has salbutamol and steroid inhalers (and knows how to use them), plus prednisolone 50 mg orally once daily reduced over 5 days.

    (ii) Admit for overnight observation if there is any doubt about discharging the patient.

COMMUNITY-ACQUIRED PNEUMONIA (CAP)

DIAGNOSIS

1 Common organisms include *Streptococcus pneumoniae* (over 50%), 'atypical' organisms such as *Legionella* spp., *Mycoplasma* and *Chlamydia*, *Haemophilus influenzae* (especially in COPD), and viruses including influenza and chickenpox.

  (i) Less common are *Staphylococcus aureus* (may follow the flu), Gram-negatives (alcoholism) and *Coxiella* (Q fever).

  (ii) Consider melioidosis in tropical areas due to *Burkholderia pseudomallei*, or in diabetics, alcoholism and chronic renal failure (CRF).

  (iii) Finally remember tuberculosis, especially in alcoholism or social deprivation and also in human immunodeficiency virus (HIV) patients, who may also get *Pneumocystis jirovecii* pneumonia. See page 156.

2 Risk factors for CAP include: age over 50 years; smoking; coexisting chronic respiratory, cardiac, renal, cerebrovascular or hepatic disease; diabetes; alcoholism; neoplasia; nursing home residency; and immunosuppression.

3 Fever, dyspnoea, productive cough, haemoptysis and pleuritic chest pain may occur.

4 Less obvious presentations include septicaemia with shock, acute confusional state particularly in the elderly, referred upper abdominal pain, or diarrhoea.

5 Examine for signs of lobar infection, with a dull percussion note and bronchial breathing. Usually there are only localized moist crepitations with diminished breath sounds.

6 Send blood for FBC, ELFTs, blood sugar, and two sets of blood cultures if require hospital admission (see below).

  (i) Only do an ABG when there are features of severe CAP (see below).

7 Perform a CXR, which may show diffuse shadowing unless there is lobar consolidation.

  (i) Look at the lateral, particularly for consolidation.

8 Features of *severe* CAP requiring hospital admission include one or more of the following:

  (i) Respiratory rate $\geq$30/min.

  (ii) Systolic BP <90 mmHg or diastolic BP <60 mmHg.

  (iii) Acute onset of confusion.

  (iv) Arterial or venous pH <7.35.

  (v) Oxygen saturation <92%, or PaO_2 <60 mmHg (below 8 kPa).

  (vi) Multilobar CXR changes.

  (vii) Urea of >7 mmol/L, or WCC $<4 \times 10^9$/L or $>30 \times 10^9$/L.

9 Otherwise, predictors of the need for intensive respiratory or vasopressor support (IRVS) are indicated by the SMART-COP score (see Table 2.7).

    (i) A score of 3–4 gives a 1:8 risk of needing IRVS.

    (ii) A score of ≥5 indicates severe CAP with a 1:3 risk of needing IRVS.

10 Alternatively use the CURB-65 scale that predicts mortality risk, hence the need for hospital admission (see Table 2.8).

    (i) A score of 2 indicates moderate risk and likely admission.

    (ii) A score of ≥3 is high risk needing inpatient care and ICU referral.

Table 2.7 SMART-COP score for assessing severity, once community-acquired pneumonia is confirmed on CXR

			Score
S Systolic BP <90 mmHg			2 points
M Multi-lobar CXR involvement			1 point
A Albumen <35 g/L			1 point
R Respiratory rate – age-adjusted cut-offs:			1 point
Age	≤50 yr	>50 yr	
RR	≥25/min	≥30/min	
T Tachycardia ≥125/min			1 point
C Confusion (new onset)			1 point
O Oxygen low – age-adjusted cut-offs:			2 points
Age	≤50 yr	>50 yr	
PaO_2	<70 mmHg	<60 mmHg	
or SaO_2	≤93%	≤90%	
or (if on O_2) PaO_2/FiO_2	<333	<250	
P Arterial pH <7.35			2 points
TOTAL SCORE			= (Max 11)

0–2 points: Low risk of needing IRVS.
3–4 points: Moderate (1 in 8) risk of needing IRVS.
5–6 points: High (1 in 3) risk of needing IRVS.
≥7 points: Very high (2 in 3) risk of needing IRVS.
A score of ≥5 indicates severe CAP.
BP, blood pressure; CAP, community-acquired pneumonia; CXR, chest x-ray; FiO_2, fractional inspired oxygen concentration; IRVS, intensive respiratory or vasopressor support; PaO_2, partial pressure of oxygen (arterial); RR, respiratory rate; SaO_2, arterial oxygen saturation.
Adapted with permission from Charles PG, Wolfe R, Whitby M et al. (2008) SMART-COP: a tool for predicting the need for intensive respiratory or vasopressor support in community-acquired pneumonia. Clinical Infectious Diseases **47**: 375–84.

Table 2.8 CURB-65 severity score to estimate mortality risk in community acquired pneumonia, and hence need for admission

		Points
C	Confusion	1
U	Urea >7 mmol/L	1
R	Resp rate ≥30/min	1
B	BP (SBP ≤90 mmHg or DBP ≤60 mmHg)	1
65	≤65 yr	1

Score 1: Low risk – 30-day mortality 2.7%. Outpatient care.
Score 2: Moderate risk – 30-day mortality 6.8%. Inpatient care (or close OP care).
Score ≥3: High risk – 30-day mortality 14–27.8%. Inpatient care / ICU referral.
BP, blood pressure; SBP, systolic blood pressure; DBP, diastolic blood pressure; OP, outpatient care; ICU, Intensive Care Unit.

MANAGEMENT

1 Give the patient high-dose oxygen, unless there is a known history of obstructive airways disease (use 28%). Aim for an oxygen saturation above 92%.

2 Start antibiotics according to the severity of the pneumonia, and/or based on local guidelines.

3 *Mild CAP*
   (i) Young, fit adults with single lobe involvement may well be able to return home on oral antibiotics:
      (a) give amoxicillin 1 g orally 8-hourly for 5–7 days, or if *Mycoplasma pneumoniae, Chlamydophila pneumoniae* or *Legionella* is suspected, give doxycycline 100 mg orally 12-hourly for 5–7 days instead, or clarithromycin 500 mg orally 12-hourly for 5–7 days particularly when pregnant
      (b) add doxycycline to the amoxicillin, if the patient fails to improve by 48 h, or if review is not going to be possible
      (c) give doxycycline or moxifloxacin 400 mg orally daily alone, if the patient has a history of immediate hypersensitivity to penicillin, depending on local practice.
   (ii) Inform the patient's GP by email or a letter if the patient is discharged, and arrange review within 1–2 days.

4 *Moderate severity CAP*
   (i) Most patients need admission to hospital and parenteral antibiotics:
      (a) give benzyl penicillin 1.2 g i.v. 6-hourly until significant improvement then change to amoxicillin 1 g orally 8-hourly for 7 days, *plus* doxycycline 100 mg orally 12-hourly for 7 days

      (b) add gentamicin 5 mg/kg i.v. daily (assuming normal renal function) if Gram-negative bacilli are identified in blood or sputum. Alternatively, change the benzyl penicillin to ceftriaxone 1 g i.v. daily

      (c) substitute ceftriaxone 1 g i.v. daily for the penicillin, or use moxifloxacin 400 mg orally daily as monotherapy, if the patient has a history of immediate hypersensitivity to penicillin, depending on local practice

      (d) in tropical areas, if the patient has risk factors for melioidosis (diabetes/alcohol/CRF) give ceftriaxone 2 g i.v. daily i.v. plus gentamicin 5 mg/kg i.v. as a single dose.

      (e) consider adding oseltamivir 75 mg orally b.d. for 5 days during any flu outbreak while awaiting nasal swab PCR result.

    (ii) Refer the patient to the medical team.

5   *Severe CAP, usually with a SMART-COP score ≥5 or CURB-65 ≥3*

    (i) Admit these patients with severe CAP to the HDU or ICU:

      (a) give ceftriaxone 1 g daily i.v. *plus* azithromycin 500 mg daily i.v.

      (b) use moxifloxacin 400 mg daily i.v. if the patient has penicillin allergy or significant renal impairment

      (c) give meropenem 1 g 8-hourly i.v. plus azithromycin 500 mg daily i.v. for severe tropical pneumonia where *B. pseudomallei* (melioidosis) or *Acinetobacter baumannii* are prevalent.

CHRONIC OBSTRUCTIVE PULMONARY DISEASE

DIAGNOSIS

1 Causes of chronic bronchitis with emphysema (COPD) include smoking, environmental pollution, occupational exposure such as silica, repeated or chronic lung infection, and α-1 antitrypsin deficiency.

2 Productive cough, dyspnoea, wheeze and reduced exercise tolerance worsen with exacerbations, until end-stage disease when there is minimal variation.

3 Ask about normal daily exercise capacity and level of dependence.

    (i) Enquire about current medication, home oxygen use, previous hospital admissions and associated cardiac disease.

4 Exacerbation of COPD.

This is usually multi-factorial, so consider the many underlying causes possible:

    (i) Infection including viral; bronchospasm; sputum retention; pneumothorax; pneumonia including aspiration; right, left or biventricular heart failure; cardiac arrhythmia including AF; myocardial infarction.

    (ii) Non-compliance with medication including steroid underdosing; iatrogenic response to excess sedatives, opiates or inadvertent β-blockade; environmental allergens or weather change; malignancy and a PE.

5   Examine for fever, lip pursing, tachypnoea, tachycardia and wheeze. Also look for:
    (i)   Cyanosis, ruddy complexion and signs of right heart failure due to cor pulmonale with a raised JVP and peripheral oedema.
    (ii) Carbon dioxide retention causing headache, drowsiness, tremor and a bounding pulse.

6   Establish venous access and send blood for FBC, ELFTs, glucose and two sets of blood cultures if pyrexial. Attach a cardiac monitor and pulse oximeter to the patient.

7   Take an ABG if patient is clearly unwell, to look for hypoxia PaO_2 <60 mmHg (8 kPa), hypercarbia $PaCO_2$ >45 mmHg (6 kPa) and a raised bicarbonate indicating compensated respiratory acidosis.

8   Perform an ECG and look for large P waves (P pulmonale), right ventricular hypertrophy or strain (cor pulmonale), and signs of ischaemia with ST and T wave changes.

9   Perform bedside lung function testing for PEF, FEV_1 and FVC to compare with previous respiratory function tests, and to follow the response to treatment.

10 Request a CXR which may show hyperinflation, bullae, atelectasis, consolidation, pneumothorax, heart failure or a lung mass.

MANAGEMENT

1   Commence controlled oxygen therapy initially at 28% via a Venturi mask if there is evidence of chronic carbon dioxide retention, with a raised $PaCO_2$ and bicarbonate. Aim for an oxygen saturation over 90%.
    (i)   Otherwise give higher dose 40–60% oxygen via face mask to treat hypoxaemia. Watch out for deterioration and a rising $PaCO_2$.

2   Give salbutamol 5 mg via a nebulizer for bronchospasm repeated as needed, and add ipratropium (Atrovent™) 500 µg to the initial nebulizer then 6-hourly.

3   Give prednisolone 50 mg orally or hydrocortisone 200 mg i.v. if unable to swallow, for bronchospasm and/or if on long-term inhaled or oral steroids.

4   Treat infection with amoxicillin 500 mg orally t.d.s., or doxycycline 200 mg orally once followed by 100 mg orally daily both for 5 days.

5   Give frusemide (furosemide) 40 mg i.v. if heart failure is suspected.

6   Admit under the medical team.

7   Call urgent senior ED doctor help if there is exhaustion, agitation or confusion; or a rising $PaCO_2$ and a falling pH. Involve the intensive care team.
    (i)   Commence bi-level non-invasive ventilation (NIV) if there are trained and experienced staff to supervise.
    (ii) Start with an inspiratory positive airways pressure (iPAP) setting of 10–12 cm H_2O and an expiratory positive airways pressure (ePAP) of 4–6 cm H_2O.

PNEUMOTHORAX

DIAGNOSIS

1 Spontaneous pneumothorax that occurs in an otherwise healthy patient with no lung disease, particularly in taller people, is designated a 'primary' pneumothorax.

2 Spontaneous pneumothorax that occurs in a patient with chronic lung disease (CLD) is termed a 'secondary' pneumothorax, and is associated with asthma, emphysema, fibrotic or bullous lung disease including cystic fibrosis and Marfan's syndrome.

    (i) In addition, this includes patients aged over 50 years who may have unrecognized underlying lung disease.

3 Spontaneous pneumothoraces are also much more common in smokers.

4 Pneumothorax may be due to both penetrating or blunt trauma.

    (i) See p. 181 for discussion on the management of traumatic pneumothorax.

5 A spontaneous primary pneumothorax may cause only slight dyspnoea and pleuritic chest pain in a fit patient, even when the whole lung is collapsed.

    (i) 'Significant' dyspnoea is considered any deterioration in usual exercise tolerance.

    (ii) Significant dyspnoea or breathlessness is more common in a secondary pneumothorax with underlying chronic lung disease, even when small.

6 Look for reduced chest expansion on the affected side, increased resonance on percussion, and diminished breath sounds. Beware that lateralizing signs may be subtle and difficult to confirm.

7 Request a standard inspiratory CXR in all cases.

    (i) Do not wait for this if there are signs of tension, but proceed immediately to insert a wide-bore cannula or intercostal drain (see p. 471).

    (ii) Assess the size of the pneumothorax on the CXR:

        (a) *small* is a visible rim of <2 cm

        (b) *large* is a visible air rim ≥2 cm around all the lung edge, that represents over 50% of lung volume lost

        (c) expiratory CXRs are no longer routine.

MANAGEMENT

This is determined by the presence or absence of chronic lung disease (i.e. a secondary or a primary pneumothorax), the degree of dyspnoea (significant or not), and by the size of the pneumothorax (large or small).

1 Discharge a patient with a small 'primary' pneumothorax <2 cm, with no CLD and no significant dyspnoea. No active interventional management is indicated.

    (i) Arrange follow-up by the GP for repeat CXR within 7–14 days, and refer to a respiratory physician.

    (ii)   Advise the patient to stop smoking, and to return immediately if they develop significant dyspnoea.

    (iii) Advise them not to fly for at least 1 week after the CXR has returned to normal, and never to go SCUBA diving (unless they have had bilateral surgical pleurectomies).

2   Also take no active intervention in a patient with underlying lung disease, i.e. a 'secondary' pneumothorax, who has a small pneumothorax <2 cm with no significant dyspnoea.

    (i)   However, admit for observation for 24 h, and start high-flow oxygen via a face mask, unless they have COPD in which case use 28%.

    (ii)   Repeat the CXR after 6–12 h and discharge after 24 h only if they remain asymptomatic and the pneumothorax is not progressing. Arrange early respiratory or medical follow-up within 7 days.

    (iii) Perform needle aspiration if the air leak has enlarged, or the patient develops significant breathlessness. Alternatively, insert a small-bore (<14 F) chest drain intercostal catheter (ICC) using a Seldinger technique, and admit the patient under the medical team (see p. 473).

3 *Needle aspiration (thoracentesis)*

Perform this for a symptomatic primary pneumothorax (no CLD) with dyspnoea, whether large or small; and in a small secondary (with CLD) pneumothorax less than 2 cm with minimal breathlessness if aged under 50 years.

    (i)   Infiltrate local anaesthetic down to the pleura in the second intercostal space in the mid-clavicular line.

    (ii)   Insert a 16-gauge cannula into the pleural cavity, withdraw the needle, and connect to a 50 mL syringe with three-way tap (see p. 471).

        (a) alternatively use a proprietary chest aspiration kit, with special fenestrated pigtail catheter and one-way valve.

    (iii) Aspirate air until resistance is felt, the patient coughs excessively, or more than 2500 mL is aspirated.

    (iv) Repeat the CXR; if the lung has re-expanded, observe and repeat the CXR again after 2–4 h:

        (a) discharge patients with a primary pneumothorax if the lung remains expanded, and arrange follow-up with the GP and give discharge advice as above

        (b) admit patients with CLD and a secondary pneumothorax overnight even if aspiration was successful, for continued observation

        (c) proceed directly to insertion of an ICC if aspiration fails, suggesting a persistent air leak, particularly with a secondary pneumothorax.

4   *Intercostal catheter*
This is therefore indicated for:
- (i)   Failed needle aspiration, e.g. with more than just a small residual rim of air around the lung.
- (ii)   Any secondary pneumothorax in a patient with CLD causing significant dyspnoea, or if aged >50 years.
- (iii)   Tension pneumothorax following initial needle thoracocentesis.
- (iv)   Traumatic pneumothorax or haemothorax (see p. 181).
- (v)   Any pneumothorax prior to anaesthesia or positive-pressure ventilation.

5   *ICC insertion* (see p. 473)
- (i)   Use a small-bore 8–14 French ICC inserted under a Seldinger technique.
- (ii)   Alternatively use a small standard size 16–22 French gauge drain directed apically for a simple pneumothorax, or a larger 28–32 French gauge directed posterior basally for any associated haemothorax.
- (iii)   Admit under the care of the medical team.

PULMONARY EMBOLUS
See page 51.

PULMONARY OEDEMA

DIAGNOSIS

1   Pulmonary oedema is usually caused by left ventricular failure due to myocardial infarction, hypertension, an arrhythmia, valvular disease, myocarditis or fluid overload.

2   Occasional non-cardiogenic causes include septicaemia, uraemia, pancreatitis, head injury, intracranial haemorrhage, near drowning, and inhalation of smoke or noxious gases.

3   The onset may be precipitate with breathlessness, cough, orthopnoea, paroxysmal nocturnal dyspnoea (PND) and dyspnoea at rest.

4   The patient is clammy, distressed and prefers to sit upright. Look for wheeze, tachypnoea sometimes with pink froth, tachycardia, basal crepitations and a triple rhythm or gallop.

5   Establish venous access and send blood for FBC, ELFTs and cardiac bio-markers, although they do not influence the initial management. Attach a cardiac monitor and pulse oximeter to the patient.

6   Perform an ECG to look for acute ischaemia, arrhythmias and evidence of underlying cardiac disease.

7   Request a CXR that shows engorged upper-lobe veins, a perihilar 'bat's wing' haze, cardiomegaly, septal Kerley B lines, and small bilateral pleural effusions.

MANAGEMENT

1   Sit the patient upright and give 40–60% oxygen, unless the patient is known to have chronic bronchitis, in which case 28% oxygen should be used. Aim for an oxygen saturation above 94%.

2   Give GTN 300–600 µg sublingually, which may be repeated every 5 min. Remove the tablet if excessive hypotension (systolic BP <100 mmHg) occurs.

3   Give frusemide (furosemide) 40 mg i.v., or twice their usual oral daily dose i.v. if already on frusemide (furosemide).

4   Get senior ED doctor help in refractory cases, repeat the frusemide (furosemide), and commence a GTN infusion, provided the patient is not hypotensive.

    (i)   Add GTN 200 mg to 500 mL of 5% dextrose, i.e. 400 µg/mL, using a glass bottle and low-absorption polyethylene infusion set.

    (ii) Infuse initially at 1 mL/h, maintaining the systolic BP above 100 mmHg. Progressively increase to ≥20 mL/h, avoiding hypotension.

5   Commence mask continuous positive airways pressure (CPAP) respiratory support:

    (i)   Use a dedicated, high-flow fresh gas circuit, tight-fitting mask and variable resistor valve, starting at 5–10 cmH$_2$O.

    (ii) A trained nurse must remain in attendance at all times, as some patients will not tolerate the mask.

    (iii) **Never** simply use wall oxygen with a black anaesthetic mask and head harness, as this will asphyxiate the patient due to inadequate fresh gas flow.

6   Morphine 0.5–2.5 mg i.v. with an antiemetic such as metoclopramide 10 mg i.v. is rarely helpful, and it may further obtund the patient particularly if the patient is tired or has COPD.

7   Admit the patient under the medical team.

ACUTE UPPER AIRWAY OBSTRUCTION

See page 13.

UPPER GASTROINTESTINAL HAEMORRHAGE

DIAGNOSIS

1   Causes of upper gastrointestinal haemorrhage include:

    (i)   Peptic ulceration (over 40% of cases):

        (a) duodenal ulcer (DU)

        (b) gastric ulcer (GU) less common.

     (ii) Gastric erosions or gastritis:
         (a) post-alcohol
         (b) drug-induced (salicylates, non-steroidal anti-inflammatory drugs [NSAIDs], steroids).
     (iii) Reflux oesophagitis.
     (iv) Bleeding oesophageal or gastric varices associated with portal hypertension (due to cirrhosis, often alcoholic).
     (v) Mallory–Weiss tear (oesophageal tear following vomiting or retching).
     (vi) Miscellaneous, including gastric neoplasm, Dieulafoy's lesion, blood coagulation disorders, angiodysplasia and aorto-enteric fistula in a patient with a past history of an abdominal aortic aneurysm (AAA) repair.

2   Mortality is 6–14%, highest with age over 60 years, re-bleeding particularly if fresh red, variceal origin (mortality over 20%), comorbid disease, shock and coagulopathy.

3   Patients can present in a variety of ways:
     (i) Haematemesis:
         (a) fresh red blood
         (b) altered blood 'coffee grounds'.
     (ii) Melaena (sticky black, tarry stool).
     (iii) Haematochezia (maroon-coloured or fresh red rectal bleeding).
     (iv) Collapse and shock.
     (v) Syncope and postural hypotension.
     (vi) Fatigue, dyspnoea, angina, etc.

4   Ask about previous gastrointestinal bleeding, recent endoscopy, medication use, alcohol, and known chronic liver disease.

5   Look for signs of volume depletion such as pallor and sweating, tachycardia, hypotension and postural hypotension.
     (i) Palpate for abdominal tenderness, organomegaly, masses, and perform a rectal examination.
     (ii) Note in particular any signs of chronic liver disease including jaundice, bruising, spider naevi, palmar erythema, clubbing, gynaecomastia, hepatomegaly and encephalopathy.
     (iii) Examine for splenomegaly and ascites as signs of portal hypertension.

6   Establish venous access with a large-bore 14-gauge i.v. cannula, and attach a pulse oximeter and cardiac monitor to the patient.
     (i) Take blood for FBC, U&Es, blood sugar, LFTs, clotting studies including a prothrombin index (PTI) and cross-match from 2 units of blood, according to the presumed aetiology and degree of shock.

MANAGEMENT

1   Commence high-dose oxygen via a face mask. Maintain the oxygen saturation above 94%.

2   Begin fluid replacement:
    (i)   Start with normal saline 10–20 mL/kg, aiming for a urine output of 0.5–1 mL/kg per hour.
    (ii)   Give cross-matched blood only for severe bleeding if the patient is shocked, or if the bleeding is continuing
           (a) if Hb drops below 70 g/L, restore to 70–90 g/L
           (b) aim for 100 g/L if active ischaemic heart disease.
    (iii) Add fresh frozen plasma 4 units and vitamin K 10 mg i.v. in chronic liver disease with abnormal coagulation.

3   Start a proton-pump inhibitor if peptic ulcer disease is likely, *and* early endoscopy (<24 h) is not feasible. Give omeprazole or pantoprazole 80 mg i.v. followed by an infusion at 8 mg/h.
    (i)   Benefit is proven only post-endoscopy for high risk non-variceal bleeding with stigmata of recent haemorrhage.
    (ii)   There is no supporting evidence at all for an H_2-antagonist.

4   Give octreotide 50 μg i.v. then 50 μg/h if varices are known, or are likely from the presence of chronic liver disease and portal hypertension. Also give ceftriaxone 1 g i.v. in chronic liver disease.
    (i)   Alternatively use terlipressin 1.7 mg i.v. every 4 h instead of octreotide for suspected bleeding varices.

5   Arrange for an urgent endoscopy, particularly in patients who have suspected varices, continue to bleed, remain unstable or are aged >60 years. Contact the intensive care team.
    (i)   Endoscopy will differentiate the cause of the bleeding and allow immediate thermal or injection therapy where appropriate, or banding for varices.

6   Otherwise admit patients who have stopped bleeding and are haemodynamically stable under the medical team, for endoscopy ideally within 24 h.

Warning: inserting a central venous pressure (CVP) line in a hypotensive, shocked patient is difficult and dangerous. Leave it until initial transfusion is under way for a skilled doctor to perform under ultrasound guidance (see p. 476).

DIABETIC COMA AND PRE-COMA

Hypoglycaemia rapidly produces coma in people with diabetes, compared with the slower onset of altered consciousness in diabetic ketoacidosis and hyperosmolar, hyperglycaemic state (HHS).

DIABETIC KETOACIDOSIS

DIAGNOSIS

1 Diabetic ketoacidosis (DKA) may occur in a known diabetic person precipitated by infection, surgery, trauma, pancreatitis, myocardial infarction, cerebral infarction or inadequate insulin therapy, e.g. insulin stopped in an unwell diabetic patient 'because he/she was not eating'!

  (i) Alternatively, it may arise *de novo* in an undiagnosed diabetic, heralded by polyuria, polydipsia, weight loss, lethargy, abdominal pain or coma.

2 DKA is defined by metabolic acidosis with pH <7.3 or bicarbonate <15 mmol/L; hyperglycaemia with blood glucose >11 mmol/L; and ketonaemia >3.0 mmol/L or marked ketonuria >2+ on dipstick.

  (i) The ketone acetone may be detected on the breath as a sickly sweet, fruity smell.

3 The predominant features arise from salt and water depletion and acidosis, hence there is dry skin, tachycardia, hypotension (especially postural) and deep sighing respirations (Kussmaul breathing).

  (i) Typical fluid and electrolyte deficits include water 100 mL/kg; sodium 7–10 mmol/kg; and potassium 3–5 mmol/kg.

4 Establish venous access and send blood urgently for FBC, ELFTs, blood glucose and blood cultures when infection is suspected. Attach a cardiac monitor and pulse oximeter to the patient.

5 Take blood for a bedside venous blood gas (VBG) or an ABG, and organize an ECG, CXR and a midstream urine (MSU).

  (i) Look at the ECG for an early indication of critical hyperkalaemia with peaked T waves, QRS widening, then absent P waves and finally a 'sine wave' trace (see p. 134).

 Tip: every patient who presents with abdominal pain, vomiting or thirst must have urine tested for sugar and ketones.

MANAGEMENT

1 Give high-dose oxygen via a face mask and aim for an oxygen saturation above 94%.

2 Start an i.v. infusion and run in normal saline 1 L in the first hour, followed by a further 500 mL/h for the next 4 h once the diagnosis is confirmed.

  (i) Aim to replace the fluid deficit gradually over the first 24 h (see Table 2.9).

  (ii) If the blood sugar drops to ≤15 mmol/L, then add 10% dextrose at 125 mL/h, but continue the insulin infusion and saline until the ketones are cleared.

Table 2.9 Replacement normal saline fluid rates in a 70 kg* patient with DKA, who is not haemodynamically compromised / shocked

Litre	Time (hours from starting treatment)
1st at 1000 mL/h	0–1
2nd at 500 mL/h + K	1–3
3rd at 500 mL/h + K	3–5
4th at 250 mL/h + K	5–9
5th at 250 mL/h + K	9–13
Reassess cardiovascular status after 12 hours and adjust rate accordingly	
6th at 166 mL/h + K	13–19

K, potassium; DKA, diabetic ketoacidosis.
* In small (<70 kg), younger adults (18–25 yr) adopt a slower rate initially with total volume replacement over 24–48 hr to reduce risk of cerebral oedema.

3   Commence short-acting soluble insulin therapy by infusion.
   (i)   Add 50 units soluble insulin to 50 mL normal saline, i.e. 1 unit/mL.
   (ii)   Run at 0.1 units/kg/h, i.e. 5–7 units/h or 5–7 mL/h via an infusion pump.

4   Add potassium to the i.v. fluid when the plasma K level is known. This should be within 30 min:
   (i)   Expect the serum potassium level to fall precipitously once insulin and fluids are commenced.
   (ii)   Replace potassium at 10–20 mmol/h, aiming to maintain serum level between 4–5 mmol/L.
   (iii)   Use pre-mixed saline with potassium solutions containing 40 mmol/L or 20 mmol/L via an infusion pump.
   (iv)   Omit the potassium if:
      (a) no urine output is established (unusual)
      (b) the serum level is >5.5 mmol/L
      (c) the ECG shows peaked T waves or QRS complex widening.

5   Refer the patient to the medical team or ICU. Remember to look for any underlying precipitating factor(s) for the DKA.

6   Do **not** give i.v. sodium bicarbonate except on the advice of the senior ED doctor.
   (i)   It may be considered if the pH remains <7.0, particularly with circulatory failure.

HYPEROSMOLAR, HYPERGLYCAEMIC STATE

DIAGNOSIS

1   HHS is more common in the elderly, non-insulin-dependent patient, with a more gradual onset than DKA.

    (i)   It is suggested by hyperglycaemia with blood glucose >30 mmol/L; hyperosmolality with serum osmolality >320 mOsm/kg; hypovolaemia; and minimal ketonaemia with pH >7.30 and bicarbonate >15 mmol/L.

    (ii) Typical fluid and electrolyte deficits include water 100–220 mL/kg; sodium 5–13 mmol/kg; and potassium 4–6 mmol/kg.

2   It may be precipitated by infection, myocardial infarction, a stroke or by thiazide diuretic use and steroids, and like DKA, may occur in a previously undiagnosed patient.

3   The patient presents with an altered level of consciousness, profound dehydration and may develop seizures or focal neurological signs. Mortality is 20–40%, compared to DKA where it has fallen to <5% in younger patients.

4   Blood glucose and serum osmolarity tend to be higher than in DKA. The osmolarity usually exceeds 350 mOsmol/L.

    (i)   Estimate the osmolarity by 2(Na + K) + urea + glucose (all units in mmol/L).

5   Make certain to do an ECG, CXR and an MSU early.

MANAGEMENT

1   This is comparable to DKA (see above).

2   Give i.v. normal saline; or 0.45% half-normal saline only when the serum osmolality *and* blood glucose are not falling, at a similar or slower rate to DKA. Beware of over-rapid rehydration causing pulmonary oedema.

3   Use a slower insulin infusion rate of 0.05 units/kg per hour, i.e. 2–3 units/h, as there is increased insulin sensitivity compared to DKA. Greater total potassium replacement amounts are also usual.

4   Commence prophylactic heparin, either unfractionated (UF) heparin 5000 units i.v. bolus then an infusion at 1000 units/h, or LMW heparin such as enoxaparin 1.5 mg/kg per day, assuming there is no active bleeding, particularly intracerebral.

5   Admit under the care of the medical team.

ALTERED CONSCIOUS LEVEL

Patients with an altered conscious level frequently present to the ED. Although history taking is compromised, a methodical, careful approach is essential using information from the family, friends, passers-by, the police, ambulance and previous medical records.

The following categories are covered, although they may overlap:

- Confused patient
- Alcohol-related medical problems
- Patient with an altered conscious level and smelling of alcohol
- Alcohol withdrawal.

The collapsed or unconscious patient in coma is covered separately in Section I on p. 24.

CONFUSED PATIENT

'Confusion' or delirium is a transient global disorder of cognition. It is a syndrome (not a diagnosis) with multiple causes that describes a state of clouding of consciousness or disturbed awareness (disorientation), which may fluctuate.

DIAGNOSIS

1 An acute confusional state may go unrecognized or be mistaken for dementia or depression particularly in the elderly (see p. 120), or for mania and even acute schizophrenia.

2 There is usually abrupt onset of:

    (i) Clouding of consciousness that may fluctuate, disorientation in time and place, impaired memory, visual, olfactory or tactile hallucinations and illusions.

    (ii) Difficulty maintaining attention, restlessness, irritability, emotional lability and poor comprehension.

    (iii) Hyperactive state with increased arousal and reversed sleep-wake cycle, or hypoactive and withdrawn.

3 Causes of confusion.

    (i) *Hypoxia*

        (a) chest infection, COPD, pulmonary embolus, cardiac failure

        (b) respiratory depression from drugs, or weakness, e.g. Guillain–Barré syndrome, myasthenia gravis or muscular dystrophy

        (c) chest injury or head injury

        (d) drowning, smoke inhalation.

    (ii) *Drugs*

        (a) intoxication or withdrawal from alcohol, sedatives, cocaine, amphetamines, phencyclidine

        (b) side effects (especially in the elderly and with polypharmacy) of analgesics, anticonvulsants, psychotropics, digoxin, anticholinergics and antiparkinsonian drugs such as benzhexol (trihexyphenidyl) and levodopa

        (c) inappropriate use, such as steroids particularly anabolic.

    (iii) *Cerebral*

        (a) meningitis, encephalitis

        (b) head injury

(c) post-ictal state, complex partial (temporal lobe) seizures

(d) cerebrovascular accident, subarachnoid haemorrhage

(e) space-occupying lesion, e.g. tumour, abscess or haematoma

(f) hypertensive encephalopathy

(g) vasculitis such as systemic lupus erythematosus (SLE).

(iv) *Metabolic*

(a) respiratory, cardiac, renal or liver failure

(b) electrolyte disorder, such as hyponatraemia, hypercalcaemia or hypernatraemia

(c) vitamin deficiency, e.g. thiamine (Wernicke's encephalopathy), nicotinic acid (pellagra) or B_{12}

(d) acute intermittent porphyria.

(v) *Endocrine*

(a) hypoglycaemia or hyperglycaemia

(b) thyrotoxicosis, myxoedema, Cushing's syndrome, hyperparathyroidism, Addison's disease.

(vi) *Septicaemia*

(a) urinary tract, biliary, meningococcaemia or malaria.

(vii) *Situational*

(a) post-operative (multi-factorial including drugs, hypoxia, infection, pain, etc.)

(b) faecal impaction, urinary retention or change in environment in the elderly (*rarely* the sole cause).

4 Build up a picture of which condition or conditions are responsible from a detailed history and examination.

5 Record the vital signs including temperature, respiratory rate, pulse, blood pressure and Glasgow Coma Scale (GCS) score.

(i) **Any** abnormality of the vital signs should be assumed to have an organic cause until proven otherwise.

6 Document a formal Mini-Mental State Examination (see Table 2.10).

(i) This records cognitive impairment by assessing orientation, attention and calculation, immediate and short-term recall, language, and ability to follow simple verbal and written commands.

(ii) A score of <24 suggests cognitive impairment, and the possibility of an organic cause.

7 Perform some or all of the following investigations based on the suspected aetiology. Always exclude hypoglycaemia first:

(i) FBC, coagulation profile.

(ii) U&Es, blood sugar, liver function tests, calcium, thyroid function tests (TFTs).

(iii) Drug screen including ethanol.

(iv) ABGs.

Table 2.10 Mini-Mental State Examination (MMSE)

Cognition tested			Score
Orientation (10 points)			
1.	What is the date?		1
	What is the day?		1
	What is the month?		1
	What is the year?		1
	What is the season?		1
2.	What is the name of this building?		1
	What floor of the building are we on?		1
	What city are we in?		1
	What state are we in?		1
	What country are we in?		1
Registration (3 points)			
3.	I am going to name three objects. After I have said them I want you to repeat them. Remember what they are because I am going to ask you to name them in a few minutes. Apple. Table. Penny. *(Code the first attempt and then repeat the answers until the patient learns all three)*	Apple	1
		Table	1
		Penny	1
Attention and calculation (5 points max)			
4.	*Either:* Can you subtract 7 from 100, and then subtract 7 from the answer you get and keep subtracting until I tell you to stop?	93	1
		86	1
		79	1
		72	1
		65	1
5.	*Or:* I'm going to spell a word forwards and I want you to spell it backwards. The word is W-O-R-L-D. Now you spell it backwards *(Repeat if necessary)*	D	1
		L	1
		R	1
		O	1
		W	1

(Continued)

Table 2.10 *(Continued)* Mini-Mental State Examination (MMSE)

Cognition tested			Score
Recall (3 points)			
6.	Now what were the three objects I asked you to remember?	Apple	1
		Table	1
		Penny	1
Language (9 points)			
7.	What is this called? *(Show wristwatch)*		1
	What is this called? *(Show pencil)*		1
8.	I'd like you to repeat a phrase after me: No ifs ands or buts		1
9.	Read the words on the bottom of this page and do what it says	Closes eyes	1
10.	*(Read the full statement below before handing the respondent a piece of paper. Do not repeat or coach)* I'm going to give you a piece of paper. What I want you to do is take the paper in you right hand, fold it in half and put the paper on your lap	Takes with right hand	1
		Folds in half	1
		Puts on lap	1
11.	Write a complete sentence on this piece of paper. The sentence should have a subject, verb and make sense. Spelling and grammatical errors are OK		1
12.	Here is a drawing. Please copy the drawing on the same piece of paper *(Hand the respondent a drawing of two intersecting pentagons)*	Correct if two five-sided pentagons intersect to make a four-sided figure	1
Total score (out of 30)			
CLOSE YOUR EYES			

A score of 23 or less indicates cognitive impairment.
Higher scores are expected in the well-educated, and lower scores in the elderly, the uneducated, and the mentally impaired.
From Folstein MF, Folstein SE, McHugh PR (1975) Mini-Mental State. A practical method for grading the cognitive state of patients for the clinician. *J Psychiatr Res* **12**:189–98.

 (v) Blood cultures, MSU.

 (vi) ECG, CXR.

 (vii) CT brain scan.

 (viii) Lumbar puncture. See page 481.

MANAGEMENT

1 Avoid the temptation to simply sedate the confused patient, without looking carefully for the underlying cause(s).

2 Admit all patients under the appropriate specialist team.

ALCOHOL-RELATED MEDICAL PROBLEMS

Acute alcohol intoxication is causally related to all types of trauma including motor vehicle crashes, incidents in the home, deliberate self-harm, assaults, drownings, child abuse and falls in the elderly. Chronic use also predisposes to a variety of medical conditions, and sudden reduction in intake causes withdrawal problems.

MEASUREMENT OF ALCOHOL LEVEL

- Various methods are available, including a breath test, a urine test, and a blood level test. None is admissible in a court of law, unless special forensic kits are used under police direction (see p. 453).
- The Australian legal limit to drive is 0.05 g/100 mL in every state or territory.
- The British legal limit for driving is a blood alcohol level below 80 mg% (0.08 g/100mL).
- Intoxication is marked above a level of 150 mg% (0.15 g/100mL), and coma usually occurs above a level of 300 mg% (0.30 g/100mL).

PATIENT WITH AN ALTERED CONSCIOUS LEVEL AND SMELLING OF ALCOHOL

DIAGNOSIS AND MANAGEMENT

Never assume that a confused, obtunded or unconscious patient smelling of alcohol is simply 'drunk' until you have considered and excluded **all** of the following:

1 *Hypoglycaemia*

 (i) Check a blood sugar, and give 50% dextrose 50 mL i.v. if it is low.

 (ii) This may precipitate worsening of the confusion due to a Wernicke's encephalopathy.

 (iii) Wernicke's is associated with alcohol abuse and malnutrition, and causes confusion, ataxia, nystagmus, and bilateral lateral rectus palsy

  (a) give thiamine 250 mg i.v. immediately

  (b) this should be routine in suspected alcoholism and in the malnourished patient receiving dextrose.

2 *Head injury*

 (i) Always remember the possibility of an extradural or subdural haematoma from a head injury.

    (ii)   Commence neurological observations and perform a CT head scan if confusion persists or there is a deteriorating conscious level (see p. 197).

        (a) a skull X-ray is reasonable **only** in the absence of a CT scan and may show a fracture, but if normal it does **not** exclude intracranial injury.

3   *Other medical problems in patients who drink*

    (i)   Epileptic seizure.

    (ii)   Acute poisoning.

    (iii)   Meningitis, chest infection, etc.

    (iv)   Cerebral haemorrhage.

    (v)   Unrecognized trauma such as a rib fracture, wrist fracture, abdominal injury.

    (vi)   Hypothermia.

    (vii) Depression and suicidal intent.

4   *Acute condition more prevalent in chronic alcoholics*

    (i)   Pneumococcal pneumonia, aspiration pneumonia or tuberculosis.

    (ii)   Cardiac arrhythmia, cardiomyopathy.

    (iii)   Gastrointestinal haemorrhage, including variceal.

    (iv)   Pancreatitis.

    (v)   Liver failure with coagulopathy and/or encephalopathy.

    (vi)   Hypokalaemia, hypomagnesaemia, hypocalcaemia.

    (vii) Withdrawal seizures or delirium tremens.

    (viii) Ketoacidosis.

    (ix)   Lactic acidosis.

    (x)   Renal failure.

    (xi)   Wernicke's encephalopathy.

    (xii) Peripheral neuropathy, cerebellar ataxia.

5   Thus, many patients smelling of alcohol will require admission to exclude the above conditions.

6   Always admit if in doubt, and do not discharge until medically well, sober and safe.

ALCOHOL WITHDRAWAL

This is caused by an absolute or relative decrease in the usual intake of alcohol, that may be intentional through lack of funds or unintentional following detention in hospital or by the police.

DIAGNOSIS AND MANAGEMENT

Two conditions are recognized: the alcohol withdrawal syndrome, and the progression to delirium tremens.

1   *Alcohol withdrawal syndrome*

(i)   This is common, occurring within 12 h of abstinence and lasting a few days. It is characterized by agitation, irritability, fine tremor, sweats and tachycardia.

(ii)   Commence diazepam 10–20 mg orally 2–6-hourly until the patient is comfortable, plus thiamine 250 mg i.v. or i.m. once daily.

(iii)   Control seizures with midazolam 0.05–0.1 mg/kg up to 10 mg i.v., or diazepam 0.1–0.2 mg/kg up to 20 mg i.v., or lorazepam 0.07 mg/kg up to 4 mg i.v., after excluding hypoglycaemia.

(iv)   Refer the patient to the medical team.

2   *Delirium tremens*

(i)   This is uncommon, occurring 48–72 h after abstinence. There is clouding of consciousness, terrifying visual hallucinations, gross tremor, autonomic hyperactivity with tachycardia and cardiac arrhythmias, dilated pupils, fever, sweating, dehydration, and grand mal seizures that may be prolonged (status epilepticus).

(ii)   Delirium tremens is a medical emergency

(a)   control seizures with midazolam, diazepam or lorazepam i.v. (see doses above)

(b)   exclude other causes of status epilepticus such as head injury and meningitis (see p. 91).

(iii)   Replace fluid and electrolyte losses, avoiding excessive normal saline in liver failure. Give thiamine 250 mg i.v. once daily.

(iv)   Refer all patients immediately to the ICU.

> **Warning:** never dispense a benzodiazepine supply or chlormethiazole (clomethiazole) capsules in the ED to take home. They are reserved for inpatient detoxification programmes only.

ACUTE NEUROLOGICAL CONDITIONS

Patients with the following neurological conditions frequently present to the ED:

- Syncope (faint)
- Seizure (fit)
- Generalized convulsive status epilepticus
- TIA
- Stroke.

Headache is covered separately on page 99.

SYNCOPE

DIAGNOSIS

1 Syncope or 'faint' is a sudden, transient loss of consciousness and postural tone due to reduced cerebral perfusion, with subsequent spontaneous recovery.

    (i) A brief tonic-clonic seizure may follow if cerebral perfusion remains impaired.

2 A faint may be difficult to distinguish from a seizure or acute vertigo, so an eye-witness account is vital. Always interview ambulance crew or accompanying adults.

3 Causes vary from benign to imminently life threatening. The aim is to always exclude the most serious conditions such as cardiac-related, hypovolaemia or subarachnoid haemorrhage:

    (i) *Cardiac*
- (a) arrhythmia either a tachycardia, or a bradycardia 'Stokes–Adams attack'
- (b) myocardial infarction
- (c) stenotic valve lesion (especially aortic stenosis)
- (d) hypertrophic cardiomyopathy
- (e) drug toxicity or side effect
  - prolonged QT from sotalol, tricyclics, erythromycin, etc.
  - calcium-channel or β-blocker.

    (ii) *Postural (orthostatic) hypotension*
- (a) haemorrhage or fluid loss:
  - vomiting and/or diarrhoea, with dehydration
  - haematemesis and melaena
  - concealed haemorrhage (such as an abdominal aortic aneurysm or ectopic pregnancy)
  - hypoadrenalism (Addison's), hypopituitarism, pancreatitis 'third spacing'
- (b) autonomic dysfunction
  - Parkinson's disease (multiple systems atrophy), diabetes
- (c) drugs:
  - antihypertensives, e.g. angiotensin-converting enzyme (ACE) inhibitors, prazosin
  - diuretics
  - nitrates
  - levodopa
  - phenothiazines
  - tricyclic antidepressants.

    (iii) *Vascular*
- (a) pulmonary embolism
- (b) carotid sinus hypersensitivity.

     (iv) *Neurological*
        (a) subarachnoid haemorrhage
        (b) vertebrobasilar insufficiency, as part of a transient ischaemic attack (TIA).
     (v) Cough, micturition or defecation syncope.
     (vi) Vasovagal (neurocardiogenic) – 'simple' faint, triggered by heat, pain or emotion. Do **not** diagnose if over 45 years old, but look first for the more sinister causes above.
     (vii) Hypoglycaemia (relative).

4 Ask about symptom patterns to suggest an underlying mechanism:
     (i) Vasovagal syncope associated with an unpleasant trigger, previous episodes, prolonged standing, and prodromal nausea and light-headedness.
     (ii) Orthostatic syncope associated with standing up, certain drugs, autonomic disease and volume depletion.
     (iii) Cardiac syncope associated with exertion, positive family history, known structural heart disease, sudden onset +/– palpitations, absence of a prodrome, sitting or supine position.
     (iv) Following sudden breathlessness (PE), or headache (SAH).

5 Examine all patients carefully, looking for hypotension (including postural drop >20 mmHg or pulse increase >20/min), a cardiac lesion, an abdominal mass or tenderness, and focal neurological signs.

6 Check the blood glucose test strip for hypoglycaemia, and perform an ECG.

7 Request other investigations *only* as indicated clinically such as FBC, U&Es, cardiac biomarkers, pregnancy test, CXR and CT scan.

MANAGEMENT

1 Refer the patient to the medical (or surgical) team for admission if a serious cardiac or orthostatic cause is possible, particularly a patient aged over 60 years. Be sure to admit patients with any one or more of the San Francisco Syncope Rule features:
     (i) History of congestive heart failure.
     (ii) Shortness of breath.
     (iii) Triage systolic BP <90 mmHg.
     (iv) Abnormal ECG.
     (v) Haematocrit <30%.

2 Refer other patients with no clear inciting history, a normal examination and a normal ECG for outpatient follow-up if no immediately life-threatening cause for syncope is found.
     (i) A 24-hour ambulatory ECG (Holter monitor) may help, particularly in unexplained recurrent syncope.

3 Inform the GP by email or letter if the patient is discharged and arrange early follow-up.

SEIZURE (FIT)

DIAGNOSIS

1 An eye-witness account is essential to establish the correct diagnosis. Helpful indicators of an epileptic seizure having occurred, rather than a faint, a fall or an episode of vertigo are:

    (i) Preceding aura, or proceeding drowsiness.

    (ii) Bitten tongue, urinary incontinence.

    (iii) Known seizure disorder.

2 The most common causes of a seizure in a known epileptic are:

    (i) Not taking their medication, or rarely medication toxicity.

    (ii) Alcohol abuse, either excess or withdrawal.

    (iii) Intercurrent infection (remember meningitis).

    (iv) Head injury.

    (v) Hypoglycaemia.

3 Exclude all the following 'acute symptomatic' secondary causes of a seizure in any patient presenting with a first seizure or a sporadic seizure:

    (i) Hypoglycaemia.

    (ii) Head injury.

    (iii) Hypoxia.

    (iv) Infection – especially meningitis, encephalitis, cerebral abscess, HIV or a febrile seizure in a child.

    (v) Acute poisoning, e.g. alcohol, tricyclic antidepressants, anticholinergics, theophylline, cocaine, amphetamine and isoniazid.

    (vi) Drug withdrawal, e.g. alcohol, benzodiazepine, narcotics, cocaine.

    (vii) Intracranial pathology:

        (a) space-occupying lesion

        (b) cerebral ischaemia

        (c) subarachnoid or intracerebral haemorrhage.

    (viii) Hyponatraemia, hypocalcaemia, uraemia and eclampsia.

4 Check a blood glucose test strip.

    (i) Give 50% dextrose 50 mL i.v. if it is low, after taking blood for a laboratory glucose estimation, or give glucagon 1 mg i.m. when venous access is impossible.

5 Insert an i.v. cannula and take blood for FBC, U&Es, LFTs, and a drug and alcohol screen.

    (i) Proceed to VBGs, β-hCG, blood cultures, ECG, CXR and CT head scan as indicated clinically, and attach a cardiac monitor and pulse oximeter to the patient.

    (ii) Send urgent anticonvulsant levels if the patient is on treatment.

MANAGEMENT

1 Give high-dose oxygen via a face mask. Aim for an oxygen saturation above 94%.

2 Make sure the head is protected from harm and turn the patient semi-prone. Do not attempt to wedge the mouth open.

3 Give midazolam 0.05–0.1 mg/kg up to 10 mg i.v., diazepam 0.1–0.2 mg/kg up to 20 mg i.v. or lorazepam 0.07 mg/kg up to 4 mg i.v. if the patient is having a seizure, or if the seizure recurs.

4 Refer the following patients for admission to the medical team:
   (i) Suspected underlying cause such as meningitis, tumour, etc.
   (ii) A seizure exceeding 5 min, or recurrent seizures, especially if there is no full recovery between them.
   (iii) Residual focal central nervous system (CNS) signs.
   (iv) Seizure following a head injury (refer to the surgeons).

5 Discharge home a previously known epileptic if:
   (i) A rapid, full recovery is made.
   (ii) The seizure lasted less than 5 min and was not associated with trauma either before or during the seizure.
   (iii) There are no residual focal CNS signs and the level of consciousness is normal.
   (iv) Their usual medication is adequate and being taken.
   (v) There is an adult to accompany the patient.

6 In addition, discharge home a patient under 40 years with a non-focal first seizure, with no serious underlying cause found (having considered the causes listed under 'acute symptomatic' on p. 91), and who makes a full recovery without focal neurology.
   (i) Perform a CT head scan first, or organize one within the next day or two.
   (ii) Confirm safe discharge with the senior ED doctor.
   (iii) Organize an outpatient EEG and medical clinic review.
   (iv) Advise the patient not to drive, operate machinery, supervise children swimming, or bathe a baby alone etc. until seen by the specialist. Record this advice in writing in the notes.

7 Always inform the GP by email or letter on discharging the patient, and if the patient was referred to the medical or neurology clinic for follow-up.

> **Warning:** *never* diagnose new-onset 'epilepsy' in a non-epileptic patient until, as a minimum, secondary causes have been excluded by a CT brain scan, and an electroencephalogram has been performed and a specialist outpatient assessment has occurred.

GENERALIZED CONVULSIVE STATUS EPILEPTICUS

DIAGNOSIS

1 Generalized convulsive, grand mal, major motor or tonic–clonic status epilepticus is defined as two or more grand mal seizures without full recovery of consciousness in between, or recurrent grand mal seizures for more than 5–10 min.

2 Over 50% patients have no prior history of seizures.
   (i) Thus it is essential to look for any of the underlying 'acute symptomatic' causes listed under point 3 on page 91.
   (ii) Therefore, perform all the tests mentioned under point 5 on p. 91, once the seizures have been terminated.

3 Attach a cardiac monitor and pulse oximeter to the patient on arrival.

MANAGEMENT

1 Give the patient oxygen via a face mask, and aim for an oxygen saturation above 94%.

2 Check the blood sugar:
   (i) Give 50% dextrose 50 mL i.v. if it is low.
   (ii) Give thiamine 250 mg i.v. in addition if chronic alcoholism or malnutrition is likely, to avoid precipitating Wernicke's encephalopathy.

3 Give midazolam 0.05–0.1 mg/kg up to 10 mg i.v., diazepam 0.1–0.2 mg/kg up to 20 mg i.v. or lorazepam 0.07 mg/kg up to 4 mg i.v.
   (i) Beware of causing respiratory depression, bradycardia and hypotension, especially in the elderly.

4 Get senior ED doctor help if the patient is still having a seizure:
   (i) Repeat the midazolam, diazepam or lorazepam i.v. until seizures cease.
   (ii) Then give phenytoin 15–18 mg/kg i.v. no faster than 50 mg/min by slow bolus, or preferably as an infusion in 250 mL normal saline (never in dextrose) over 30 min under ECG monitoring, or
   (iii) Give the pro-drug fosphenytoin at an equivalent dose but faster rate.

5 Other drugs that may be used include phenobarbitone (phenobarbital) 10–20 mg/kg i.v. no faster than 100 mg/min, or sodium valproate 10 mg/kg slowly i.v. over 5 min, followed by 1–2 mg/kg/h infusion to maximum 2500 mg/day.
   (i) By now, make sure the ICU team is involved if seizures continue.
   (ii) All patients will require admission, possibly to a high-dependency area.

6 Occasionally, if i.v. access is impossible, give:
   (i) Rectal diazepam, especially in children, using parenteral diazepam solution 0.5 mg/kg given through a small syringe (see p. 312) or midazolam 0.5 mg/kg p.r. or via the buccal route.

7 Consider the following underlying reasons when a patient fails to regain consciousness, despite the seizures stopping:
  - (i) Medical consequences of the seizures:
    - (a) hypoxia
    - (b) hypo- or hyperglycaemia
    - (c) hypotension
    - (d) hyperpyrexia
    - (e) cerebral oedema
    - (f) lactic acidosis
    - (g) iatrogenic over-sedation.
  - (ii) Progression of an underlying disease process:
    - (a) head injury, e.g. extradural or subdural
    - (b) meningitis or encephalitis
    - (c) cerebral hypoxia
    - (d) drug toxicity, e.g. theophylline.
  - (iii) Subtle generalized convulsive status epilepticus.
  - (iv) Non-convulsive status epilepticus:
    - (a) complex–partial (temporal lobe) seizures
    - (b) absence status.

TRANSIENT ISCHAEMIC ATTACK

DIAGNOSIS

1 TIAs are episodes of sudden transient focal neurological deficit, maximal at the outset and lasting for <24 h, usually <1 hour.
  - (i) They may recur and are important in that they are part of a spectrum that can progress to a full-blown stroke.
  - (ii) Thus they may be followed by a major ischaemic stroke or other serious vascular event:
    - (a) 2.5–5% at 2 days
    - (b) 5–10% at 30 days
    - (c) 10–20% at 90 days.

2 The causes may be considered in three groups.
  - (i) *Embolic*
    - (a) extracranial vessels – carotid stenosis, narrowed vertebral artery
    - (b) cardiac – AF, post-myocardial infarction, mitral stenosis, valve prosthesis.
  - (ii) *Reduced cerebral perfusion*
    - (a) hypotension from hypovolaemia, drugs or a cardiac arrhythmia
    - (b) hypertension (especially in hypertensive encephalopathy)
    - (c) polycythaemia, paraproteinaemia, or a hypercoagulable state such as protein C, protein S or antithrombin III deficiency, and with antiphospholipid antibodies
    - (d) vasculitis, e.g. temporal arteritis, SLE, polyarteritis nodosa, or syphilis.

    (iii) *Lack of nutrients*
      (a) anaemia
      (b) hypoglycaemia.

3 TIAs present clinically as:
    (i) Carotid territory dysfunction causing hemiparesis, hemianaesthesia, homonymous hemianopia, dysphasia, dysarthria and amaurosis fugax (transitory monocular blindness).
    (ii) Vertebrobasilar territory dysfunction (posterior circulation) causing combinations of bilateral limb paresis, crossed sensory symptoms, diplopia, nystagmus, ataxia, vertigo and cortical blindness.

4 Examine the pulse rhythm, heart sounds, blood pressure (in both arms and postural), listen for carotid bruits and perform a full neurological assessment.

5 Risk stratify the patient using the $ABCD^2$ scoring system (see Table 2.11).
    (i) $ABCD^2$ score of ≥ 4 points is considered 'high-risk', with a 7-day risk of completed stroke of 5.9–11.7%.
    (ii) $ABCD^2$ score of 0–3 points is considered 'low-risk', with a 7-day risk of completed stroke of 1.2%.

Table 2.11 $ABCD^2$ score for early risk stratification in transient ischaemic attack

	Score
Age ≥ 60 years	1 point
Blood pressure ≥ 140 mmHg (SBP) and/or ≥ 90 mmHg (DBP)	1 point
Clinical signs	
Unilateral weakness	2 points
Speech disturbance *without* weakness	1 point
Other	0 points
Duration	
≥ 60 min	2 points
10–59 min	1 point
<10 min	0 points
Diabetes	1 point
TOTAL	= (Max 7)

High risk ≥ 4 points: with a 7-day risk of completed stroke of 5.9–11.7%.
Low risk 0–3 points: with a 7-day risk of completed stroke of 1.2%.
DBP, diastolic blood pressure; SBP, systolic blood pressure.
Adapted with permission from Johnston C, Rothwell P, Nguyen-Huynh M *et al.* (2007) Validation and refinement of scores to predict very early stroke risk after transient ischaemic attack. *Lancet* **369**: 283–92.

5   Check a bedside blood glucose test strip. Send blood for FBC, ESR, coagulation profile, blood sugar, ELFTs and a lipid profile in all patients.

6   Perform an ECG and request a CXR.

7   Arrange an urgent CT brain scan to differentiate haemorrhage from infarction, and to look for a structural, non-vascular lesion.

8   Organize a duplex carotid ultrasound for a suspected carotid territory ischaemic event as soon as possible, certainly for the high-risk patient with an ABCD^2 score of ≥4 points.

MANAGEMENT

1   Give aspirin 300 mg orally, then 75–150 mg once daily as soon as the CT scan has excluded haemorrhage.

2   Deciding who to admit can be difficult. Refer the patient for immediate medical admission if:

   (i)   High-risk patient with an ABCD^2 score of ≥4 points.
   (ii)   The ECG is abnormal, and a cardiac embolic source is suspected, particularly new or untreated atrial fibrillation.
   (iii) TIAs are recurring over a period of hours or are progressing in severity and intensity (known as crescendo TIAs).
   (iv)   There are residual neurological findings.
   (v)   The patient has new or poorly controlled diabetes.
   (vi)   The patient has poorly controlled hypertension with systolic BP ≥180 mmHg, or diastolic BP ≥100 mmHg.
   (vii) Carotid territory disease, particularly in an otherwise healthy patient with an audible carotid bruit and possible high-grade stenosis, or a history of known carotid stenosis.

3   Refer the remaining patients to medical or neurology outpatients within 7 days, if complete recovery has occurred, and the patient is low-risk with an ABCD^2 score of 0–3 points.

   (i)   Arrange an echocardiogram (if cardiac cause suspected) as an outpatient.
   (ii)   Inform the GP by email and by letter.

> **Warning:** remember that patients can present with the consequences of their TIA, e.g. a head injury, Colles' fracture, or fracture of the neck of femur. Do not fail to investigate for these, or to look for the true precipitating event (i.e. the TIA).

STROKE

These are due to a vascular disturbance producing a focal neurological deficit for over 24 h.

DIAGNOSIS

1 The causes include:
 (i) *Cerebral ischaemia or infarction (80%)*
  (a) cerebral thrombosis from atherosclerosis, hypertension or rarely arteritis, etc.
  (b) cerebral embolism from atheromatous plaques in a neck vessel, AF, post-myocardial infarction or mitral stenosis
  (c) hypotension causing cerebral hypoperfusion.
 (ii) *Cerebral haemorrhage (20%)*
  (a) intracerebral haemorrhage associated with hypertension or rarely intracranial tumour and bleeding disorders including anticoagulation
  (b) subarachnoid haemorrhage from ruptured berry aneurysm or arteriovenous malformation.

2 Presentation may give a clue to aetiology:
 (i) Cerebral thrombosis is often preceded by a TIA and the neurological deficit usually progresses gradually. Headache and loss of consciousness are uncommon.
 (ii) Cerebral embolism causes a sudden, complete neurological deficit.
 (iii) Intracerebral haemorrhage causes sudden onset of headache, vomiting, stupor or coma with a rapidly progressive neurological deficit.
 (iv) Subarachnoid haemorrhage is heralded by:
  (a) sudden, severe 'worst headache ever', sometimes following exertion, associated with meningism, i.e. stiff neck, photophobia, vomiting and Kernig's sign (see p. 100)
  (b) confusion or lethargy, which are common, or focal neurological deficit and coma, which are rare and serious.

3 Record the vital signs, including the temperature, pulse, blood pressure, respiratory rate and GCS score (see p. 30).

4 Perform a full neurological examination, recording any progression of symptoms and signs.

5 Gain i.v. access and send blood for FBC, ESR, coagulation profile, ELFTs and blood sugar. Attach a cardiac monitor and pulse oximeter to the patient, and catheterize the bladder.

6 Obtain an ECG and CXR, and arrange an immediate CT brain scan.
 (i) Request a CT brain urgently if thrombolysis is possible for symptom onset within 4.5 h.
 (ii) This CT scan is to exclude cerebral haemorrhage or a structural brain lesion stroke mimic.
 (iii) CT angiogram of brain and neck, and CT perfusion brain scan are not considered routine, but are requested according to availability and local policy.

MANAGEMENT

1 This is now time critical to obtain CT scanning when thrombolysis is being considered.

  (i) Make certain a bedside blood glucose test strip has been done and give 50% dextrose 50 mL i.v. if it is low.

2 If the patient is unconscious:

  (i) Open the airway by tilting the head and lifting the chin, insert an oropharyngeal airway, give high-dose oxygen via a face mask and pass a nasogastric tube (NGT).

  (ii) Place the patient in the left lateral position. Get a senior ED doctor help.

  (iii) Consider endotracheal intubation if there is respiratory depression, deteriorating neurological status and/or signs of raised intracranial pressure. Discuss this with the intensive care team.

3 Otherwise, commence oxygen, and aim for an oxygen saturation above 94%.

4 Refer the patient to the medical team or stroke unit for admission and definitive management.

  (i) Give aspirin 300 mg orally daily or via NGT within 48 h, once CT scan has excluded haemorrhage, unless thrombolysis is used (withold for 24 h).

  (ii) Select patients suitable for thrombolysis if symptom onset is less than 4.5 h, there is a measurable and clinically significant deficit on NIH Stroke Scale examination, CT scan excludes haemorrhage or non-vascular cause, and age is over 18 yr

  (a) NIH Stroke Scale is a 15-item neurologic examination to evaluate and document neurological status, determine appropriate treatment and predict patient outcome.

  (iii) Get senior ED doctor help and carefully follow local thrombolysis guidelines such as 'Code Stroke'.

  (iv) Give alteplase 0.9 mg/kg up to 90 mg i.v. over 1 h, with 10% as an initial bolus, having excluded absolute contraindications (see Table 2.12) and considered relative contraindications.

5 **Avoid** the temptation to treat acutely raised blood pressure unless aortic dissection (see p. 57) or subarachnoid haemorrhage (see p. 101) are found.

  (i) In an ischaemic stroke if the BP is acutely raised >220/120 mmHg, reduction by 10–20% may be performed (i.e. no lower than 180/95 mmHg initially).

6 Keep nil by mouth (NBM) until a swallowing assessment is completed within the first 24 h.

7 Seek an urgent neurosurgical opinion for any of: a younger patient with extensive hemispheric infarction, acute hydrocephalus associated with large cerebellar infarct, or a cerebellar haematoma >3 cm presenting with headache, dizziness, vertigo, truncal or limb ataxia, gaze palsy and a diagnostic CT brain scan.

Table 2.12 Absolute contraindications for thrombolysis in stroke

Uncertainty about time of stroke onset (i.e. patient awaking from sleep)
Coma or severe obtundation with fixed eye deviation and complete hemiplegia
Minor stroke deficit that is rapidly improving
Seizure observed or known to have occurred at onset of stroke
Hypertension: systolic blood pressure ≥185 mmHg, or diastolic blood pressure >110 mmHg on repeated measures
Clinical presentation suggestive of subarachnoid haemorrhage (even if the CT scan is normal)
Presumed septic embolus
Patient has received heparin within the last 48 h and has elevated APTT; or has a known hereditary or acquired haemorrhagic diathesis (i.e. PT or APTT greater than normal)
INR >1.5
Platelet count <100 x 10⁹/L
Plasma glucose concentration <2.8 mmol/L or >22 mmol/L

If any of the above apply, do NOT use alteplase (or other lytic agent).
CT, computed tomography; APTT, activated partial thromboplastin time;
PT, prothrombin time; INR, international normalized ratio.

HEADACHE

DIFFERENTIAL DIAGNOSIS

Consider the serious or life-threatening diagnoses first:
- Meningitis
- Subarachnoid haemorrhage
- Space-occupying lesion
- Temporal arteritis (age >50 years; erythrocyte sedimentation rate [ESR] >50 mm/h)
- Acute narrow-angle glaucoma
- Hypertensive encephalopathy.

The majority, however, will be due to:
- Migraine
- Tension or muscle contraction headache
- Post-traumatic headache
- Disease in other cranial structures.

The history is vital as physical signs may be minimal or lacking, even in the serious group. A new headache or a change in quality of a usual one must be evaluated carefully, especially in the elderly.

MENINGITIS

DIAGNOSIS

1 Causes include meningococcus, *Streptococcus pneumoniae, Listeria monocytogenes* (adults over 50 years, in alcoholism, pregnancy, immunosuppression or cancer), group B streptococcus and *Escherichia coli* (infants <3 months), viruses, and *Cryptococcus neoformans* and tuberculosis (immunosuppression including HIV).

   (i) *Haemophilus influenzae* is now becoming rare following vaccination programmes.

2 Prodromal malaise is followed by generalized headache, fever and vomiting, with altered mental status, irritability and drowsiness progressing to confusion or coma.

3 Pyrexia, photophobia and neck stiffness are found. Localized cranial nerve palsies or seizures may occur.

4 Eliciting signs of meningeal irritation are rarely positive (<10%):

   (i) Kernig's sign: pain and spasm in the hamstrings on attempted knee extension, with a flexed hip.

   (ii) Brudzinski's sign: involuntary flexion of both hips and knees on passive neck flexion.

5 Always consider meningitis in the confused elderly, sick neonate, in generalized convulsive status epilepticus, and in coma of unknown cause.

6 A petechial rash, impaired consciousness and meningism are features of meningococcal septicaemia (meningococcaemia), but are relatively late signs. Therefore look out for the earlier signs of possible meningococcaemia such as:

   (i) Muscle pain including leg pains, abnormal skin colour with pallor or mottling, and cold hands and feet.

   (ii) Rigors, vomiting, headache or abdominal pain and a rapid evolution of illness within 24 h.

   (iii) Progression to shock and obtundation indicate fulminant meningococcal disease.

7 Gain i.v. access and send blood for FBC, coagulation profile, ELFTs, blood sugar, viral studies and two sets of blood cultures (from different venepuncture sites).

8 Attach a cardiac monitor and pulse oximeter to the patient, and perform a CXR.

MANAGEMENT

1 Give the patient oxygen and commence a normal saline infusion.

2 Seek immediate senior ED doctor help, and give antibiotics as soon as the diagnosis is suspected.

   (i) Give ceftriaxone 4 g i.v. daily, or 2 g i.v. 12-hourly; or cefotaxime 2 g i.v. then 6-hourly.

(ii) Add benzylpenicillin 2.4 g i.v. 4-hourly if *Listeria* is possible, such as in immunosuppression, adults >50 years, chronic alcohol abuse, pregnancy or debilitation.

(iii) Add vancomycin 1.5 g i.v. 12-hourly, if patient has known or suspected otitis media or sinusitis, or Gram-positive diplococci are seen in the cerebrospinal fluid (CSF), or a pneumococcal antigen assay on CSF is positive.

3 Give dexamethasone 0.15 mg/kg up to 10 mg i.v. then 6-hourly at the same time as the antibiotics, if bacterial meningitis is strongly suspected, particularly when ill or obtunded, although its efficacy is unclear.

4 Then perform a CT scan to look for a cerebral mass lesion, especially if there are focal neurological signs, papilloedema, seizures, or mental obtundation.

(i) Even if this CT scan is normal, omit the lumbar puncture until these signs improve or disappear.

5 Consider lumbar puncture (LP) without CT when there are no focal neurological signs and the patient has a normal mental state, particularly if a CT scan is unavailable.

6 Admit the patient under the medical team, or to the ICU if altered mental status or haemodynamically unstable.

SUBARACHNOID HAEMORRHAGE

DIAGNOSIS

1 The majority of cases are associated with a ruptured berry aneurysm, some of which occur in patients who have a family history, hypertension, polycystic kidneys or coarctation of the aorta.

(i) The remainder are due to an arteriovenous malformation, or rarely coagulopathy and vasculitis.

2 Ask about any prodromal episodes of headache or diplopia due to a 'warning leak'. These may precede a sudden, severe *'worst headache ever'*, sometimes following exertion.

3 Lethargy, nausea, vomiting and meningism with photophobia and neck stiffness occur, although fever is usually absent or is low grade.

(i) A IIIrd nerve oculomotor palsy suggests bleeding from a posterior communicating artery aneurysm.

4 Less typical presentations include acute confusion, transient loss of consciousness with recovery, or coma when a stiff neck and sub-hyaloid (pre-retinal) haemorrhage are useful diagnostic pointers on examination.

5 Gain i.v. access and send blood for FBC, coagulation profile, U&Es, blood sugar and a group and hold. Attach a cardiac monitor and pulse oximeter to the patient.

6 Perform an ECG and request a CXR.

MANAGEMENT

1 Give the patient oxygen and nurse head upwards. Aim for an oxygen saturation above 94%.

2 Give midazolam 0.05–0.1 mg/kg up to 10 mg i.v., or diazepam 0.1–0.2 mg/kg up to 20 mg i.v., or lorazepam 0.07 mg/kg up to 4 mg i.v. for seizures or severe agitation.

3 Give paracetamol 500 mg and codeine phosphate 8 mg two tablets orally or rarely morphine 2.5–5 mg i.v. for pain relief, with an antiemetic such as metoclopramide 10 mg i.v.

4 Arrange a CT brain scan urgently to confirm the diagnosis.
   (i) A normal non-contrast CT brain scan performed within 6 h of headache onset effectively excludes the diagnosis.
   (ii) CT scan sensitivity then drops after 6 h, and reaches as low as 50% by day 7.

5 Proceed to perform a lumbar puncture if the CT brain scan is negative but the patient presented after 6 h.
   (i) Wait until ideally 12 h have passed since headache onset and make sure there are no focal neurological signs or papilloedema.
   (ii) Request xanthochromia studies by spectrophotometry of the CSF to differentiate a traumatic tap (absent) from a true subarachnoid haemorrhage (positive).

6 Refer the patient to ICU for admission, or to a neurosurgical unit.
   (i) Seek specialist consultation and commence nimodipine 60 mg orally 4-hourly or an infusion at 1 mg/h if comatose, increased to 2 mg/h after 2 h if the blood pressure is stable, when the diagnosis is confirmed.

SPACE-OCCUPYING LESION

DIAGNOSIS

1 Causes include an intracranial haematoma, cerebral tumour, or cerebral abscess.

2 The headaches become progressively more frequent and severe, worse in the mornings and exacerbated by coughing, bending or straining.

3 Vomiting without nausea occurs, and focal neurological signs develop, ranging from subtle personality changes, ataxia, and visual problems to cranial nerve palsies, hemiparesis and seizures.

4 Papilloedema may be seen, with loss of venous pulsation and blurring of the disc margin with filling in of the optic cup as the earliest signs on funduscopy.

5 Perform a CXR to look for a primary tumour and arrange an immediate CT head scan.

MANAGEMENT

1 Give oxygen, and treat seizures with midazolam 0.05–0.1 mg/kg up to 10 mg i.v., or diazepam 0.1–0.2 mg/kg up to 20 mg i.v., or lorazepam 0.07 mg/kg up to 4 mg i.v.

2 Refer a patient with an extradural or subdural haematoma to the neurosurgical team.

3 Otherwise refer the patient to the medical team for full investigation.

TEMPORAL ARTERITIS

DIAGNOSIS

1 This occurs in patients over 50 years, with relentless, diffuse or bitemporal headache often associated with a history of fatigue, malaise, weight loss and fever.

    (i) Occasionally there is pain on chewing (jaw claudication).

    (ii) Polymyalgia rheumatica (PMR) with shoulder girdle weakness and aching stiffness coexists in >30% of patients.

2 Look for localized scalp tenderness, hyperaesthesia and decreased temporal arterial pulsation.

3 Send blood for an urgent ESR (one of the few times this is actually indicated in the ED!).

4 The immediate danger is sudden visual loss due to ophthalmic artery involvement, which may affect both eyes if steroid treatment is delayed.

MANAGEMENT

1 Commence prednisolone 60 mg orally if the ESR is raised >50 mm/h, or if the result is not available immediately.

2 Refer the patient to the medical or ophthalmology team for admission for urgent temporal artery biopsy and continued high-dose steroid therapy.

ACUTE NARROW-ANGLE GLAUCOMA

See page 355.

HYPERTENSIVE ENCEPHALOPATHY

DIAGNOSIS

1 This is due to an acute accelerated or malignant hypertensive crisis, related to rapid onset hypertension with headache, nausea and vomiting, confusion, and blurred vision.

2 Ask about drug non-compliance if known hypertension, renal disease, autoimmune disease such as SLE or scleroderma, recreational drug use such as cocaine or amphetamines, and the possibility of pregnancy.

3 Examine for focal neurological signs. Seizures and coma may develop later.

    (i) Look for papilloedema, retinal haemorrhages, exudates and cotton-wool spots on funduscopy (grade IV retinal changes).

4 Gain i.v. access and send blood for FBC, ELFTs, blood sugar and cardiac biomarker such as troponin if there are chest pains or ECG changes. Attach a cardiac monitor and pulse oximeter to the patient.

5 Perform an ECG and request a CXR.

6 Check an MSU for proteinuria and send it for microscopy to look for evidence of renal disease, with casts or abnormal urinary red blood cells (>70% dysmorphic).

  (i) Perform a urinary β-human chorionic gonadotrophin (hCG) pregnancy test (qualitative and immediate) or send blood (quantitative but takes time).

7 Arrange an urgent CT brain scan.

MANAGEMENT

1 Give the patient oxygen, and aim for an oxygen saturation above 94%.

2 Get senior ED doctor help and take expert advice.

  (i) Aim to reduce mean arterial pressure (MAP) initially by no more than 25%, or aim for a diastolic BP of 100–110 mmHg within the first 24 h.

  (ii) Use oral treatment with labetalol 100 mg, atenolol 100 mg, or amlodipine 5–10 mg or felodipine sustained-release 5–10 mg.

  (iii) *Avoid* more potent i.v. agents such as sodium nitroprusside 0.25–10 μg/kg per min i.v., unless intra-arterial blood pressure monitoring is in place. ICU admission is indicated.

3 Refer the patient to the medical team for blood pressure control and to observe for the complications of heart failure, aortic dissection, intracranial haemorrhage and renal impairment (cause or effect).

MIGRAINE

DIAGNOSIS

1 'Common' migraine or migraine without aura (66–75% migraineurs). This is diagnosed by a history of at least five previous attacks that:

  (i) Last 4–72 h if untreated.

  (ii) Have at least two of the following headache characteristics:

    (a) unilateral
    (b) pulsating or throbbing
    (c) moderate to severe
    (d) aggravated by movement.

  (iii) Have at least one associated symptom of:

    (a) nausea and/or vomiting
    (b) photophobia
    (c) phonophobia.

2   'Classic' migraine, or migraine with aura, is less common (25–30% migraineurs). It has similar features to those above, plus a history of at least two previous attacks that:
    (i)   Have a typical aura:
          (a) fully reversible visual, sensory or speech symptoms (or mixed), but *not* motor weakness
          (b) visual symptoms can be uni- or bilateral flashing lights, zig-zag lines (teichopsia), fortification spectra and a central scotoma, or transient hemianopia
          (c) sensory symptoms are unilateral positive or negative
          (c) these symptoms develop over 5 min, or each symptom lasts ≥5 min but <60 min.
    (ii) Headache precedes, accompanies, or follows the aura within 60 min, although up to 40% can have an aura with no headache, or
    (iii) Have a less typical aura (these are all rare):
          (a) hemiplegic (sporadic or familial)
          (b) basilar (ataxia, vertigo, tinnitus, nystagmus, diplopia, confusion)
          (c) ophthalmoplegic.

3   Therefore it is not possible to diagnose the first episodes of migraine, without initially excluding a more serious cause such as a subarachnoid haemorrhage, space-occupying lesion or other intracranial haemorrhage.
    (i)   Also do not diagnose a 'migraine' when the headache is different from a typical attack, was sudden or precipitate in onset, is more longer lasting, if the aura is prolonged and/or if there is residual neurology.
    (ii) Get senior ED doctor help and arrange investigations including a CT brain scan.

MANAGEMENT

1   Nurse the patient in a darkened room, give oxygen by face mask and an oral analgesic such as aspirin 300 mg three tablets, ibuprofen 200 mg two or three tablets, or paracetamol 500 mg and codeine phosphate 8 mg two tablets.

2   Give an antiemetic with antidopaminergic effects, such as metoclopramide 10–20 mg i.v.

3   Give chlorpromazine 0.1–0.2 mg/kg i.v. if the above fail, with a fluid bolus of normal saline 10 mL/kg, or

4   Consider a triptan such as sumatriptan 6 mg s.c. for resistant headache:
    (i)   Side effects of tingling, heat and flushing may occur, or rarely chest pain and tightness.

     (ii)   Sumatriptan is contraindicated in known coronary artery disease (CAD), previous myocardial infarction, and in patients with possible unrecognized coronary artery disease, such as men over 40 years or post-menopausal women, with CAD risk factors.

     (iii) Sumatriptan is also contraindicated within 24 h of ergotamine-containing therapy.

5   Discharge the patient back to the GP, after a discussion of precipitating factors such as emotional stress, menstruation, alcohol, caffeine, hunger, etc.

TENSION (MUSCLE CONTRACTION) HEADACHE

DIAGNOSIS

1   This is a 'featureless headache' with none of the above associated symptoms as for migraine, and that lacks a family history or trigger factors other than stress, or some craniocervical musculoskeletal problems.

     (i)   It can become episodic or chronic.

2   Women are more commonly affected and the pain comes on gradually, is bilateral, mild to moderate, dull, constant and band-like.

3   Mild nausea, phonophobia and photophobia can occur, but are uncommon and vomiting is absent.

MANAGEMENT

1   Give the patient an analgesic such as paracetamol 500 mg and codeine phosphate 8 mg two tablets orally 6-hourly.

2   Reassure the patient and discharge back to the care of the GP.

POST-TRAUMATIC HEADACHE

DIAGNOSIS

1   Headache following head injury may begin immediately or after a few days, and is present in up to 30% of patients at 6 weeks after mild concussion.

2   Inability to concentrate, irritability, dizziness, insomnia and emotional lability may develop, known as the 'post-concussion syndrome'.

3   Request an urgent CT head scan if there is persistent worsening of headache, recurrent vomiting, clouding of consciousness, or focal neurological signs, to exclude a subdural haematoma.

MANAGEMENT

1   Treatment is supportive including analgesics, rest, and reassurance that complete recovery is the rule.

     (i)   Instruct the patient to avoid all contact sport until symptoms are fully resolved, usually 2 weeks minimum.

2   Refer the patient back to the GP, as symptoms may persist for some months.

3   Discuss patients with an abnormal CT scan with the neurosurgeons.

DISEASE IN OTHER CRANIAL STRUCTURES

DIAGNOSIS AND MANAGEMENT

1   Iritis (see p. 354), otitis media (see p. 365), sinusitis or dental caries may all present with headache.

2   Treatment is aimed at the underlying condition.

ACUTE ARTHROPATHY

Acute joint pain in the ED may be divided into three main types:
• Acute monoarthritis
• Acute polyarthritis
• Periarticular swellings.

ACUTE MONOARTHRITIS

DIFFERENTIAL DIAGNOSIS

It is important to distinguish between:
• Septic arthritis
• Gout or pseudogout
• Trauma and haemarthrosis
and occasionally:
• Rheumatoid arthritis
• Osteoarthritis.
though these last two are more commonly polyarticular.

SEPTIC ARTHRITIS

DIAGNOSIS

1   This may occur with any penetrating trauma, even trivial such as a rose thorn, or following arthrocentesis.

2   Most cases, however, develop from haematogenous spread. This is predisposed to by:
    (i)   Rheumatoid arthritis.
    (ii)   Osteoarthritis, particularly in the elderly.
    (iii) Intravenous drug abuse.
    (iv)   Diabetes mellitus.
    (v)   Immunosuppression.
    (vi)   Disseminated gonococcal or meningococcal infection.
    (vii) Sickle cell disease, often from *Salmonella*.

3   Check temperature, pulse and blood pressure. There is localized joint pain, warmth, erythema and severely restricted range of active and passive movement, but with a less precipitate onset than with gout.

4   Send blood for two sets of blood cultures, FBC, ESR and C-reactive protein (CRP).

5   Request an X-ray which will initially be normal, but subsequently may show destruction of bone with loss of the joint space.

6   Or arrange an ultrasound scan, which is most helpful in demonstrating an effusion in joints such as the hip (see p. 317), or even a CT scan for the sterno-clavicular joint.

MANAGEMENT

1   Give an analgesic such as paracetamol 500 mg and codeine phosphate 8 mg two tablets orally.

2   Refer the patient immediately to the orthopaedic team for joint aspiration under sterile conditions, i.v. antibiotics, rest and repeated operative drainage.
   (i)   Joint aspiration should yield turbid, yellow fluid with a polymorph WCC >50 000/mL. A fluid culture is positive in >50%.

GOUTY ARTHRITIS

DIAGNOSIS

1   Gout is much more common in men, and is associated with diabetes, hypertension, hypercholesterolaemia and myeloproliferative disease (especially following treatment), renal failure (cause or effect), thiazide diuretic therapy, or dietary excess, alcohol and trauma.

2   It is most common in the metatarsophalangeal joint of the great toe or in the ankle, wrist and knee, sometimes with a precipitate onset waking the patient from sleep.

3   Chronic cases may be associated with gouty tophi on the ear and around the joints, polyarthropathy and recurrent acute attacks.

4   The patient may be mildly pyrexial with a red, shiny 'angry' joint.

5   Send blood for FBC, ELFTs, and ESR plus CRP if septic arthritis is as likely.
   (i)   Laboratory blood results may show a mild leucocytosis, with a raised uric acid level (>0.4 mmol/L), but the serum uric acid may be normal in up to 40% of acute attacks.

6   Definitive diagnosis is by joint aspiration and polarizing light microscopy showing strongly negative birefringent crystals.
   (i)   Joint aspiration yields cloudy yellow fluid, with a WCC of 2000–50 000/mL. Polarizing microscopy is diagnostic.

MANAGEMENT

1   Give the patient an NSAID in a known relapsing case, or if there is strong clinical suspicion of gout, such as ibuprofen 600 mg orally once, then 200–400 mg orally t.d.s. or naproxen 500 g orally, followed by 250 mg orally t.d.s.

2 Give prednisone 50 mg orally daily for 3 days instead, then tapered over 10–14 days in patients with renal or gastrointestinal disease unable to take NSAIDs.

3 Reserve colchicine 1 mg orally then 0.5 mg orally up to 1 h later, if the patient cannot tolerate either steroids (heart failure or diabetes) or NSAIDs (renal or gastrointestinal disease).

    (i) Do not repeat the colchicine dose for at least 3 days.

4 Refer the patient back to the GP or to medical outpatients.

5 Refer the patient immediately to the orthopaedic team for joint aspiration if septic arthritis cannot be excluded (see p. 107).

PSEUDOGOUT

1 This is much less common than gout, typically affecting the knee, wrist or shoulder, and is associated with diabetes, osteoarthritis, hyperparathyroidism, haemochromatosis and many other rare conditions.

2 X-ray may show chondrocalcinosis (streaking of the soft tissues with calcium), and joint aspiration shows weakly positive birefringent calcium pyrophosphate crystals under polarizing light microscopy.

3 Treatment is as for acute gout, with referral back to the GP or to medical outpatients for follow-up.

TRAUMATIC HAEMARTHROSIS

DIAGNOSIS

1 Severe joint pain is usually associated with obvious trauma, although occasionally the trauma is mild or even forgotten.

2 Haemarthroses may also occur spontaneously in haemophilia A (factor VIII deficiency), haemophilia B (Christmas disease with factor IX deficiency) or severe von Willebrand's disease (with deficiency of both von Willebrand's factor and factor VIII).

3 Request an X-ray, although it may not always demonstrate an obvious fracture.

    (i) Suspect a fracture when there is supporting evidence of a haemarthrosis with a joint effusion or periosteal elevation (e.g. scaphoid or radial head fracture).

4 Arrange joint aspiration performed by a senior ED doctor to look for a haemorrhagic joint effusion, with fat globules floating on the surface in cases of intra-articular fracture, if there is doubt about the diagnosis.

    (i) Also perform joint aspiration when septic arthritis cannot be excluded, or refer the patient directly to the orthopaedic team.

MANAGEMENT

1 Give analgesia and refer the patient to the orthopaedic team as necessary. Management varies according to the joint involved (see Section VI, Orthopaedic Emergencies).

2 Give factor VIII to a patient with known haemophilia A, factor IX to a known haemophilia B patient and von Willebrand's factor plus factor VIII to a patient with von Willebrand's.

    (i) Organize this as *rapidly* as possible in consultation with the haematology team.

ACUTE POLYARTHRITIS

DIAGNOSIS

1 There are many causes, including:

    (i) Rheumatoid arthritis.

    (ii) SLE.

    (iii) Psoriatic arthritis.

    (iv) Ankylosing spondylitis.

    (v) Reiter syndrome.

    (vi) Viral illness, e.g. hepatitis B, rubella, alphavirus such as Ross River, parvovirus B19, and HIV.

    (vii) Sarcoid.

    (viii) Ulcerative colitis, Crohn's disease, gonococcus (early bacteraemic phase), Behçet's disease, and Henoch–Schonlein purpura.

    (ix) Gout and pseudogout.

    (x) Rheumatic fever, or bacterial endocarditis.

    (xi) Osteoarthritis, haemochromatosis, acromegaly (all non-inflammatory).

2 Send blood for FBC, ESR, CRP, ELFTs, uric acid, rheumatoid factor and anti-CCP (anticyclic citrullinated peptide), anti-nuclear antibody (ANA) and DNA antibodies, viral titres and blood cultures according to the suspected cause.

3 Request X-rays of the affected joints.

MANAGEMENT

1 Refer to the medical team for admission, bed rest, drug treatment and definitive diagnosis if the patient is systemically unwell.

2 Otherwise, commence an NSAID analgesic such as ibuprofen 200–400 mg orally t.d.s. or naproxen 250 mg orally t.d.s. and refer the patient to medical or rheumatology outpatients.

RHEUMATOID ARTHRITIS

DIAGNOSIS

1 This occasionally presents as a monoarthritis, although usually it causes a symmetrical polyarthritis affecting the metacarpophalangeal and proximal interphalangeal joints in particular, initially with morning stiffness.

    (i) Other joints affected include the elbows, wrists, hips and knees.

2 Systemic involvement may occur with malaise, weight loss, fever, myalgia, nodules, pleurisy, pericarditis, vasculitis, splenomegaly, episcleritis and pancytopenia.

3 Check FBC, ESR, rheumatoid factor and anti-CCP, ANA and DNA antibodies.

4 X-rays initially show soft-tissue swelling only and juxta-articular osteoporosis, followed by joint deformity.

MANAGEMENT

1 Refer the patient to the medical team for admission if systemically unwell.

2 Refer the patient to the orthopaedic team if septic arthritis cannot be excluded, remembering that rheumatoid arthritis predisposes to septic arthritis.

3 Otherwise commence an NSAID analgesic such as ibuprofen 200–400 mg orally t.d.s. or naproxen 250 mg orally t.d.s. and refer the patient to medical outpatients or the GP.

OSTEOARTHRITIS

DIAGNOSIS

1 This usually presents as a polyarthritis of insidious onset, typically affecting the distal interphalangeal joints, hips and knees with pain and stiffness on movement, but no systemic features.

2 However, occasionally an acute monoarthritis exacerbation may be seen associated with marked joint crepitus.

3 Request an X-ray that may show loss of joint space, osteophyte formation and bony cysts.

MANAGEMENT

1 Refer the patient to the orthopaedic team if septic arthritis cannot be excluded.

2 Otherwise, give the patient an NSAID analgesic and return to the care of the GP.

PERIARTICULAR SWELLINGS

See pp. 275–279 in Section VII, Musculoskeletal and Soft-Tissue Emergencies.

ALLERGIC OR IMMUNOLOGICAL CONDITIONS

The following immunological conditions may present, ranging from those that are socially inconvenient to imminently life-threatening:

- Urticaria (hives)
- Angioedema
- Anaphylaxis – see page 27 (Section I, Critical Care).

URTICARIA (HIVES)

DIAGNOSIS

1 There are many immunological and non-immune causes, including:
- (i) Foods – nuts, shellfish, eggs, strawberries, chocolate, food dyes or preservatives.
- (ii) Drugs – penicillin, sulphonamide, aspirin, NSAIDs, codeine, morphine.
- (iii) Insect stings, animals, parasitic infections including nematodes (in children).
- (iv) Physical – cold, heat, sun, pressure, exercise, water and vibratory.
- (v) Systemic illness – malignancy including Hodgkin's lymphoma, vasculitis, viruses including picornavirus, respiratory syncytial, hepatitis A or Epstein–Barr virus (EBV) and serum sickness.
- (vi) Idiopathic (in >90% of chronic cases).

2 Itchy, oedematous, transient skin swellings are seen, which may occur in crops lasting several hours.
- (i) Urticaria may be acute, or chronic arbitrarily defined as present for over 6 weeks.
- (ii) It may be accompanied by angioedema, and be part of anaphylaxis.

MANAGEMENT

1 Give the patient a less sedating H_1 histamine antagonist such as cetirizine 10 mg or fexofenadine 180 mg orally daily. These are minimally sedating, unlike promethazine.
- (i) Refractory cases may respond to the addition of an H_2 histamine antagonist such as ranitidine 150 mg orally b.d.

2 Attempt to identify the likely cause from the recent history. Most reactions occur within minutes but may be delayed for up to 24 h.

3 Observe for any multi-system involvement suggesting progression to anaphylaxis (see p. 27).

ANGIOEDEMA

DIAGNOSIS

1 This is an urticarial reaction involving the deep tissues of the face, eyelids, lips, tongue and occasionally the larynx, often without pruritus.
- (i) Other sites include the hands, feet and genitalia.

2 The causes are as for urticaria, especially aspirin or a bee sting, or in particular ACE inhibitors when itch and urticaria are absent.

3 It may cause facial, lip and tongue swelling, progressing to laryngeal oedema with hoarseness, dysphagia, dysphonia and stridor.

4 Attach a cardiac monitor and pulse oximeter to the patient.

5   A rare autosomal dominant hereditary form is due to C1 esterase inhibitor deficiency. A family history of attacks without urticaria, often following minor trauma, and recurrent abdominal pain are suggestive.

MANAGEMENT

1   Commence high-dose oxygen aiming for an oxygen saturation above 94%.

2   Give 1 in 1000 adrenaline (epinephrine) 0.3–0.5 mg (0.3–0.5 mL) i.m. into the upper outer thigh, repeated as necessary.

3   Call the senior ED doctor urgently if airway obstruction persists. Prepare for intubation.

        (i)   Give 1 in 1000 adrenaline (epinephrine) 2–4 mg (2–4 mL) nebulized, repeated as necessary.

        (ii)   Change to 1 in 10 000 or 1 in 100 000 adrenaline (epinephrine) 0.75–1.5 µg/kg i.v., i.e. 50–100 µg or 0.5–1.0 mL of 1 in 10 000 or 5–10 mL of 1 in 100 000 adrenaline (epinephrine) slowly over 5 min i.v., if rapid deterioration occurs with imminent airway obstruction. The ECG **must** be monitored.

4   Give H_1 and H_2 blockers and steroids, only after cardiorespiratory stability has been achieved.

        (i)   Cetirizine 10 mg orally or fexofenadine 180 mg orally, or chlorphenamine 10–20 mg i.v. slowly, plus ranitidine 50 mg i.v.

        (ii)   Hydrocortisone 200 mg i.v.

5   Hereditary angioedema responds poorly to adrenaline (epinephrine). Give urgent C1 esterase inhibitor i.v., or fresh frozen plasma if this is unavailable.

6   Admit the patient when stable for 6–8 h observation, as late deterioration may occur in up to 5% with anaphylaxis (known as a biphasic reaction).

7   Then discharge home on prednisolone 50 mg once daily, cetirizine 10 mg or fexofenadine 180 mg once daily plus ranitidine 150 mg b.d., all orally for 3 days.

        (i)   Inform the GP by email or letter.

        (ii)   Refer all significant or recurrent attacks to the allergy clinic, especially if the cause is unavoidable or unknown.

SKIN DISORDERS

The vast majority of skin disorders are managed by GPs and the dermatology department. However, some patients may present as emergencies with blistering, itching or purpuric conditions. Exanthematous diseases are common in children and young adults, and malignant melanoma particularly in areas of high sunshine.

BLISTERING (VESICOBULLOUS) CONDITIONS

DIAGNOSIS

1 Common causes:
- (i) Viral:
  - (a) herpes zoster
  - (b) herpes simplex.
- (ii) Impetigo.
- (iii) Scabies.
- (iv) Insect bites and papular urticaria.
- (v) Bullous eczema and pompholyx.
- (vi) Drugs – sulphonamides, penicillin, barbiturates.
- (vii) Contact dermatitis.

2 Less common causes:
- (i) Erythema multiforme minor (1–2 cm 'target lesions' only) or erythema multiforme major ('target lesions' rash, plus one mucous membrane involved) due to:
  - (a) *Mycoplasma pneumonia*
  - (b) herpes simplex
  - (c) drugs – sulphonamides and penicillins
  - (d) idiopathic (50%).
- (ii) Stevens–Johnson syndrome (SJS) and toxic epidermal necrolysis (TEN) causing epidermal detachment with mucosal erosions due to:
  - (a) drugs such as anticonvulsants, sulphonamides, NSAIDs and penicillins.
- (iii) Staphylococcal scalded-skin syndrome (SSSS) usually in children.
- (iv) Dermatitis herpetiformis (gluten sensitivity).
- (v) Pemphigus and pemphigoid.

3 Rare causes:
- (i) Porphyria cutanea tarda.
- (ii) Epidermolysis bullosa (congenital).

MANAGEMENT

1 Refer patients with widespread or potentially life-threatening blistering immediately to the dermatology team or medical team.
- (i) This should include any patient with SJS, TEN, SSSS, pemphigus and pemphigoid, who may die from intercurrent infection and multi-organ failure.

2 Otherwise give symptomatic treatment including:
- (i) Antihistamine orally such as promethazine 10 mg t.d.s. if there is associated pruritus, with a warning about drowsiness.
- (ii) Antibiotics orally such as flucloxacillin 500 mg q.d.s. or cephalexin 500 mg q.d.s. for secondary staphylococcal

infection in herpes zoster, impetigo, insect bites and eczema. Give clindamycin 450 mg t.d.s. for patients with severe penicillin allergy.
   (iii) Parasiticidal preparation for scabies (see p. 116).
   (iv) Antiviral agent orally such as famciclovir 1500 mg once, valaciclovir 2 g twice 12 h apart, or aciclovir 400 mg five times a day for 5 days for severe herpes simplex; or famciclovir 250 mg t.d.s., valaciclovir 1 g t.d.s, or aciclovir 800 mg five times a day all for 7 days for severe herpes zoster.
   (v) Topical steroid antiseptic such as 1% hydrocortisone with 1% clioquinol cream t.d.s. for papular urticaria and bullous eczema.

3 Return the patient to the care of their GP.

PRURITUS (ITCHING CONDITIONS)

DIAGNOSIS

1 Causes of pruritus *with* skin disease:
   (i) Scabies, pediculosis, insect bites, parasites (roundworm).
   (ii) Eczema and psoriasis.
   (iii) Contact dermatitis.
   (iv) Urticaria.
   (v) Lichen planus (pruritic, planar, purple, polygonal papules with chronic oral mucous membrane involvement).
   (vi) Pityriasis rosea (upper respiratory infection preceding 'herald' patch, followed after 7–14 days by a pink or red, flaky, oval-shaped rash).
   (vii) Drugs, which may cause any of the conditions (ii)–(vi) above.
   (viii) Dermatitis herpetiformis (chronic itchy, papulovesicular eruptions, usually distributed symmetrically on extensor surfaces, associated with gluten sensitivity).

2 Causes of pruritus *without* skin disease:
   (i) Hepatobiliary – jaundice, including primary biliary cirrhosis.
   (ii) Chronic renal failure.
   (iii) Haematological:
     (a) lymphoma
     (b) polycythaemia rubra vera
     (c) leukaemia – CLL.
   (iv) Endocrine:
     (a) myxoedema
     (b) thyrotoxicosis.
   (v) Carcinoma:
     (a) lung
     (b) stomach.
   (vi) Drugs.

3 Take a general medical history, and ask in particular about medications.

MANAGEMENT

1 Refer patients unable to sleep with intractable pruritus to the dermatology team or medical team.

2 Otherwise give symptomatic treatment including:
  - (i) Antipruritic drug orally:
    - (a) promethazine 10 mg t.d.s. with a warning about drowsiness.
  - (ii) Scabies:
    - (a) scabies is suggested by itch worse at night that does not involve the head, a close partner affected, and finding burrows (often excoriated) in interdigital webs, around the genitalia, or on the nipples
    - (b) treat the patient and close contacts with 5% permethrin aqueous lotion over the whole body including the face and hair, washed off after 8–24 h; all clothes should also be washed
    - (c) arrange repeat treatment in 7 days
    - (d) explain to the patient that although itching may persist, it is no longer contagious
    - (e) advise the patient to attend a genitourinary medicine clinic to exclude an associated sexually transmitted disease if the scabies followed casual sex.
  - (iii) Urticaria, see page 112.
  - (iv) Cease any recent drug therapy considered causal, including non-prescription drugs.

4 Return the patient to the care of their GP.

PURPURIC CONDITIONS

DIAGNOSIS

1 Petechiae and purpura are non-blanching, cutaneous areas of bleeding that may be non-palpable or palpable.

2 Causes of non-palpable purpura include:
  - (i) Thrombocytopenia, with splenomegaly:
    - (a) normal marrow:
      - – liver disease with portal hypertension
      - – myeloproliferative disorders
      - – lymphoproliferative disorders
      - – hypersplenism
    - (b) abnormal marrow:
      - – leukaemia
      - – lymphoma
      - – myeloid metaplasia.

(ii) Thrombocytopenia, without splenomegaly:
- (a) normal marrow:
  - immune: idiopathic thrombocytopenic purpura (ITP), drugs, infections including HIV
  - non-immune: vasculitis, sepsis, disseminated intravascular coagulation (DIC), haemolytic–uraemic syndrome (HUS), thrombotic thrombocytopenic purpura (TTP)
- (b) abnormal marrow:
  - aplasia, fibrosis or infiltration
  - cytotoxics
  - alcohol, thiazides.

(iii) Non-thrombocytopenic:
- (a) cutaneous disorders:
  - trauma, sun
  - steroids, old age
- (b) systemic disorders:
  - uraemia
  - von Willebrand's disease
  - scurvy, amyloid.

3 Causes of palpable purpura include:
- (i) Vasculitis:
  - (a) polyarteritis nodosa
  - (b) leucocytoclastic (hypersensitivity), Henoch–Schönlein purpura.
- (ii) Emboli:
  - (a) meningococcaemia
  - (b) gonococcaemia
  - (c) other infections: *Staphylococcus*, Rickettsia (Rocky Mountain spotted fever), enteroviruses.

4 Ask about any drugs taken, systemic symptoms, bleeding tendency, travel history, alcohol use and HIV disease or risk behaviour.

5 Check the temperature, pulse, blood pressure, SaO_2 and examine for lymphadenopathy and hepatosplenomegaly. Perform a urinalysis for casts.

6 Send blood for FBC and film, coagulation profile, ELFTs and blood cultures according to the likely aetiology.

MANAGEMENT

1 Management is of the underlying cause.

2 This is urgent for suspected meningococcaemia with ceftriaxone 2 g i.v. and for Rocky Mountain spotted fever with doxycycline 100 mg orally b.d.

EXANTHEMATOUS DISEASES

DIAGNOSIS

1   Exanthems are generalized erythematous, often blanching, maculopapular eruptions secondary to viral or bacterial infection.

    (i)   Some have 'classic' clinical presentations such as chickenpox, fifth disease, glandular fever, measles, rubella and scarlet fever (see Table 2.13).

Table 2.13 Common exanthematous diseases

Disease	Incubation period (days)	Prodrome	Rash	Other features and infectivity
Chickenpox	10–20	None	Macules, papules, vesicles and pustules of differing ages	Infective until all vesicles are crusted over (usually 6 days after last crop)
Fifth disease (erythema infectiosum)	7–10	Fever, malaise	Raised red 'slapped cheeks', diffuse maculopapular	Transient arthralgia, then relapsing rash; infective *before* onset of rash. Fetal abnormality
Glandular fever	5–14	Fever, sore throat, malaise	Transient maculopapular (rare); itchy drug rash with ampicillin (common)	Tonsillar exudate, cervical lymphadenopathy; hepatosplenomegaly; infective for many months by close physical contact
Measles	9–14	3 days of cough, cold, conjunctivitis	Red, confluent, maculopapular; lasts 7–11 days	Koplik's spots; cough predominates; may be quite ill; infective for 5 days after rash appears
Rubella	14–21	None	Pink, maculopapular, discrete; lasts 3–5 days	Occipital and pre-auricular lymphadenopathy; infective until rash disappears. Fetal abnormality
Scarlet fever	2–5	1–2 days of sore throat, fever, vomiting	Minute, red punctuate papules; last 7 days	Unwell; circumoral pallor; 'strawberry tongue'; infective until negative throat swabs following penicillin

(ii) Others are non-specific rashes, secondary to enteroviruses or respiratory viruses.

2 Ask about recent known contacts, particularly at childcare or in school, as well as any constitutional symptoms such as fever and malaise.

3 Most are diagnosed on clinical features, but serology for antibody titres may aid confirmation, particularly when there is concern following contact in a pregnant person.

MANAGEMENT

1 Give symptomatic treatment, or phenoxymethylpenicillin 500 mg orally b.d. for 10 days in the case of streptococcal scarlet fever.

2 Isolate the patient at home until non-infectious.
   (i) Rarely admission is indicated in the immunosuppressed, or patients with severe systemic features.

3 Discuss pregnant contacts of a rubella or fifth disease patient with an infectious disease specialist or obstetrician.

MALIGNANT MELANOMA

The incidence of malignant melanoma has doubled in many countries over the past decade.

DIAGNOSIS AND MANAGEMENT

1 Look for the following suspicious signs when a malignant melanoma is possible:
   (i) ABCDE features:
      (a) asymmetry
      (b) border irregularity
      (c) colour variation
      (d) diameter ≥ 5 mm
      (e) elevation, enlargement, evolution ie. bleeding.

2 Refer a patient with any suspicious lesion urgently to the dermatology team.

3 Remember that the most common sites for melanoma are on the back and on the legs.

ELDERLY PATIENT

1 An increasing number of patients over the age of 75 years attend the ED and pose unique problems of their own.

2 These problems begin in the waiting area, where old people may become frightened or confused due to their inability to see, hear or move easily, and understand instructions.

3 Always consider all of the following factors **before** discharging an elderly patient:

  (i) Can the patient walk safely with or without a stick?

  (ii) Can the patient understand new or existing medication?

  (iii) Can the patient get home safely and easily?

  (iv) Once home, can the patient cope with dressing, washing, using the toilet, shopping, cooking, cleaning or relaxing?

  (v) Can relatives or friends cope any more?

4 Do **not** discharge the patient without seeking help from the following people, if any factor above is present. Keep the patient in overnight to facilitate arrangements, when there is any doubt:

  (i) General practitioner:

   (a) the key person to coordinate the care of the patient at home

   (b) always contact by email as well as by letter.

  (ii) 'Hospital in the Home', or 'Hospital in the Nursing Home' service.

  (iii) District or community nursing service.

  (iv) Social worker (hospital- or community-based), who can offer:

   (a) home help

   (b) 'meals on wheels'

   (c) lunch and recreational clubs

   (d) voluntary visiting services

   (e) laundry service

   (f) chiropody service

   (g) home adaptation service

   (h) emergency accommodation.

  (v) Domiciliary physiotherapist or occupational therapist.

DISORDERED BEHAVIOUR IN THE ELDERLY

A breakdown in a patient's normal, socially acceptable behaviour is best considered in three broad categories, that can overlap and/or be mistaken for each other:

- Delirium – acute transient organic brain syndrome with global disorder of cognition
- Dementia – progressive intellectual decline
- Depression – pathological, unrelenting and disabling low mood.

DIAGNOSIS

1 *Delirium* (see p. 82)

  (i) This includes clouding of consciousness, inattention and failure of recent memory.

  (ii) It results in an acute or fluctuating confusional state associated with restless sometimes aggressive behaviour and non-auditory hallucinations. It is often worse at night.

    (iii) Causes are many, including:
- (a) infection – pneumonia, urinary tract infection (UTI), cholecystitis, septicaemia
- (b) hypoxia – respiratory disease, heart failure, anaemia
- (c) cerebral lesion – haematoma, tumour, infection, stroke
- (d) iatrogenic – many drugs (remember poisoning, both accidental and deliberate), alcohol
- (e) metabolic – including dehydration, electrolyte imbalance, hypoglycaemia or hyperglycaemia and thyroid disease
- (f) urinary retention, faecal impaction, pain, cold or change in environment (these are *rarely* the sole cause).

2 Dementia

    (i) This includes disorientation in place, time and person, abnormal or antisocial behaviour, short-term memory loss, loss of intellect, and loss of insight. There is no clouding of consciousness.

    (ii) The causes are many, although a definitive new diagnosis is seldom made in the ED.

    (iii) However, look for and exclude the causes listed in 1 (iii) above if a known demented patient is brought into the ED with a recent deterioration.

3 Depression

    (i) This includes difficulty in sleeping, demanding, anxious or withdrawn behaviour, hypochondriasis, a loss of self-interest and a sense of futility.

    (ii) Suicide is a particular risk, especially if the patient lives alone and is physically incapacitated, or has made previous attempts at suicide.

MANAGEMENT

1 Delirium and acutely decompensated dementia require hospital admission (do not simply sedate).

2 Depression and a high suicide risk require urgent referral to a psychiatrist and possible hospital admission.

FALLS IN THE ELDERLY

DIAGNOSIS

Always consider the underlying cause as well as the potential result following any fall in the elderly:

1 Cause of the fall:
    (i) Accidental:
- (a) obstacles in the home, such as a trailing flex, the edge of a carpet, poor lighting, or no handrails
- (b) inappropriate footwear.

  (ii) Musculoskeletal:
    (a) arthritis
    (b) obesity
    (c) weakness
    (d) physical inactivity.
  (iii) Visual failure:
    (a) cataracts
    (b) senile macular degeneration
    (c) glaucoma.
  (iv) Sedating drugs:
    (a) benzodiazepines
    (b) antihistamines
    (c) psychotropics
    (d) alcohol.
  (v) Postural hypotension:
    (a) occult bleeding
    (b) autonomic failure
    (c) drug-induced.
  (vi) Syncopal episode:
    (a) cardiac arrhythmia, myocardial infarction, heart block
    (b) vertebrobasilar insufficiency.
  (vii) Cerebral disorder:
    (a) Parkinson's disease
    (b) ataxia
    (c) seizure
    (d) stroke.
  (viii) Balance disorder:
    (a) inner ear disease
    (b) impaired proprioception.

2 Result of the fall:
  (i) Fracture:
    (a) Colles'
    (b) neck of femur or pelvis
    (c) neck of humerus
    (d) ribs
    (e) skull.
  (ii) Hypothermia.
  (iii) Hypostatic pneumonia.
  (iv) Pressure sore, rhabdomyolysis.
  (v) Fear, loss of confidence and independence, loss of mobility.

3 All falls in the elderly, particularly if recurrent, must be diagnosed and managed correctly, otherwise ultimately a fatal outcome will occur.

MANAGEMENT

1 Refer the patient to the medical or geriatric team for admission if acute care is needed, or if there is any doubt about their ability to cope at home.

2 Otherwise, refer to outpatients, physiotherapy, occupational therapy or social services and liaise closely with the GP.

FURTHER READING

American Heart Association (2015) Part 9: Acute coronary syndromes: 2015 American Heart Association guidelines update for cardiopulmonary resuscitation and emergency cardiovascular care. *Circulation* **132**: S483–S500.

American Heart Association/American Stroke Association (2013) Guidelines for the early management of patients with acute ischemic stroke. *Stroke* **44**: 870–947.

British Infection Association. http://www.britishinfection.org/guidelines-resources/ (meningitis and meninogococcaemia).

British Society of Gastroenterology. http://www.bsg.org.uk/ (gastrointestinal bleeding).

British Thoracic Society. http://www.brit-thoracic.org.uk/ (pulmonary embolus, pneumonia, chronic obstructive pulmonary disease, pneumothorax).

Diabetes UK. http://www.diabetes.org.uk/ (diabetic ketoacidosis).

European Resuscitation Council (2015) European Resuscitation Council Guidelines for Resuscitation 2015 Section 8. Initial management of acute coronary syndromes. *Resuscitation* **95**: 264–77.

Heart Foundation (Australia). http://www.heartfoundation.org.au/ (acute coronary syndromes)

Meningitis Research Foundation. http://www.meningitis.org/ (meningitis and septicaemia).

National Health and Medical Research Council (Australia). http://www.nhmrc.gov.au/guidelines/search

National Institute for Health and Care Excellence, NHS UK. http://www.nice.org.uk/guidance/published

Scottish Intercollegiate Guidelines Network. http://www.sign.ac.uk/

Stroke Foundation (Australia). http://www.strokefoundation.com.au/ (stroke and TIA).

Therapeutic Guidelines. eTG complete 2015. http://www.tg.org.au/

Section III

ACID–BASE, ELECTROLYTE AND RENAL EMERGENCIES

ACID–BASE DISTURBANCES

ARTERIAL BLOOD GAS INTERPRETATION

Blood gas analysis provides information regarding potential primary and compensatory processes that affect the body's acid–base buffering system.

Acidosis is an abnormal process that increases the serum hydrogen ion concentration, lowers the pH, and results in *acidaemia*.

Alkalosis is an abnormal process with decrease in the hydrogen ion concentration, resulting in *alkalaemia*.

1   Blood gas analysis is used to:
   (i)   Determine the adequacy of oxygenation and ventilation.
   (ii) Assess the respiratory function.
   (iii) Determine the acid–base balance.

2   Interpret the arterial blood gas result in a stepwise manner as follows (see Table 3.1):
   (i)   Determine the adequacy of oxygenation (PaO_2):
      (a) normal range 80–100 mmHg (10.6–13.3 kPa)
      (b) provides direct evidence of hypoxaemia
      (c) determine if there is a raised A-a gradient due to VQ mismatch/shunting, if there is a lower than expected PaO_2

Table 3.1 Determining the likely acid–base disorder from the pH, $PaCO_2$ and HCO_3

pH	$PaCO_2$	HCO_3	Acid–base disorder
↓	N	↓	**Primary metabolic acidosis**
↓	↓	↓	Metabolic acidosis with respiratory compensation
↓	↑	N	**Primary respiratory acidosis**
↓	↑	↑	Respiratory acidosis with renal compensation
↓	↑	↓	**Mixed metabolic and respiratory acidosis**
↑	↓	N	**Primary respiratory alkalosis**
↑	↓	↓	Respiratory alkalosis with renal compensation
↑	N	↑	**Primary metabolic alkalosis**
↑	↑	↑	Metabolic alkalosis with respiratory compensation
↑	↓	↑	**Mixed metabolic and respiratory alkalosis**

Note: respiratory compensation occurs rapidly by changes in $PaCO_2$. Renal compensation occurs more slowly by changes in HCO_3.
N, normal.

        (d) assuming 100% humidity at sea level, the A-a gradient can be calculated by:
  - A-a gradient = $P_AO_2 - P_aO_2$
    where $P_AO_2 = (F_iO_2 \times (760 - 47)) - (P_aCO_2/0.8)$
        (e) normal A-a gradient is <10 torr (mmHg), or approximately < (age/4) + 4.

  (ii) Review the pH or hydrogen ion status:
        (a) normal range pH 7.35–7.45 (H+ 35–45 nmol/L)
        (b) *acidaemia* is a pH <7.35 (H+ >45 nmol/L)
        (c) *alkalaemia* is a pH >7.45 (H+ <35 nmol/L).

  (iii) Determine the respiratory component ($PaCO_2$):
        (a) normal range 35–45 mmHg (4.7–6.0 kPa)
        (b) $PaCO_2$ >45 mmHg (6.0 kPa):
  - acidaemia indicates a primary respiratory acidosis
  - alkalaemia indicates respiratory compensation for a metabolic alkalosis
        (c) $PaCO_2$ <35 mmHg (4.7 kPa):
  - alkalaemia indicates a primary respiratory alkalosis
  - acidaemia indicates respiratory compensation for a metabolic acidosis

  (iv) Determine the metabolic component (bicarbonate, HCO_3):
        (a) HCO_3 normal range 22–26 mmol/L
        (b) HCO_3 <22 mmol/L:
  - acidaemia indicates a primary metabolic acidosis
  - alkalaemia indicates renal compensation for a respiratory alkalosis
        (c) HCO_3 >26 mmol/L:
  - alkalaemia indicates a primary metabolic alkalosis
  - acidaemia indicates renal compensation for a respiratory acidosis.

3 This approach will determine most primary acid–base disturbances and their associated renal or respiratory compensatory changes.

4 Remember:
  (i) Renal or respiratory compensation is always a secondary process and should really **not** then be described in terms of an 'acidosis' or 'alkalosis':
        (a) rather, in the presence of metabolic acidaemia, think of the respiratory compensation as 'compensatory hyperventilation' rather than a 'secondary respiratory alkalosis'.
  (ii) Chronic compensation returns the pH value towards normal, but overcompensation never occurs.

   (iii)   The presence of a normal pH with abnormal HCO_3 and $PaCO_2$ suggests both a primary respiratory *and* a primary metabolic process are present:
   (a)   pH normal: $PaCO_2$ >45 mmHg (6.0 kPa), HCO_3 >26 mmol/L
      – dual primary process involving a primary respiratory acidosis and a primary metabolic alkalosis
   (b)   pH normal: $PaCO_2$ <35 mmHg (4.7 kPa), HCO_3 <22 mmol/L
      – dual primary process involving a primary respiratory alkalosis and a primary metabolic acidosis.

5   Alternatively, for simplicity, use an acid–base nomogram to plot and read off the interpretation of the arterial blood gas abnormality (see Fig. 3.1)!

METABOLIC ACIDOSIS

DIAGNOSIS

1   An abnormal process or condition leading to the increase of fixed acids in the blood, best determined by a fall in plasma bicarbonate to less than 22 mmol/L.

2   Metabolic acidosis may be associated with a high, normal, or low anion gap.
   (i)   The anion gap is calculated from the equation $[Na^+] - ([Cl^-] + [HCO_3^-])$ with all units in mmol/L.
   (ii)   A normal anion gap is 8–16.

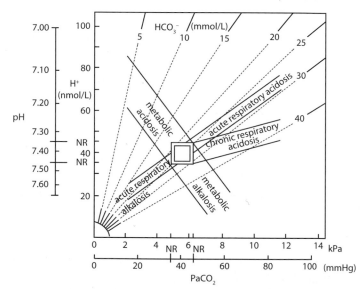

Figure 3.1 Acid–base nomogram for plotting interpretation of the arterial blood gas (NR is normal range)

3 Causes of a *high* anion gap metabolic acidosis (anion gap >16) include:
- (i) Increased acid production:
  - (a) ketoacidosis, e.g. diabetes, alcoholism, starvation
  - (b) lactic acidosis (serum lactate >2.5 mmol/L):
    - – type A: impaired tissue perfusion in cardiac arrest, shock, hypoxia, sepsis, mesenteric ischaemia
    - – type B: impaired carbohydrate metabolism in hepatic or renal failure, lymphoma, pancreatitis and drugs such as metformin and salbutamol.
- (ii) Decreased acid excretion, as in renal failure.
- (iii) Exogenous acid ingestion:
  - (a) methanol, ethylene glycol, iron, cyanide and salicylates.

4 Causes of a *normal* anion gap metabolic acidosis (anion gap 8–16) include:
- (i) Renal:
  - (a) renal tubular acidosis
  - (b) carbonic anhydrase inhibitors.
- (ii) Gastrointestinal:
  - (a) severe diarrhoea
  - (b) small bowel fistula
  - (c) drainage of pancreatic or biliary secretions.
- (iii) Other:
  - (a) rapid large volume sodium chloride infusion, ammonium chloride
  - (b) recovery from ketoacidosis.

5 The body compensates to reduce the acid load by hyperventilation. The expected compensatory reduction in $PaCO_2$ may be calculated (see Table 3.2):
- (i) The acidosis is only partially compensated if the $PaCO_2$ value is higher than predicted.
- (ii) A primary respiratory alkalosis coexists if the $PaCO_2$ value is lower than predicted.

6 There are few specific clinical features due to an acute metabolic acidosis itself, other than hyperventilation known as Kussmaul breathing.

7 Urea and electrolytes (U&Es) confirm a primary fall in plasma bicarbonate below 22 mmol/L and usually show an associated rise in plasma potassium from an extracellular shift.

MANAGEMENT

1 Provide supportive treatment with oxygen, i.v. fluids and treat symptomatic hyperkalaemia (see p. 134).

2 Correct any reversible underlying disorder:
- (i) Administer fluid and insulin, and replace potassium in diabetic ketoacidosis.

Table 3.2 Predicting the expected compensatory changes in $PaCO_2$ and HCO_3

	Metabolic acidosis	Metabolic alkalosis
Predicted $PaCO_2$ (kPa)	$0.2 \times [HCO_3] + 1$ kPa $(+/-0.25)$	$\dfrac{[HCO_3]}{10} + 2.5$ kPa $(+/-0.7)$
Predicted $PaCO_2$ (mmHg)	$1.5 \times [HCO_3] + 8$ mmHg $(+/-2)$	$0.7 \times [HCO_3] + 20$ mmHg $(+/-5)$

	Respiratory acidosis		Respiratory alkalosis	
	Acute	**Chronic**	**Acute**	**Chronic**
Predicted HCO_3 (kPa)	$24 + (PaCO_2 - 5.33) \times 0.75$	$24 + (PaCO_2 - 5.33) \times 3$	$24 - (5.33 - PaCO_2) \times 1.5$	$24 - (5.33 - PaCO_2) \times 3.75$
Predicted HCO_3 (mmHg)	$24 + \dfrac{PaCO_2 - 40}{10}$	$24 + \left(\dfrac{PaCO_2 - 40}{10}\right) \times 4$	$24 - \left(\dfrac{40 - PaCO_2}{10}\right) \times 2$	$24 - \left(\dfrac{40 - PaCO_2}{10}\right) \times 5$

(ii) Ensure adequate oxygenation and restore the intravascular volume to improve peripheral perfusion in lactic acidosis.

3 Refer the patient to the medical team. Dialysis will be necessary for renal failure and severe methanol or salicylate poisoning.

METABOLIC ALKALOSIS

DIAGNOSIS

1 An abnormal process or condition leading to a serum bicarbonate level of >28 mmol/L.

2 Causes include:
- (i) Addition of base to extracellular fluid:
  - (a) recovery from organic acidosis secondary to metabolism of lactate and acetate
  - (b) milk-alkali syndrome (excess antacids)
  - (c) massive blood transfusion (metabolism of citrate).
- (ii) Chloride depletion:
  - (a) loss of gastric acid from vomiting or gastric aspiration
  - (b) diuretics.
- (iii) Potassium depletion:
  - (a) primary (Conn's) and secondary hyperaldosteronism
  - (b) Cushing's or Bartter's syndromes
  - (c) severe hypokalaemia.
- (iv) Other:
  - (a) laxative abuse
  - (b) severe hypoalbuminaemia.

3 The body compensates to reduce the bicarbonate load by hypoventilation. The expected compensatory rise in $PaCO_2$ may be calculated (see Table 3.2).
- (i) This effect can be pronounced. Compensatory arterial $PaCO_2$ levels as high as 86 mmHg (11.5 kPa) have been recorded.
- (ii) However, this compensatory $PaCO_2$ elevation is variable:
  - (a) pain or hypoxia cause the respiratory rate to rise and the $PaCO_2$ to fall, thereby worsening the alkalosis.

4 There are few specific clinical features other than hypoventilation. Symptoms relating to associated hypocalcaemia (tetany) and hypokalaemia (weakness) may be present.

MANAGEMENT

1 Give high-flow oxygen to reduce complications associated with hypoventilation. Try to avoid hyperventilation, as this worsens the alkalaemia.

2 Correct any reversible underlying disorder.

3 Administer normal saline at 500 mL/h i.v to replace lost chloride, restore intravascular volume, and enhance renal bicarbonate excretion.

4   Replace potassium with potassium chloride 10–20 mmol/h i.v. if the potassium is low.

5   Consider the use of acetazolamide 250 mg orally to increase the rate of bicarbonate elimination.

RESPIRATORY ACIDOSIS

DIAGNOSIS

1   A primary acid–base disorder associated with respiratory failure, inadequate alveolar ventilation and an arterial $PaCO_2$ >45 mmHg (6.0 kPa).

2   Causes include:
   (i)   Loss of central respiratory drive:
      (a) drugs, e.g. opiates, sedatives, anaesthetic agents
      (b) cerebral trauma, tumour, haemorrhage or stroke.
   (ii) Neuromuscular disorders:
      (a) Guillain–Barré syndrome, myasthenia gravis
      (b) toxins, e.g. organophosphate poisoning and snake venom.
   (iii) Respiratory compromise:
      (a) chronic obstructive pulmonary disease (COPD), critical asthma, restrictive lung disease
      (b) pulmonary oedema, aspiration, pneumonia
      (c) upper airway obstruction and laryngospasm
      (d) thoracic trauma, pneumothorax, diaphragm splinting
      (e) high thoracic or cervical spinal cord trauma
      (f) morbid obesity.

3   Clinical manifestations of respiratory acidosis are secondary to the hypercapnoea. Look for the following:
   (i)   The patient is usually warm, flushed, sweaty and tachycardic with 'bounding' peripheral pulses, from cardiovascular stimulation.
   (ii) Acute confusion, mental obtundation, somnolence and occasionally focal neurological signs from increased cerebral blood flow, cerebral vasodilation and raised intracranial pressure.

4   The body compensates to reduce acidaemia by minimizing the excretion of bicarbonate by the kidneys. However, this renal compensatory response is slow.
   (i)   There is no time for any significant renal compensatory response in an acute respiratory acidosis.
   (ii) The kidneys are able to retain bicarbonate in chronic respiratory acidosis lasting over a few days, so the plasma bicarbonate level rises and the pH returns towards normal.
   (iii) The expected compensatory rise in plasma bicarbonate in acute and chronic respiratory acidosis may be calculated (see Table 3.2, p. 130).

MANAGEMENT

1 Give oxygen and commence assisted ventilation by bag-mask ventilation. Call for senior emergency department (ED) doctor help and prepare for emergency endotracheal intubation, or non-invasive ventilation such as continuous positive airway pressure (CPAP), for instance in acute pulmonary oedema.

2 Correct any reversible underlying disorder, e.g. naloxone for opiate poisoning.

> **Warning:** the pulse oximeter may record a normal oxygen saturation in a patient receiving supplemental oxygen, despite the presence of dangerous hypercapnoea from hypoventilation.

RESPIRATORY ALKALOSIS

DIAGNOSIS

1 A primary acid–base disturbance, associated with increased alveolar ventilation and an arterial $PaCO_2$ of <35 mmHg (4.7 kPa).

2 Causes include:
    (i) Asthma, pneumonia, pulmonary embolus, pulmonary oedema and pulmonary fibrosis (mediated by intrapulmonary receptors).
    (ii) Hypoxia (mediated by peripheral chemoreceptors).
    (iii) Centrally induced hyperventilation secondary to respiratory centre stimulation:
        (a) head injury, stroke
        (b) fever (cytokines), pregnancy (progesterone), thyrotoxicosis, liver disease
        (c) drugs, e.g. salicylate poisoning
        (d) pain, fear, stress, psychogenic, voluntary.
    (iv) Iatrogenic from excessive artificial ventilation.

3 Clinical manifestations are secondary to hypocapnoea, hypokalaemia and hypocalcaemia. Look for the specific effects of hypocapnoea:
    (i) Circumoral paraesthesia, carpopedal spasm and tetany from neuromuscular irritability.
    (ii) Light-headedness and confusion from cerebral vasoconstriction (usually adapts in 6–8 h).
    (iii) Cardiac arrhythmias and decreased myocardial contractility.

4 The body compensates to reduce alkalaemia by excreting or buffering bicarbonate ions.
    (i) A moderate compensatory response via a non-renal-mediated buffering process can reduce plasma bicarbonate levels to 18–20 mmol/L in an acute respiratory alkalosis within hours.

(ii) The kidneys increase the rate of bicarbonate excretion in chronic respiratory alkalosis, and reduce serum bicarbonate levels to as low as 12–15 mmol/L returning the pH towards normal

(a) this renal compensatory response is slow. The maximal effect takes 2–3 days to occur.

(iii) The expected compensatory fall in plasma bicarbonate in acute and chronic respiratory alkalosis may be calculated (see Table 3.2, p. 130).

MANAGEMENT

1 Give oxygen to treat any coexistent hypoxia.

2 Look for and correct any reversible underlying disorder.

3 Never diagnose 'hysterical' hyperventilation until subtle presentations of pneumonia, pulmonary embolism, pneumothorax, fever, etc., have been actively excluded.

4 Otherwise if no significant underlying cause for hyperventilation is likely, reassure the patient and/or ask them to rebreathe into a paper bag.

ELECTROLYTE DISORDERS

Electrolyte disturbances are commonly associated with cardiovascular emergencies and may cause cardiac arrhythmias and cardiopulmonary arrest. Prompt recognition and immediate treatment of electrolyte disorders can prevent cardiac arrest.

POTASSIUM DISORDERS

The potassium gradient across the cellular membrane is essential to maintain excitability of nerve and muscle cells, including the myocardium.

Extracellular potassium levels are strictly regulated between 3.5 and 5.0 mmol/L and may be affected by many processes including serum pH.

As the pH rises, serum potassium falls as potassium is shifted intracellularly; when serum pH decreases, serum potassium increases as intracellular potassium shifts into the vascular space.

HYPERKALAEMIA

DIAGNOSIS

1 This is the most common electrolyte disturbance associated with cardiac arrest.

2 Causes include:

(i) Increased potassium intake:

(a) oral or i.v. potassium supplements, transfusion of stored blood.

(ii) Increased production:

(a) burns, ischaemia, haemolysis

      (b) rhabdomyolysis, tumour lysis syndrome

      (c) intense physical activity.

  (iii) Decreased renal excretion:

      (a) acute or chronic renal failure

      (b) drugs, e.g. potassium-sparing diuretics, angiotensin-converting enzyme (ACE) inhibitors, non-steroidal anti-inflammatory drugs (NSAIDs)

      (c) Addison's disease, hypoaldosteronism.

  (iv) Transcellular compartmental shift:

      (a) acidosis (metabolic or respiratory)

      (b) hyperglycaemia

      (c) digoxin poisoning, suxamethonium.

  (v) Factitious:

      (a) haemolysed specimen, thrombocytosis, massive leucocytosis.

3 The risk of adverse events associated with hyperkalaemia increases with the serum concentration level. The severity of hyperkalaemia may be defined by the serum potassium level:

  (i) Mild hyperkalaemia: potassium >5.5 mmol/L.

  (ii) Moderate hyperkalaemia: potassium 6.0–6.5 mmol/L.

  (iii) Severe hyperkalaemia: potassium >6.5 mmol/L.

4 Patients may present with weakness, ascending paralysis, loss of deep tendon reflexes, and respiratory failure.

5 Gain i.v. access and attach an electrocardiography (ECG) monitor and pulse oximeter to the patient.

6 Look for the characteristic ECG changes that are usually progressive and determined by the absolute serum potassium, as well as its rate of increase:

  (i) Tall, peaked (tented) T waves.

  (ii) Prolonged PR interval with flattened P waves.

  (iii) ST segment depression.

  (iv) QRS widening, absent P waves and sinusoidal wave pattern.

  (v) Ventricular tachycardia and cardiac arrest from ventricular fibrillation, pulseless electrical activity (PEA) or asystole.

 Tip: consider hyperkalaemia in any patient with an arrhythmia or in cardiac arrest.

MANAGEMENT

1 Give high-flow oxygen via face mask. Cease any exogenous sources of potassium supplementation.

2 *Severe hyperkalaemia* (>6.5 mmol/L) or hyperkalaemia with life-threatening ECG changes.

Provide immediate cardioprotection to prevent cardiac arrest:

(i) Give 10% calcium chloride 10 mL i.v. over 2–5 min, repeated until the ECG and cardiac output normalize

    (a) this does not lower the potassium level, but antagonizes the deleterious effects of hyperkalaemia on the myocardium, reducing the risk of ventricular fibrillation (onset of protection in 1–3 min).

(ii) Use the other therapies outlined below to shift potassium into the cells, and eliminate potassium from the body.

3 *Moderate hyperkalaemia* (6.0–6.5 mmol/L).

Shift potassium intracellularly with:

(i) 50% dextrose 50 mL i.v. with 10 units of soluble insulin over 20 min (onset of action 15 min, with maximal effect within 1 h).

    (a) beware more rapid delivery of the 50% dextrose with the insulin as it may paradoxically release intracellular potassium due to its hypertonicity

    (b) give the soluble insulin alone in hyperglycaemic patients with a blood sugar of >12 mmol/L (i.e. without the dextrose).

(ii) Salbutamol 10–20 mg nebulized. Several doses may be required (onset of action 15 min).

(iii) 8.4% sodium bicarbonate 50 mL i.v. over 5 min, provided there is no danger of fluid overload, as it contains 50 mmol sodium

    (a) less effective as a sole agent, but works well in combination with salbutamol and dextrose/insulin (onset of action 15–30 min), and if a metabolic acidosis is present.

4 *Mild hyperkalaemia* (5.5–6.0 mmol/L).

Remove potassium from the body with:

(i) Frusemide (furosemide) 40–80 mg i.v. (onset of action with diuresis, provided not anuric).

(ii) Potassium-exchange resin: calcium resonium 30 g orally or by enema (onset of action 1–3 h after administration).

5 Refer the patient to the medical team, and according to the potassium level and underlying cause, organize urgent haemodialysis or peritoneal dialysis as needed, particularly in known renal failure.

HYPOKALAEMIA

DIAGNOSIS

1 Hypokalaemia is associated with an increased incidence of cardiac arrhythmias especially in those patients with pre-existing heart disease, and in those treated with digoxin.

2 Causes include:

(i) Inadequate intake of potassium, e.g. alcoholism, starvation.

(ii) Abnormal gastrointestinal losses from vomiting, diarrhoea and laxative abuse.

    (iii) Abnormal renal losses:
        (a) Cushing's, Conn's and Bartter's syndromes
        (b) ectopic adrenocorticotrophic hormone (ACTH) production
        (c) drugs, e.g. diuretics and steroids
        (d) hypomagnesaemia.
    (iv) Compartmental shift:
        (a) metabolic alkalosis
        (b) insulin
        (c) drugs, e.g. salbutamol, terbutaline, aminophylline
        (d) hypomagnesaemia.

3 Hypokalaemia occurs when serum potassium level is <3.5 mmol/L and is defined as severe if the serum potassium is <2.5 mmol/L.

4 Look for weakness, fatigue, leg cramps and constipation.
    (i) Polydipsia, polyuria, rhabdomyolysis, ascending paralysis and respiratory compromise may develop as the potassium level falls.

5 Gain i.v. access and attach an ECG monitor. Non-specific ECG changes include:
    (i) Flat or inverted T waves, prominent U waves.
    (ii) Prolonged PR interval.
    (iii) ST segment depression.
    (iv) Ventricular arrhythmias, including torsades de pointes.

 Tip: consider hypokalaemia in any patient with an arrhythmia or in cardiac arrest.

MANAGEMENT

1 Replace potassium immediately in the following situations:
    (i) Serum potassium <3.0 mmol/L.
    (ii) Serum potassium 3.0–3.5 mmol/L in patients with chronic heart failure or cardiac arrhythmias, particularly if on digoxin or following myocardial infarction.

2 Give potassium 10–20 mmol/h i.v. under ECG control using a fluid infusion device, but do **not** exceed 40 mmol/h.

3 Give magnesium sulphate 10 mmol (2.5 g) diluted in 100 mL normal saline over 30–45 min in severe or intractable hypokalaemia, as magnesium enhances potassium uptake and helps maintain intracellular potassium levels.

4 Change to oral supplements or maintenance i.v. replacement when the serum potassium is >3.5 mmol/L.

5 Refer the patient to the medical team as necessary for treatment of the underlying condition.

SODIUM DISORDERS

Sodium is the most common intravascular cation. It has a major influence on serum osmolality and determines the volume of the extracellular fluid.

HYPERNATRAEMIA

DIAGNOSIS

1 Hypernatraemia is defined as a serum sodium level of >145–150 mmol/L.

2 Causes include:
    (i) Decreased fluid intake with normal fluid loss:
        (a) disordered thirst perception, e.g. hypothalamic lesion
        (b) inability to communicate water needs, e.g. cerebrovascular accident, infants, intubated patients.
    (ii) Hypotonic fluid loss, with water loss in excess of salt loss:
        (a) skin loss from excessive sweating in hot climates, dermal burns
        (b) gastrointestinal loss from diarrhoea or vomiting
        (c) renal loss from impaired salt-concentrating ability, e.g. diabetes insipidus, osmotic diuretic agents, hyperglycaemia, hypercalcaemia, chronic renal disease.
    (iii) Increased salt load:
        (a) hyperaldosteronism or Cushing's syndrome
        (b) ingestion of seawater, salt tablets, and administration of sodium bicarbonate or hypertonic saline.

3 Symptoms and signs of hypernatraemia are progressive and directly related to the serum osmolality level. Look for:
    (i) Increased thirst, weakness, lethargy and irritability (>375 mOsm/kg).
    (ii) Altered mental status, ataxia, tremor and focal neurological signs (>400 mOsm/kg).
    (iii) Seizures and coma (>430 mOsm/kg).

4 Assess the underlying volume status. Look at the skin turgor, jugular venous pressure (JVP), measure lying and sitting blood pressures, listen for basal crackles.

5 Send blood for full blood count (FBC), U&Es, liver function tests (LFTs), and serum osmolality.

6 Perform an ECG and request a chest radiograph (CXR).

MANAGEMENT

1 Give high-flow oxygen via a face mask.

2 Replace fluid orally, or via a nasogastric tube in stable asymptomatic patients.

3 Give hypovolaemic patients volume replacement with i.v. normal saline without causing too rapid a reduction in the serum sodium.
    (i) Aim to reduce serum sodium by 0.5–1.0 mmol/L per h.

HYPONATRAEMIA

DIAGNOSIS

1 Hyponatraemia is defined by a serum sodium level <130 mmol/L.

2 Causes include:

  (i) *Factitious 'pseudohyponatraemia'*
  (a) associated with hyperglycaemia, hyperlipidaemia, hyperproteinaemia
  (b) correct the sodium for hyperglycaemia by adjusting the serum sodium up by 1 mmol/L for every 3 mmol/L elevation in blood sugar.

  (ii) *Hypovolaemic hyponatraemia*
  (a) urinary sodium >20 mmol/L: renal causes including diuretics, Addison's disease, salt-losing nephropathy, glycosuria, ketonuria
  (b) urinary sodium <20 mmol/L: extrarenal losses such as vomiting, diarrhoea, burns, pancreatitis.

  (iii) *Normovolaemic hyponatraemia*
  (a) urine osmolality > serum osmolality:
    – syndrome of inappropriate antidiuretic hormone secretion (SIADH) due to head injury, meningoencephalitis, CVA, pneumonia, COPD, neoplasia, human immunodeficiency virus (HIV) infection, drugs such as carbamazepine, NSAIDs and antidepressants such as SSRIs
    – positive-pressure ventilation, porphyria
  (b) urine osmolality < serum osmolality:
    – hypotonic post-operative fluids such as 5% dextrose or 4% dextrose 1/5 normal saline, transurethral resection of the prostate (TURP) irrigation fluid, psychogenic polydipsia, 'tea and toast' diet, beer potomania.

  (iv) *Hypervolaemic hyponatraemia*
  (a) urinary sodium <20 mmol/L: congestive cardiac failure, cirrhosis, nephrotic syndrome, hypoalbuminaemia, hepatorenal syndrome
  (b) urinary sodium >20 mmol/L: steroids, cerebral salt wasting, chronic renal failure, hypothyroidism.

3 Clinical features progress as the serum sodium level drops, but depend also on the rate of fall, i.e. the more rapid the fall the greater the symptoms:

  (i) Na >125 mmol/L: usually asymptomatic.
  (ii) Na 115–125 mmol/L: lethargy, weakness, ataxia, and vomiting.
  (iii) Na <115 mmol/L: confusion, headache, convulsions, and coma.

4 Assess the underlying volume status:

  (i) Look at the skin turgor, jugular venous pressure (JVP), measure lying and sitting blood pressure (BP), listen for basal crackles.

5   Send blood for FBC, U&Es, LFTs, thyroid function and serum osmolality. Send urine for sodium and osmolality.

6   Perform an ECG and request a CXR.

MANAGEMENT

1   Commence high-flow oxygen by face mask.

2   Asymptomatic patients:
    (i)   Discontinue implicated drug therapy and treat the underlying medical condition, e.g. antibiotics for sepsis.
    (ii)   Restrict fluid intake to 50% of estimated maintenance fluid requirements in SIADH, i.e. around 750 mL/day.
    (iii) Aim to increase the serum sodium gradually by 0.5 mmol/L per h, to a maximum rate of 12 mmol/L per 24 h.

3   Get senior ED doctor help if the patient has neurological symptoms.
    (i)   Administer 3% hypertonic saline at 1–2 mL/kg/h to raise serum sodium levels by 1 mmol/L/h.
    (ii)   Aim to initially raise the serum sodium level by no more than 4–6 mmol/L.
    (iii) Consult with the intensive care team if the patient develops seizures or coma.

Warning: too rapid correction of hyponatraemia may cause coma associated with osmotic demyelination syndrome or central pontine demyelinosis, or the underlying disease process itself.

CALCIUM DISORDERS

Calcium is the most abundant mineral in the body and essential for bone strength, neuromuscular function and a myriad of intracellular processes. Minor degrees of hypercalcaemia may be the first clue to an underlying diagnosis of malignancy or hyperparathyroidism.

HYPERCALCAEMIA

DIAGNOSIS

1   Hypercalcaemia is defined by a serum calcium level of >2.6 mmol/L after correction for albumin.

2   Causes include:
    (i)   Malignancy, myeloma, sarcoidosis, thyrotoxicosis and tuberculosis.
    (ii)   Primary or tertiary hyperparathyroidism.
    (iii) Drugs, e.g. thiazides.
    (iv)   Addison's disease.

3   Patients present with anorexia, thirst, weakness, abdominal pain, constipation, lethargy and confusion or psychosis. Coma may occur at serum calcium levels of >3.5 mmol/L.

4   Insert a large-bore i.v. cannula and send blood for FBC, U&Es, LFTs, calcium, lipase and thyroid function.

5   Perform an ECG. Typical changes include:
    (i)   Bradycardia.
    (ii)   Short QT interval with a widened QRS.
    (iii) Flattened T waves, atrioventricular block and cardiac arrest.

6   Request a CXR that may show an underlying cause.

MANAGEMENT

1   Commence rehydration with 0.9% normal saline i.v. at 500 mL/h.

2   Give frusemide (furosemide) 20–40 mg i.v. once urine output is established to maintain a diuresis.

3   Refer the patient to the medical team for longer-term therapy with steroids, bisphosphonates or dialysis.

HYPOCALCAEMIA

DIAGNOSIS

1   Hypocalcaemia is defined by a serum calcium level of <2.1 mmol/L after correction for albumin.

2   Causes include:
    (i)   Chronic renal failure, acute pancreatitis.
    (ii)   Rhabdomyolysis, tumour lysis syndrome, whole blood transfusion and toxic shock syndrome.
    (iii) Primary respiratory alkalosis (hyperventilation).
    (iv)   Post-parathyroidectomy or thyroid surgery; autoimmune hypoparathyroidism.

3   Patients present with paraesthesiae of the extremities and face, muscle cramps, carpopedal spasm, stridor, tetany, seizures and cardiac failure.

4   Look for hyper-reflexia and a positive Chvostek's or Trousseau's sign:
    (i)   Chvostek's sign: facial twitching from percussing the facial nerve in front of the ear.
    (ii)   Trousseau's sign: carpal spasm after 3 min of inflation of a BP cuff above systolic pressure.

5   Insert a large-bore i.v. cannula and send blood for FBC, U&Es, LFTs, creatine kinase (CK), magnesium and lipase.

6   Perform an ECG and look for:
    (i)   QT interval prolongation, T wave inversion.
    (ii)   AV block, torsades de pointes (cardiac arrest may ensue).

MANAGEMENT

1 Commence rehydration with 0.9% normal saline i.v. at 250 mL/h.

2 Look for and treat the underlying cause.

3 Give calcium i.v. in symptomatic patients:
   (i) 10% calcium chloride 10–40 mL i.v.
   (ii) discuss further elemental calcium infusion with the medical team or intensive care unit (ICU) admitting team.

4 Give calcium by oral calcium supplements, or vitamin D-rich milk in asymptomatic patients.

MAGNESIUM DISORDERS

Magnesium is the second most abundant intracellular cation and essential for stabilizing excitable cellular membranes and facilitating the movement of calcium, potassium and sodium into and out of cells.

HYPERMAGNESAEMIA

DIAGNOSIS

1 Hypermagnesaemia occurs at a serum level of >1.1 mmol/L.

2 Causes include:
   (i) Renal failure.
   (ii) Iatrogenic magnesium administration i.v.
   (iii) Rhabdomyolysis and tumour lysis syndrome.

3 Patients present with muscular weakness, respiratory depression, confusion, ataxia and hypotension.
   (i) Extreme magnesium toxicity >5.0 mmol/L may be associated with bradycardia, respiratory depression, altered conscious level and cardiac arrest.

4 Insert a large-bore i.v. cannula and send blood for FBC, U&Es, LFTs, magnesium and thyroid function.

5 ECG changes are similar to hyperkalaemia.

MANAGEMENT

1 Commence i.v. rehydration with normal saline at 500 mL/h.

2 Give 10% calcium chloride 10 mL i.v. for life-threatening arrhythmias and severe magnesium toxicity.

3 Otherwise give a combination of normal saline i.v. and frusemide (furosemide) 1 mg/kg i.v. to increase the renal excretion of magnesium, provided the urine output is normal.
   (i) Check calcium levels regularly to prevent hypocalcaemia, which will worsen the symptoms of magnesium toxicity.

4 Refer the patient to the medical team or ICU for consideration of dialysis in severe toxicity with levels >5.0 mmol/L.

HYPOMAGNESAEMIA

DIAGNOSIS

1 Hypomagnesaemia occurs at a serum level of <0.6 mmol/L.
2 Causes include:
   - (i)   Increased magnesium losses:
     - (a) gastrointestinal loss from vomiting, diarrhoea, pancreatitis
     - (b) acute tubular necrosis (ATN) or chronic renal failure
     - (c) drugs, e.g. alcohol, diuretics, gentamicin, cisplatin.
   - (ii) Reduced magnesium intake in starvation, malnutrition, chronic alcoholism.
   - (iii) Metabolic with low levels of calcium, phosphate and potassium.
   - (iv) Endocrine such as diabetic ketoacidosis (DKA), thyrotoxicosis, hyperparathyroidism, hypothermia.
3 Clinical manifestations are non-specific and may mimic hypocalcaemia and hypokalaemia. Look for tremor, paraesthesiae, tetany, altered mental state, ataxia, nystagmus and seizures.
4 Insert a large-bore i.v. cannula and send blood for FBC, U&Es, LFTs, CK, magnesium, lipase and thyroid function.
5 Perform an ECG and look for:
   - (i)   Prolongation of PR and QT intervals.
   - (ii) ST segment depression.
   - (iii) Widened QRS and torsades de pointes.

MANAGEMENT

1 Commence rehydration with 0.9% normal saline i.v. at 250 mL/h.
2 Look for and treat the underlying cause.
3 Administer oral magnesium supplements to asymptomatic patients.
4 Start parenteral magnesium in more severe cases:
   - (i)   Give patients with seizures, torsades de pointes, or cardiac arrest 50% magnesium sulphate 8 mmol or 2 g i.v. over 2–5 min.
   - (ii) Give other symptomatic patients 50% magnesium sulphate 8 mmol (2 g) i.v. at a slower rate over 10–15 min.
5 Refer the patient to the medical team and discuss further elemental mag-nesium treatment.

ACUTE RENAL FAILURE

ACUTE KIDNEY INJURY

Acute renal failure is now encompassed in the term 'acute kidney injury' (AKI) that denotes the spectrum of rapid loss of kidney function from minor changes to the requirement for renal replacement therapy.

The RIFLE classification is used for diagnostic staging of acute kidney injury and allows differentiation between mild and severe, as well as early and late cases.

RIFLE criteria refer to:

Risk: serum creatinine $\uparrow \times 1.5$; or urine production <0.5 mL/kg per hour for 6 h

Injury: serum creat $\uparrow \times 2$; or urine production <0.5 mL/kg per hour for 12 h

Failure: serum creat $\uparrow \times 3$ or >355 μmol/L (with acute rise >44); or urine output <0.3 mL/kg per hour for 24 h 'oliguria', or anuria for 12 h

Loss: persistent AKI with complete loss of kidney function for >4 weeks

End-stage kidney disease: complete loss of kidney function for >3 months.

DIAGNOSIS

1 Acute renal failure leads to an abrupt, sustained increase in serum urea and creatinine secondary to decreased glomerular filtration rate (GFR), usually associated with oliguria or anuria.

2 Causes include:
- (i) *Pre-renal failure* (decreased renal perfusion):
  - (a) shock, burns, sepsis, dehydration, low-output cardiac failure
  - (b) renovascular disease: renal artery stenosis, renal artery emboli.
- (ii) *Intrinsic renal failure*:
  - (a) acute tubular necrosis (ATN): following prolonged pre-renal hypoperfusion, ischaemia, sepsis, toxins, e.g. gentamicin, radiographic contrast, myoglobin, ethylene glycol
  - (b) acute interstitial nephritis: drugs (including antibiotics and NSAIDs), infection, sarcoidosis, autoimmune disease, e.g. systemic lupus erythematosus
  - (c) acute glomerulonephritis: post-infectious, vasculitis, autoimmune disease, complement-related
  - (d) acute cortical necrosis: profound hypoperfusion, e.g. obstetric complication with haemorrhage
  - (e) miscellaneous: ACE inhibitors, thrombotic microangiopathy, malignant hypertension, renal vein thrombosis.
- (iii) *Post-renal failure*:

  Obstruction may be extramural, intramural or intraluminal at any point from the renal tubule to the distal urethra. Causes include:
  - (a) ureteric obstruction to a single kidney, or bilateral ureteric obstruction to both kidneys
  - (b) retroperitoneal fibrosis; ureteric strictures, calculi or crystal deposition; tumours such as uterine cancer; prostatic disease such as benign prostatic hypertrophy or malignancy.

3 Take a thorough history, including a drug history for potential nephrotoxic agents, and obtain an accurate weight on arrival as this will help monitor treatment progress.

4 As acute kidney injury is associated with multiple pathologies it may present in a variety of ways.

  (i) Pre-renal failure with symptoms and signs of hypovolaemia such as confusion, dehydration, orthostatic hypotension, oliguria and anuria.

  (ii) Nephritic syndrome with acute hypertension, haematuria with red cell casts and dysmorphic red cells, and generalized oedema from acute glomerular disease.

  (iii) Flank pain, loin pain and microscopic or macroscopic haematuria.

5 Examine patients systematically. Look for:

  (i) Volume status

    (a) signs of volume depletion: hypotension, tachycardia, decreased skin turgor, dry mucous membranes in a patient with decreased renal perfusion associated with a pre-renal condition

    (b) signs of volume overload: raised JVP, peripheral oedema and respiratory crepitations in intrinsic renal disease.

  (ii) Clinical manifestations of acute uraemia: sallow complexion, asterixis (flap), pericardial or pleural rub, pulmonary oedema or pleural effusion, altered mental status, confusion, seizures.

  (iii) Signs of post-renal obstruction: enlarged prostate on per rectal (p.r.) examination, cervical or uterine mass lesion on vaginal examination, and an enlarged palpable bladder.

6 Insert an i.v. cannula and send bloods for FBC, U&Es, LFTs, blood sugar, CK, calcium and uric acid. Take an arterial or venous blood gas analysis. Attach a cardiac monitor to the patient.

7 Organize a bedside bladder scan to determine the presence of urinary retention, which may signal a post-renal obstruction cause.

8 Insert an indwelling catheter and send a midstream urine sample for urinary osmolality and electrolyte screen to help distinguish a pre-renal from an intrinsic renal cause of renal failure.

  (i) Request microscopy for signs of glomerulonephritis such as red cell casts or >70% dysmorphic red cells, and for myoglobinuria, haemoglobinuria (absent red cells) or evidence of infection.

9 Take an ECG to look for signs of hyperkalaemia, or an arrhythmia such as atrial fibrillation which may, for instance, be associated with renal embolic disease.

10 Request a CXR to look for volume overload, metastatic disease and pulmonary–renal syndromes such as Wegener's granulomatosis.

11 Arrange an urgent renal tract ultrasound to look at the size of the kidneys, particularly looking for evidence of obstruction anywhere from the renal pelvis to the bladder outlet.

  (i) Shrunken kidneys suggest an acute on chronic process.

    (ii)   **Exceptions** are polycystic kidneys, amyloid or HIV nephropathy, and diabetic nephropathy, which are associated with enlarged or preserved renal size even with chronic renal failure.

MANAGEMENT

1   Determine the need for urgent treatment.

    (i)   Treat severe hyperkalaemia with 10% calcium chloride 10 mL i.v. over 2–5 min, repeated until the ECG and cardiac output normalize (see p. 134).

    (ii)   Treat accelerated hypertension and any suspected sepsis including urinary tract.

    (iii)   Avoid nephrotoxic drugs such as NSAIDs and iodinated contrast.

    (iv)   Arrange early haemodialysis for patients with volume overload and refractory pulmonary oedema, pericarditis, uraemic encephalopathy or if a dialysable drug is responsible such as lithium or salicylate.

2   Commence fluid resuscitation with caution.

    (i)   Aim to optimize renal perfusion by treating hypovolaemia, but take care not to precipitate acute volume overload.

    (ii)   Closely monitor urine output.

3   Refer the patient to the medical, renal or urology team depending on the suspected underlying pathology, response to resuscitation, and any urgent requirement for dialysis.

FURTHER READING

American Heart Association (2015) Part 10. Special circumstances of resuscitation: 2015 American Heart Association guidelines update for cardiopulmonary resuscitation and emergency cardiovascular care. *Circulation* **132**: S501–S518.

European Resuscitation Council (2015) European Resuscitation Council Guidelines for Resuscitation 2015 Section 4. Cardiac arrest in special circumstances. *Resuscitation* **95**: 148–201.

Lopes J, Jorge S (2013) The RIFLE and AKIN classifications for acute kidney injury: a critical and comprehensive review. *Clin Kidney J* **6**: 8–14.

Therapeutic Guidelines. eTG complete 2015. http://www.tg.org.au/

Section IV

INFECTIOUS DISEASE AND FOREIGN TRAVEL EMERGENCIES

FEBRILE NEUTROPENIC PATIENT

Neutropenia has a significant generalized infection risk with a temperature >38°C (100°F) in patients with an absolute neutrophil count <0.5 × 10⁹/L, or <1.0 × 10⁹/L if the count is rapidly falling.

DIAGNOSIS

1 Neutropenic patients may already know their diagnosis and/or be receiving treatment, or can present as a new case.

2 Causes of neutropenia include:
  (i) Reduced neutrophil production:
    (a) aplastic anaemia
    (b) leukaemia, lymphoma
    (c) myeloproliferative syndrome
    (d) metastatic bone marrow disease
    (e) drug-induced agranulocytosis, including chemotherapy
    (f) megaloblastic anaemia crisis.
  (ii) Reduced neutrophil survival:
    (a) systemic lupus erythematosus (SLE)
    (b) immune-mediated
    (c) drug-related
    (d) Felty syndrome.
  (iii) Reduced neutrophil circulation:
    (a) septicaemia
    (b) hypersplenism.

3 Ask about constitutional symptoms including fever and malaise, plus organ-specific features such as cough, frequency and dysuria, diarrhoea or headache and confusion.
  (i) Take a detailed drug history, contact and travel history.

4 Record the vital signs and note any focal sources of sepsis including the skin, ears, throat and perineum, indwelling catheters, and for evidence of anaemia or bruising suggesting a pancytopenia.

5 Establish venous access with strict asepsis, and send blood for full blood count (FBC), coagulation profile, electrolyte and liver function tests (ELFTs) and two sets of blood cultures from different venepuncture sites.

6 Request a chest radiograph (CXR) and send a midstream urine (MSU) sample.

MANAGEMENT

1 Start empirical antibiotic therapy initially, unless there is a clear focus of infection, and discuss with an infectious disease physician or microbiologist.

      (i) Urgent empirical i.v. therapy with broad-spectrum antimicrobials is universal, although the optimal regimen will depend on local bacteriological susceptibilities and preference. Give:

         (a) piperacillin 4 g with tazobactam 0.5 g i.v. 6-hourly, *plus* gentamicin 4–7 mg/kg i.v. once daily when critically ill

         (b) ceftazidime 2 g i.v., t.d.s. if penicillin-sensitive, *plus* gentamicin 4–7 mg/kg i.v. once daily when critically ill

         (c) add vancomycin 1.5 g i.v. 12-hourly for possible line sepsis, MRSA or if the patient is shocked.

2 Admit the patient under the medical team, even if the patient looks well with only a fever, as rapid deterioration may occur.

      (i) Refer haemodynamically unstable patients to the intensive care unit (ICU).

HEPATITIS

DIAGNOSIS

1 Causes of hepatitis include:

      (i) Viruses such as enterically transmitted hepatitis A or E, or parenterally spread hepatitis B, C, D or G, and infectious mononucleosis, cytomegalovirus (CMV) or herpes simplex virus (HSV).

      (ii) Toxins and drugs such as alcohol, antibiotics, methyldopa, statins, chlorpromazine, isoniazid and paracetamol (remember the possibility of acute poisoning), herbal medication and *Amanita* mushrooms.

      (iii) Bacteria such as leptospirosis, or amoebae.

2 Hepatitis presents with anorexia, malaise, nausea, vomiting, abdominal pain and joint pain.

3 Look for a raised temperature, jaundice, tender hepatomegaly and splenomegaly. Assess for confusion or an altered conscious level.

4 Send blood for serology for hepatitis A, B or C, plus FBC, coagulation profile, ELFTs and lipase.

      (i) AST is two to three times higher than ALT in alcoholic hepatitis.

5 Test the urine for bilirubin and urobilinogen.

MANAGEMENT

1 Admit unwell patients to the medical team.

      (i) This should include those with fever and malaise, persistent vomiting, dehydration, encephalopathy or a bleeding tendency with a prolonged prothrombin time.

2 Otherwise, discharge the well patient with advice to avoid preparing food for others and to use their own knife, fork, spoon, cup and plate (assuming the patient could have hepatitis A or E).

3 Advise the patient to avoid alcohol and cigarettes.

4 Give the patient a referral letter to medical outpatients or to their general practitioner (GP) for definitive diagnosis and follow-up.

GASTROINTESTINAL TRACT INFECTION

DIAGNOSIS

1 The most common manifestation is sudden acute diarrhoea, often with vomiting.

2 Causes of infectious diarrhoea include:

(i) *Toxin-related* diarrhoea from staphylococcal food poisoning which has a precipitate onset in hours, as does *Bacillus cereus* enterotoxin from rice, in which vomiting and abdominal cramps predominate.

(ii) *Viral* diarrhoea from the rotavirus in young children, and norovirus in older children and adults with an incubation period of 1–2 days, sometimes occurring in outbreaks of non-bloody diarrhoea. Other viral causes include enteric adenovirus and astrovirus.

(iii) *Salmonella* with an incubation period of 6–72 h and *Shigella* infections with an incubation period of 1–3 days result in fever, malaise, diarrhoea (which may be blood-stained), vomiting and abdominal pain.

(iv) *Campylobacter* infection has an incubation period of 2–5 days and presents with colicky abdominal pain, which may precede the onset of diarrhoea, that is watery and offensive, and sometimes blood-stained.

(v) 'Traveller's diarrhoea' is most often due to enterotoxigenic *Escherichia coli*, and is usually self-limiting over 2–5 days, causing watery stools and occasionally vomiting

(a) fever is unusual, and may indicate a more serious infection that needs active investigation, including malaria or even epidemic influenza.

(vi) *Amoebiasis* may cause an acute, relapsing diarrhoea, with stools containing blood and mucus. Ask about travel to Africa, Asia or Latin America.

(vii) *Giardiasis* with an incubation period of 3–25 days causes explosive watery diarrhoea, which often persists for weeks. Chronic infection may eventually cause malabsorption with steatorrhoea. Ask about travel to Russia or North America, and contact with children in day care who have had recent diarrhoea.

3 The most important feature in all cases, after establishing any contact or travel history, is clinical evidence of dehydration.

   (i) Dehydration causes thirst, lassitude, dry lax skin, tachycardia and postural hypotension, leading to oliguria, confusion and coma when critical.

4 Also consider other causes of acute diarrhoea including drug-related, *Clostridium difficile* antibiotic-related diarrhoea (CDAD), Crohn's disease, ulcerative colitis, ischaemic colitis, irritable bowel syndrome, and 'spurious' from faecal impaction.

5 Send blood for FBC and ELFTs, and commence an i.v. infusion of normal saline in all dehydrated, febrile or toxic patients.

   (i) Send a stool specimen for *C. difficile* toxin assay, if antibiotic-associated diarrhoea is suspected following any antibiotic use in the previous 12 weeks.

MANAGEMENT

1 Admit dehydrated, toxic, very young or elderly, and immunosuppressed patients for rehydration.

2 Allow other patients home and encourage them to drink plenty of fluid.

   (i) Alternatively, give the patient an oral glucose and electrolyte rehydration solution, which may also be purchased over the counter.

   (ii) Give an antimotility agent such as loperamide 4 mg initially, followed by 2 mg after each loose stool to a maximum of 16 mg/day (not in children, and not with fever or bloody diarrhoea).

3 Ask the patient to return within 24–48 h if symptoms persist:

   (i) Send stools for microscopy and culture then.

   (ii) Consider empirical treatment for moderate to severe systemic illness with bloody diarrhoea or for associated rigors
       (a) give ciprofloxacin 500 mg orally b.d. for 2–3 days (not in children).

   (iii) Give tinidazole 2 g orally once if *Giardia* is suspected.

4 Arrange follow-up in medical outpatients or by the local GP.

   (i) Stop any antibiotics if CDAD is confirmed and give metronidazole 400 mg orally t.d.s. for 10 days, with a reminder to avoid alcohol.

SEXUALLY TRANSMITTED DISEASES

DIAGNOSIS

1 A sexually transmitted disease (STD) may be caused by non-specific infection, *Chlamydia*, gonococcus, HSV, human papilloma virus, *Trichomonas*, scabies or lice, syphilis, and of course human immunodeficiency virus (HIV).

2 Males may present with dysuria, urethral discharge, penile ulceration, warts, epididymo-orchitis and balanitis.

3 Females may present with vaginal discharge, vaginal pruritus, ulceration, warts, menstrual irregularities and abdominal pain.
   (i) Pelvic inflammatory disease is commonly sexually acquired (see p. 325).

4 Take swabs for bacterial, viral and chlamydial studies for microscopy, culture and nucleic acid amplification, if you intend to commence treatment.
   (i) Discuss the swabs and transport medium with your microbiology lab if you are unsure
   (ii) Arrange a first-voided urine specimen for PCR nucleic acid testing for *Chlamydia trachomatis* or *Neisseria gonorrhoeae*.

MANAGEMENT

1 All STDs deserve expert diagnosis, treatment, follow-up and partner-contact tracing most readily available from the local GP, or in a genitourinary medicine clinic (Special Clinic).

2 As patients are reluctant to attend these clinics, explain carefully the local appointment system, what to expect, and how to locate the clinic, and refer the patient on.
   (i) Advise males not to empty the bladder for at least 4 h before attendance.

3 Commence empirical antibiotic treatment in the homeless or itinerant patient considered unlikely to attend any clinic.
   (i) Give azithromycin 1 g orally as a single dose **plus** ceftriaxone 500 mg i.m. for urethritis.

4 In addition, consider treating the patient with an immediately painful condition such as genital herpes simplex:
   (i) Give aciclovir 400 mg orally t.d.s., famciclovir 250 mg orally t.d.s. or valaciclovir 500 mg b.d. all for 5 days.

5 Admit a patient under the medical or gynaecology team for treatment of the acute manifestations of HIV infection, secondary syphilis, acute Reiter's syndrome, disseminated gonococcal infection, severe primary genital herpes, or acute severe salpingitis.

NEEDLESTICK AND SHARPS INCIDENTS

INOCULATION INCIDENT WITH HIV RISK

DIAGNOSIS

1 The risk of seroconversion is 0.1–0.5% following accidental inoculation of blood or infectious material from a suspected HIV-positive person.

2   This risk depends on the nature and extent of the inoculation, and the viral disease activity of the HIV-positive source.

3   Take 10 mL clotted blood from the injured person, and if possible 10 mL with consent from the source. Send for HIV, hepatitis B and C testing, clearly marking the specimen as 'needlestick/sharps injury'.

MANAGEMENT

1   Wash wounds, and clean and flush mucous membranes immediately after exposure. Use a skin antiseptic such as 0.5% chlorhexidine in 70% alcohol and encourage bleeding by local venous occlusion.

2   When the source is known to be HIV-positive with a high viral load or late-stage disease, and higher-risk exposure has occurred, e.g. a deep needlestick or laceration with blood inoculated, proceed as follows:
    (i)   Discuss the situation immediately with an infectious diseases specialist.
    (ii) On their advice, commence (within hours) antiretroviral therapy such as lamivudine 150 mg with zidovudine 300 mg orally b.d., plus lopinavir 400 mg with ritonavir 100 mg orally b.d. usually for 4 weeks. Check your local policy for regional variations.
    (iii) The side effects of these drugs are complex and significant, including rash, malaise, fatigue, headache, nausea, vomiting, diarrhoea, hepatitis, pancreatitis and blood dyscrasias.

3   When the source is HIV-positive with a low viral load and lower-risk exposure has occurred, e.g. superficial scratch or mucous membrane contamination, commence zidovudine and lamivudine alone, or according to local policy.

4   Refer the injured person to Occupational Health for follow-up with repeat serology and monitoring blood tests, advice and ongoing counselling with psychological support.
    (i)   Report the incident to the senior ED doctor and infection control officer.
    (ii) The exposed person requires follow-up for up to 6 months, should practise safe sex, should not donate blood, and should avoid pregnancy.
    (iii) Assure confidentiality and sensitivity for all concerned.

5   Consider the additional possibility of transmission of hepatitis B and the need for tetanus prophylaxis (see p. 269).

INOCULATION INCIDENT WITH HEPATITIS RISK

DIAGNOSIS

1   The risk of seroconversion in a non-immunized person following a needlestick injury with HBV-positive blood is 5–40%, and following injury with hepatitis C virus-positive blood is <3%.

2   Take 10 mL clotted blood from the injured person, and if possible 10 mL with consent from the source. Send for hepatitis B and C and HIV testing, clearly marking the specimen as 'needlestick/sharps injury'.

Table 4.1 Hepatitis B prophylaxis following significant percutaneous, ocular or mucous membrane exposure for persons without adequate immunity

Exposure source	Exposed person
Test for HBsAg	Test for anti-HBs (unless recent satisfactory level of ≥10 IU/mL is known)
HBsAg +ve, or cannot be identified and tested rapidly	**anti-HBs** –ve or <10 IU/mL, give: **HBIG**[a] **HB vaccine**[b]
HBsAg –ve	**anti-HBs** –ve offer **HB vaccine**[c]

anti-HBs, antibody to HBsAg; HB vaccine, hepatitis B vaccine; HBIG, hepatitis B immunoglobulin; HBsAg, hepatitis B surface antigen.
[a] HBIG: 400 IU i.m. for adults, or 100 IU i.m. for children <30 kg, within 72 hours.
[b] HB vaccine: 1 mL i.m. within 7 days, then at 1–2 months, and a third dose at 6 months.
[c] Injury indicates evidence that the work area represents a significant exposure risk, so full vaccination is encouraged for the injured (exposed) person.

MANAGEMENT

1 Wash the area with soap and water, dress the wound, and give tetanus prophylaxis.

2 Use Table 4.1 to determine the need for hepatitis B prophylaxis following significant percutaneous, ocular or mucous membrane exposure in persons without adequate immunity, i.e. anti-HBs levels unrecordable or <10 IU/mL. Check your local policy for regional variations.

3 Refer the injured person to Occupational Health for follow-up, with repeat serology and monitoring blood tests for up to 6 months.
    (i) Inform the senior ED doctor and infection control officer.
    (ii) The exposed person requires follow-up for 6 months, should practise safe sex, should not donate blood and should avoid pregnancy.
    (iii) Assure confidentiality and sensitivity for all concerned.

HUMAN IMMUNODEFICIENCY VIRUS INFECTION

DIAGNOSIS

1 HIV is a cytopathic RNA retrovirus. It is transmitted by sexual contact, by syringe sharing in i.v. drug abusers, transplacentally and rarely now by blood transfusion.
    (i) Remember acute HIV infection may present after international travel.

2   HIV risk groups include:
    (i)   Men who have sex with men.
    (ii) Intravenous drug users.
    (iii) Heterosexual partners of HIV/AIDS patients.
    (iv) Children of HIV/AIDS affected mothers.
    (v) Blood product recipients in the early 1980s.

3   The *Revised Surveillance Case Definition for HIV Infection – United States, 2014* was published by the US Centers for Disease Control and Prevention in 2014. It is designed for use in all age groups, and is adapted to recent changes in diagnostic criteria.
    (i)   Four stages of CD4+ count are recognized for medical management purposes:
        (a) Stage 1. CD4 count $\geq$500/mm^3
        (b) Stage 2. CD4 count 200–499/mm^3
        (c) Stage 3. CD4 count <200/mm^3
        (d) Unknown Stage. No information available on CD4 count or percentage.
    (ii) A CD4+ count <200/mm^3 or <14% can be used to define HIV infection stage 3 or acquired immune deficiency syndrome (AIDS).

4   Presentation varies according to the disease stage and progression.
    (i)   *Acute infection*:
        (a) 50–70% of patients infected with HIV develop an acute illness with lethargy, fever, pharyngitis, myalgia, maculopapular rash and lymphadenopathy about 2 weeks after exposure. Acute meningitis or encephalitis are occasionally seen
        (b) although the patient is infectious, serology for HIV antibodies at this early stage will be negative
        (c) if the HIV test remains negative at 6 months, this is then termed stage 0.
    (ii) *Asymptomatic infection*:
        (a) the acute infection symptoms usually resolve by 3 weeks
        (b) infected patients seroconvert to HIV-positive over the next 6 months, most within 2–12 weeks of exposure
        (c) 50% of these patients used to have fully developed AIDS by 8–10 years, although disease progression has now slowed to an almost normal life expectancy with modern highly active anti-retroviral therapy (HAART).
    (iii) *Persistent generalized lymphadenopathy/intermediate phase*:
        (a) enlarged nodes in two or more non-contiguous extra-inguinal sites for at least 3 months and not due to a disease other than HIV
        (b) apparently minor but debilitating complaints such as recalcitrant dermatitis, oral candida, extensive warts, varicella zoster and thrombocytopenia may occur

  (c) otherwise the patient is relatively well usually with a CD4 count >500/mm^3, and enters a latency period of 2–10 years or more.

 (iv) *Symptomatic infection* (delayed and less common now with HAART):

  (a) subgroup A: constitutional disease with persistent fever, unexplained weight loss of 10% body mass or diarrhoea for over 1 month

  (b) subgroup B: neurological disease, including encephalopathy, myelopathy and peripheral neuropathy

  (c) subgroup C: secondary infectious diseases due to opportunistic infections usually as the CD4+ count drops below 200/mm^3. These include *Pneumocystis jirovecii* pneumonia, recurrent pneumonia, *Mycobacterium tuberculosis*, atypical mycobacteria, toxoplasmosis, cryptosporidiosis, isosporiasis, strongyloidosis, cytomegalovirus, systemic candidiasis, cryptococcosis and many others

  (d) subgroup D: secondary cancers including Kaposi's sarcoma, high-grade non-Hodgkin's lymphoma, primary lymphoma of the brain and invasive cervical cancer

  (e) subgroup E: other conditions such as the HIV-wasting syndrome and chronic lymphoid interstitial pneumonitis in adults.

5 AIDS-defining illnesses in an HIV-positive patient are in subgroups B to E, most commonly *P. jirovecii* pneumonia and *Cryptococcus neoformans* meningitis.

6 Thus, patients encountered in the ED infected with HIV range from the asymptomatic carrier state in the majority to non-specific illness or to acute problems as varied as collapse, cardiac disease, respiratory failure, gastrointestinal bleeding, skin disorders, depression, dementia, stroke and coma.

 (i) Alternatively those on HAART may present with side effects of these drugs ranging from rashes including hypersensitivity reactions to hepatitis, pancreatitis, lactic acidosis and marrow suppression.

7 Always maintain a high index of suspicion to identify an HIV-risk patient, if necessary by direct questioning.

8 Send blood for HIV antigen if the patient is acutely unwell with a possible new HIV illness, requesting nucleic acid amplification (NAA) testing such as a polymerase chain reaction (PCR) assay for HIV RNA, viral load and p24 antigen, as well as standard 4th generation ELISA antibody testing.

9 'Routine' HIV antibody testing in the ED is inappropriate if skilled counselling and follow-up are not available.

 (i) Also relying on a single serum test for HIV antibody to establish or exclude HIV infection is unwise as:

  (a) occasional false positives occur

  (b) false negatives occur in those infected due to:

   – early infection

   – lack of seroconversion in the first few months.

MANAGEMENT

1 Consider every patient to be potentially infectious and adopt standard infection control precautions including designated hospital hand hygiene practice, and the use of personal protective equipment to minimize body substance exposure.

    (i) Precautions must be consistently observed with **every** ED patient in order to prevent any HIV dissemination and consequent exposure to disease risk.

    (ii) Always wash hands before and after contact with a patient.

    (iii) Wear gloves when handling blood specimens and body fluids.

    (iv) Wear a disposable apron if there is likely to be contamination of clothing (e.g. from bleeding), and a face mask and goggles if splashing is even a small possibility.

    (v) Take great care handling needles or scalpel blades, particularly on disposal.

    (vi) Clean blood spills immediately with a suitable chlorine-based disinfectant.

2 Refer the patient to the medical team in the usual way if he or she is acutely ill.

    (i) Otherwise refer the patient to infectious disease, genitourinary medicine (special clinic), or to the medical outpatient service for complete and ongoing care.

TUBERCULOSIS

DIAGNOSIS

1 Tuberculosis is an unusual diagnosis in the ED, particularly in developed countries such as Australia and the UK. However, as tuberculosis is a treatable and potentially curable disease its diagnosis must be considered.

2 Pulmonary tuberculosis has a significant risk of secondary transmission. Although the risk to staff and other patients in the ED is small, the patient should be isolated and wear a face mask.

3 Request an acid-fast stain for *Mycobacteria* in the following clinical settings, even though their differential diagnosis is wide-ranging and obviously includes malignancy:

    (i) Family history of tuberculosis.

    (ii) Previous migration from overseas, particularly Africa, Asia and southern Europe.

    (iii) Fever and cough in a patient with HIV/AIDS, or risk behaviour.

    (iv) Fever, productive cough and haemoptysis, particularly if immunosuppressed, diabetic, homeless or indigenous.

    (v) Otherwise unexplained fever, chronic cough, weight loss and night sweats.

4   Perform a chest X-ray, although the appearances are not diagnostic.

   (i)   Radiographic presentations include apical shadowing, hilar lymphadenopathy, consolidation, cavitation, effusion, fibrosis and calcification, or a miliary pattern.

5   Send blood and sputum for microscopy with Ziehl–Neelsen staining, culture and polymerase chain reaction (PCR) assay for *M. tuberculosis.*

   (i)   An acid-fast smear is rapid but less sensitive than culture, although culture may take several weeks to produce a definitive result.

   (ii)   A negative sputum smear does not rule out pulmonary tuberculosis, and a positive smear does not confirm *M. tuberculosis*, as atypical mycobacteria have the same appearance.

MANAGEMENT

1   Assess any patient with suspected pulmonary tuberculosis in a separate room (isolation room), and not in a standard ED resuscitation or observation cubicle.

2   Pulmonary tuberculosis is rarely severe enough to warrant commencing immediate antimycobacterial therapy. Rather ensure that you:

   (i)   Send a series of sputum samples for microscopy and culture.

   (ii)   Liaise with the on-call infectious disease team or respiratory medicine team to determine the best treatment course and area for admission:

      (a)   standard short-course therapy consists of 2 months treatment with daily isoniazid, rifampicin, pyrazinamide and ethambutol followed by 4 months of daily isoniazid and rifampicin

      (b)   starting therapy in the ED is rarely ever indicated.

   (iii)   Contact the infection control service for a patient with suspected pulmonary tuberculosis to determine an infection control risk assessment and to initiate contact tracing.

3   Tuberculosis is a notifiable disease to the relevant public health authority.

BITES WITH RABIES OR OTHER LYSSAVIRUS RISK

RABIES AND LYSSAVIRUS RISK

DIAGNOSIS

1   Transmission of rabies or other lyssaviruses usually occurs from the bite of a dog, other canids such as foxes and wolves, cats, monkeys, bats, raccoons and skunks.

2 Rabies is endemic in most continents apart from Australia, but several cases of a similar disease caused by the Australian bat lyssavirus (ABLV), a zoonotic virus closely related to rabies virus, have occurred following a bat bite or scratch.

3 The incubation period is 3–8 weeks, but may be 3 months or more, by which time a travel history and animal or bat bite history may have been forgotten.

4 Clinical signs of infection include anorexia, fever, pain at the bite site and headache, progressing to confusion and agitation from encephalitis with pre-fatal hypersalivation, hyperthermia and hydrophobia.

5 Discuss any laboratory test with the infectious diseases team or pathology laboratory prior to sample collection.
    (i) Laboratory confirmation includes immunofluorescent stain of a skin biopsy from the nape of the neck, antibody detection in blood or CSF, or PCR assay of saliva, blood or CSF.

MANAGEMENT

1 Established rabies is inevitably fatal. All cases of rabies exposure that have survived have been vaccinated before the onset of clinical disease.

2 Immediately wash and flush all bite wounds and scratches for at least 5 min. Check the patient's tetanus immunization status, and give adsorbed diphtheria and tetanus toxoid (ADT) as required.

3 Try to evaluate the exposure risk:
    (i) Category I – touching or feeding animals, licks on intact skin.
    (ii) Category II – nibbling of uncovered skin, minor scratches or abrasions without bleeding.
    (iii) Category III – single or multiple transdermal bites or scratches, contamination of mucous membrane with saliva from licks, licks on broken skin.

4 Discuss post-exposure rabies and ABLV prophylaxis (post-exposure prophylaxis [PEP]) immediately with an infectious diseases specialist or the on-call population health unit specialist.
    (i) PEP is a combination of human rabies immunoglobulin (HRIG) and rabies vaccine, and should be given within 48 h of the bite:
        (a) category I exposure – no further treatment required
        (b) category II exposure – administer rabies vaccine i.m.
        (c) category III – administer rabies vaccine and HRIG i.m.
    (ii) Depending on the vaccine type, PEP in the previously unvaccinated immunocompetent person includes rabies vaccine 1 mL i.m. in the deltoid muscle to a total of four doses over two weeks on day 0, 3, 7 and 14. In addition, HRIG 20 IU/kg is infiltrated around the wound site on the first day.

- Ask any patient who has been travelling abroad specifically about the time, place and type of travel. Ask how long they spent in each foreign country and when they arrived back.

- Enquire specifically about malaria prophylaxis and whether it was taken for 4 weeks after leaving a malarial zone, and about immunizations before going abroad.

- The CDC Travelers' Health website (see http://wwwnc.cdc.gov/travel/) has information to assist travellers and their healthcare providers in deciding on the vaccines, medications, and other measures necessary to prevent illness and injury during international travel. It covers all aspects of foreign travel, including lists of recent disease outbreaks, and information on illnesses in alphabetical order from African tick-bite fever to yellow fever.

- Remember that the returned traveller may well have a condition that is not considered 'tropical', such as an STD including HIV infection, meningococcal infection, pneumonia, pyelonephritis, and enteric infection other than traveller's diarrhoea.

- Some of the tropical diseases discussed below can be endemic, but mostly are contracted abroad.

MALARIA

DIAGNOSIS

1   Falciparum malaria is the most dangerous form of malaria. Cases are imported to Australia from Africa, Asia and Papua New Guinea, but other tropical sources include the western Pacific, Amazon basin and Oceania.

   (i)   Malaria is a potentially fatal infection. Survivors may experience damage to the brain, kidneys, liver, heart, gastrointestinal tract and lungs.

   (ii) Cerebral malaria is an abrupt onset of encephalopathy with headache that can progress rapidly to confusion, seizures and coma.

   (iii) Other malaria presentations include an influenza-like illness, diarrhoea and vomiting, jaundice, acute renal failure, acute respiratory distress, postural hypotension or shock, progressive anaemia and thrombocytopenia.

   (iv) The patient may not look ill in the first few days, but the non-immune or splenectomized patient may then deteriorate rapidly over a few hours and die.

2   The patient usually presents within 4 weeks of returning from a malarious area with fever, rigors, nausea, vomiting, diarrhoea, and headache. Hepatosplenomegaly is common.

3 Infection may persist for months due to the release of parasites from the hepatic extra-erythrocytic phase in the liver, even after apparently successful treatment.

    (i)   Late onset acute presentation can occur months or even more than a year after return from overseas.

    (ii)   This relapse due to persistent dormant hepatic hypnozoites does **not** occur in falciparum malaria.

4 Send blood for FBC, coagulation profile, ELFTs, two sets of blood cultures and:

    (i)   Request at least two sets of thick and thin blood films for malarial parasites in *every* patient returning from abroad with fever and with any of the above symptoms or signs.

    (ii)   Perform a PCR test when available particularly for mixed infection, or if microscopy is negative.

5 Request an MSU.

MANAGEMENT

1 Falciparum malaria is a medical emergency requiring prompt treatment with oral or i.v. artemisinin derivative therapy.

    (i)   Call the senior ED doctor if you suspect falciparum malaria.

    (ii)   Give immediate artesunate 2.4 mg/kg i.v. repeated at 12 and 24 h, then once daily, if there is an altered conscious level, jaundice, oliguria, severe anaemia, hypoglycaemia, vomiting, acidosis or respiratory distress, or if over 2% red cells are parasitized. Admit these *severe* cases to the ICU

        (a) give quinine 20 mg/kg up to 1.4 g infused over 4 h if artesunate is not immediately available, with BP, blood sugar (risk of hypoglycaemia) and electrocardiographic monitoring.

    (iii) Admit other less severe patients under the medical team when falciparum malaria is even considered possible, and begin treatment immediately – if necessary before definitive blood results are available

        (a) give those who can tolerate oral treatment artemether-lumefantrine combination therapy.

2 Refer patients with other types of malaria (*P. vivax*, *P. ovale*, *P. malariae* and *P. knowlesi*) to the medical team; some may be suitable for treatment as an outpatient.

3 Ask a patient with two sets of negative thick and thin blood films, but a suggestive history, to return for repeat malaria blood films in 48 h or earlier if symptoms persist.

    (i)   Inform the GP of the possibility of malaria by email and letter.

Warning: do not diagnose the flu in a febrile patient without asking about recent foreign travel and considering malaria.

TYPHOID

DIAGNOSIS

1 The incubation period is up to 3 weeks following travel to India, Latin America, the Philippines and South-East Asia. There is an initial insidious onset of fever, malaise, headache, anorexia, dry cough, and constipation in the first week.

2 The illness then progresses to abdominal distension and pain associated with diarrhoea, splenomegaly, a relative bradycardia, bronchitis, confusion or coma.

    (i)   The characteristic crop of fine rose-pink macules on the trunk is rare.

3 Send blood for FBC that may show a leucopenia with a relative lymphocytosis. Send ELFTs and two sets of blood cultures in all suspected cases.

4 Request an MSU and a stool culture if diarrhoea is prominent.

    (i)   Blood cultures are positive in up to 90% in the first week.

    (ii)   Stool culture becomes positive in 75% and urine culture in 25% in the second week.

MANAGEMENT

1 Commence i.v. rehydration with normal saline or Hartmann's.

2 Refer all suspected cases to the medical team for azithromycin 1 g i.v. or orally daily for 5 days.

    (i)   Or give ciprofloxacin 400 mg i.v. 12-hourly or ciprofloxacin 500 mg b.d. orally for 7–10 days, if the infection was not acquired in the Indian subcontinent or South-East Asia.

DENGUE

DIAGNOSIS

1 Dengue occurs after a short 1-week incubation period from infection by one of four serotypes of mosquito-borne flavivirus, particularly in Central or South America and South-East Asia.

2 There are abrupt fever, chills, retro-orbital or frontal headache, myalgia, back pain, lymphadenopathy and rash.

    (i)   The initial rash is a transient, generalized, blanching macular rash in the first 1–2 days.

    (ii)   A secondary maculopapular rash with areas of sparing occurs lasting 1–5 days.

    (iii)   A later haemorrhagic rash may be associated with thrombocytopenia.

3 Dengue haemorrhagic fever (DHF) and dengue shock syndrome (DSS) occur in repeat infections with a different serotype.

4 Send blood for FBC, coagulation profile, ELFTs, two sets of blood cultures and dengue IgM serology and/or PCR.

MANAGEMENT

1 Admit the patient under the medical team for supportive care with i.v. fluids and antipyretic analgesics.

2 Admit patients with DHF or dengue shock syndrome to the ICU.

TYPHUS AND SPOTTED FEVERS

DIAGNOSIS

1 Typhus includes several diseases caused by *Rickettsiae*, such as epidemic and murine (endemic) typhus.

2 Scrub typhus is one of the spotted fevers, and is caused by an acute bacterial infection by *Orientia tsutsugamushi*, transmitted by trombiculid mites ('chiggers'). Foci of scrub typhus occur in South-East Asia, northern Japan and northern Australia.

    (i) Other tick-borne spotted fevers include Queensland tick typhus, Rocky Mountain and Mediterranean.

3 Infection is characterized by high fevers, headache, lymphadenopathy and a fine vasculitic maculopapular rash, with a characteristic black necrotic eschar at the site of the original chigger bite in scrub typhus.

4 Potential complications include pneumonitis, encephalitis and myocarditis, which usually occur in the late phase of the illness.

5 Send blood for FBC, coagulation profile, ELFTs, blood cultures and serology.

    (i) Leucopenia and deranged LFTs are common in the early phase of infection.

6 Scrub typhus can be confirmed by PCR assay on ethylenediaminetetraacetic acid (EDTA) blood in its early stages, or serological tests in the later or convalescent stage.

MANAGEMENT

1 Give doxycycline 100 mg orally b.d. for 7–10 days.

2 Refer the patient to an infectious disease specialist for exclusion of additional travel-related infections, and follow up.

HELMINTH INFECTIONS

DIAGNOSIS

1 *Schistosomiasis* (bilharzia) caused by fresh-water trematodes (flukes) rarely presents acutely, but should be suspected in acute cases from endemic areas such as Africa, South America, the Middle East and Asia presenting with fever, urticarial rash, hepatosplenomegaly and diarrhoea associated with eosinophilia (Katayama fever).

    (i) Chronic infection may present up to years later with painless terminal haematuria or obstructive uropathy, portal or pulmonary hypertension and seizures.

2 *Roundworm* infection (ascariasis) is discovered when the adult worm is passed in the stool, although occasionally allergic pneumonitis, abdominal pain, diarrhoea or urticaria occur.

3 *Tapeworm* infection usually presents with lassitude, weight loss and anaemia or with disease-specific complications such as seizures in cysticercosis, and mass effects in hydatid disease (*Echinococcus*).

MANAGEMENT

1 Discuss your suspicions with an infectious disease specialist and take advice about which laboratory tests are indicated.

PANDEMIC INFLUENZA

- A pandemic is a global outbreak of a new type of infection in susceptible individuals, with rapid person-to-person spread and the potential to affect millions.
- International travel is the main reason for the speed of pandemic spread, so international travellers are among the first cases of a variant of influenza to be seen in any new location.
- World Health Organisation website has the latest influenza updates (http://www.who.int/influenza/en/), as well as the Centers for Disease Control and Prevention (CDC).

DIAGNOSIS

1 Influenza is an acute illness with an abrupt onset and peak symptoms in the first 24–48 h.
   (i) These most commonly include sudden fever, chills, headache, dry cough, sore throat and muscle aches.
   (ii) Diarrhoea can be a presenting complaint.

2 Ask patients presenting with fever or respiratory symptoms specifically about interstate and international travel, or about contact with anyone who has an acute respiratory illness ideally at triage, **before** entering the ED.
   (i) Check the status of the current 'at-risk' countries at http://wwwnc.cdc.gov/travel/ or refer to local policy information concerning global infection threats.

MANAGEMENT

1 Place a suspected case of influenza in isolation, preferably a negative-pressure room, and give him or her a surgical mask to wear.

2 All attending staff must wear a correctly fitted, high-filtration mask (N95), long-sleeved gown, gloves, and full eye protection.

3 Inform the senior ED doctor, the local infectious disease physician, and hospital infection control officer.

    (i) Call the clinical microbiologist and take FBC, ELFTs, blood cultures and 30 mL serology including for atypical pneumonia.

    (ii) Send a nose/throat swab and arrange a chest X-ray:

        (a) alert the radiographer to the infection risk.

    (iii) A nasopharyngeal aspirate (NPA) has a higher risk to staff and is not recommended.

4 Specialist consultation and local policy will determine further management.

FURTHER READING

Australian Government Department of Health (2013). *The Australian Immunisation Handbook*, 10th edn. http://www.health.gov.au/internet/immunise/publishing.nsf/Content/Handbook10-home (hepatitis B, HIV, rabies).

Australian Prescriber (2012). http://www.australianprescriber.com/magazine/35/1/article/1248.pdf (fever in the returned traveller).

CDC Travelers' Health. http://wwwnc.cdc.gov/travel/ (travellers' health).

Department of Health UK. Immunisation Against Infectious Disease 2013. 'The Green Book'. www.gov.uk/government/collections/immunisation-against-infectious-disease-the-green-book#the-green-book (immunisation).

Public Health England. https://www.gov.uk/government/organisations/public-health-england (infectious diseases).

Therapeutic Guidelines. eTG complete 2015. http://www.tg.org.au/

World Health Organization. http://www.who.int/rabies/human/postexp/en/ (rabies).

SURGICAL EMERGENCIES

OVERVIEW

The management of **every** severely injured patient requires a coordinated approach, such as that taught in Advanced Trauma Life Support (ATLS™, American College of Surgeons) and the equivalent Early Management of Severe Trauma (EMST™, Royal Australasian College of Surgeons) courses.

This involves a rapid primary survey, resuscitation of vital functions, a detailed secondary survey and the initiation of definitive care.

1 *Primary survey*

   Rapid patient assessment to identify life-threatening conditions and establish immediate priorities.

2 *Resuscitation phase*

   Optimizes the patient's respiratory and circulatory status. The response to resuscitation is recorded with comprehensive non-invasive monitoring.

   (i)   Once resuscitation is under way, a trauma series of X-rays is taken, bloods are sent, and additional procedures such as a rapid bedside ultrasound, nasogastric tube insertion and urinary catheterization are performed.

3 *Secondary survey*

   Commences after the primary survey is complete and the resuscitation phase well under way:

   (i)   A detailed head-to-toe examination is made.

   (ii)   Special X-rays, repeat ultrasound, computed tomography (CT) scan and angiographic studies are performed as indicated.

4 *Definitive care*

   Management of all the injuries identified, including surgery, fracture stabilization, hospital admission or preparation of the patient for transfer, if required.

5 Expect serious injuries in patients presenting with altered physiology, or after the following high-risk mechanisms:

   (i)   Abnormal vital signs: systolic blood pressure <90 mmHg, Glasgow Coma Scale (GCS) score ≤12, respiratory rate <10/min or >30/min.

   (ii)   Motorcyclist or pedestrian struck.

   (iii) Fall >5 m (15 ft).

   (iv)   Entrapment.

   (v)   High-speed impact, ejection or death of another vehicle occupant.

6 Call senior Emergency Department (ED) staff immediately for any multiple-injury patient, to organize an integrated team response incorporating anaesthetic, intensive care, surgical and orthopaedic colleagues.

7 The time-honoured mnemonic for the initial sequence of care is ABCDE (see Table 5.1).

Table 5.1 Mnemonic for initial sequence of care of the multiply-injured patient during the primary survey and resuscitation phases

A	**A**irway maintenance with cervical spine control
B	**B**reathing and ventilation
C	**C**irculation with haemorrhage control
D	**D**isability: brief neurological evaluation
E	**E**xposure/**E**nvironmental control: completely undress the patient, but prevent hypothermia

IMMEDIATE MANAGEMENT

1 *Airway*

    (i)   Assess the airway to ascertain patency and identify potential obstruction:

        (a) clear the airway of loose or broken dentures and suck out any debris

        (b) insert an oropharyngeal airway if the patient is unconscious

        (c) give 100% oxygen by tight-fitting mask with reservoir bag

        (d) aim for an oxygen saturation above 94%.

    (ii)   *Intubation*

        (a) a definitive procedure to protect and maintain the airway is indicated if the patient is unconscious, or has a reduced or absent gag reflex

        (b) take great care to minimize neck movements in the unconscious head injury or suspected neck injury by maintaining in-line manual immobilization during airway assessment and endotracheal intubation

        (c) *rapid sequence induction (RSI) intubation*

          – this is the airway technique of choice, provided the operator is skilled in the technique

          – confirm correct tube placement using capnography to measure end-tidal carbon dioxide ($ETCO_2$) (see p. 467)

          – normoventilate aiming for a $PaCO_2$ 37.5–41 mmHg (5.0–5.5 kPa).

 Warning: never attempt RSI unless you have been trained. Use a bag-valve mask technique instead while awaiting help.

    (iii) Surgical airway: proceed directly to cricothyrotomy if endotracheal intubation is impossible due to laryngeal injury or severe maxillofacial injury (see p. 380).

2   Maintain the integrity of the cervical spine

    (i)   Place the unconscious head injury and the patient with suspected neck injury in a semi-rigid collar.

    (ii)   Minimize head movement. When the patient requires turning, the body should be 'log-rolled', holding the head in the neutral position at all times.

3   Breathing and ventilation

Look for and treat the following critical conditions:

    (i)   *Tension pneumothorax*

        (a) suspect a tension pneumothorax in a patient with extreme dyspnoea, if there is tachycardia, hypotension, unequal chest expansion, absent or decreased breath sounds and distended neck veins

        (b) insert a wide-bore cannula into the second intercostal space in the mid-clavicular line on the affected side. Following initial decompression, proceed to formal intercostal tube drainage (see p. 473).

    (ii)   *Sucking chest wound with open pneumothorax*

        (a) cover with an occlusive dressing such as paraffin gauze under an adhesive film dressing, secured along three sides only. Leave the fourth side open for air to escape

        (b) proceed to formal intercostal catheter drainage (see p. 473).

    (iii) *Flail chest*

        (a) causes paradoxical movement of part of the chest wall and compromised ventilation

        (b) an associated haemothorax or pneumothorax will require an intercostal catheter chest drain to prevent the development of a tension pneumothorax, if positive-pressure ventilation is needed.

4   Circulation with haemorrhage control

    (i)   Apply a bulky sterile dressing to compress any external bleeding point

        (a) leave a tourniquet applied pre-hospital to stop life-threatening haemorrhage from an open extremity injury, until urgent surgical control of bleeding can be achieved.

    (ii)   Monitor the pulse, blood pressure, pulse oximetry and electrocardiogram (ECG).

    (iii) *Establish an i.v. infusion*

        (a) insert two large-bore (14- or 16-gauge) cannulae into the antecubital veins

        (b) one cannula should be below the diaphragm in mediastinal or neck injuries, e.g. in the femoral vein

        (c) although a central venous (CVP) line is useful both to administer fluids and to monitor the response to resuscitation, only senior ED staff should perform this under ultrasound guidance to minimize the potential complications of arterial puncture and pneumothorax. See page 476.

(iv) *Infusion fluid*
- (a) infuse warmed normal saline or Hartmann's (compound sodium lactate) in 250–500 mL amounts and assess the response
- (b) remember that in healthy adults the only signs associated with the loss of up to 30% of the circulatory blood volume (1500 mL) may be tachycardia with a narrowed pulse pressure
- (c) a consistent fall in systolic blood pressure potentially indicates that *at least* 30% of the blood volume may already have been lost
- (d) change infusion fluid to blood if the normal saline or Hartmann's (compound sodium lactate) fails to reverse hypotension, whilst early surgical intervention is considered
- (e) full cross-match takes 45 min, a type-specific cross-match takes 10 min, and O rhesus-negative blood is available immediately
- (f) use a blood warmer and macropore blood filter for multiple transfusions
  - give fresh frozen plasma 8–10 units and platelets after transfusing 8–10 units of blood or more, i.e. in a 1:1 ratio for a 'massive blood transfusion'.

(v) Give tranexamic acid 1 g i.v. over 10 min to the bleeding patient within 3 h after injury
- (a) follow by infusion of tranexamic acid 1 g over 8 h.

(vi) Send blood for haemoglobin, urea and electrolytes (U&Es), liver function tests (LFTs), lactate and blood sugar, and cross-match at least 4 units of blood according to the suspected injuries. Save serum for a drug screen in case alcohol or drug intoxication is subsequently suspected.

(vii) *Cardiac tamponade*
- (a) consider cardiac tamponade if there is persistent hypotension with distended neck veins that fill on inspiration (Kussmaul's sign), particularly following penetrating chest trauma
- (b) arrange an immediate focused ultrasound to look for pericardial fluid (blood)
- (c) call the surgical and/or cardiothoracic team for an urgent thoracotomy if there is persistent haemodynamic compromise (see p. 187).

5 *Disability: brief neurological evaluation*
(i) Assess the level of consciousness using the GCS (see p. 30).
(ii) Examine the eye movements, pupil size, shape and reactivity.

(iii) Assess for abnormal tone, weakness and gross sensory loss, or an asymmetrical response to pain if the patient is unconscious. Check the limb reflexes, including the plantar responses.

(iv) Examine the face and scalp for injuries.

6 Exposure: completely undress the patient

(i) Request a chest radiograph (CXR) and pelvic X-ray as part of a 'trauma series'. Perform these in the resuscitation bay without interrupting patient care
  (a) lateral cervical spine X-ray has now largely been replaced by incorporating the cervical spine with CT scanning of the head
  (b) or it should be part of a full series including AP and open-mouth views performed when all major life threats have been dealt with.

(ii) Examine the front of the abdomen, including the perineum, for evidence of blunt or penetrating trauma, e.g. seat-belt bruising or a tyre mark on the skin. Cover any exposed abdominal viscera with saline-soaked packs.

(iii) Assess for a major pelvic injury suggested by a urethral injury, limb length discrepancy or a rotational deformity without leg fracture, and/or on gentle palpation
  (a) make sure a pelvic binder is in place at the level of the greater trochanters for a major pelvic ring disruption.

(iv) Look for associated urethral injury. Suspect urethral transection if there is any bleeding from the urethral meatus, a scrotal haematoma or a high-riding prostate
  (a) do not attempt urethral catheterization if any of these are present
  (b) otherwise, insert a urethral catheter and measure the urine output, which should be at least 0.5 mL/kg per hour in the adult, and 1 mL/kg per hour in a child.

(v) Log-roll the patient and examine the back for evidence of blunt or penetrating trauma. Palpate the spine for deformity and widened interspinous gaps.

(vi) Perform a rectal examination to assess the anal sphincter tone, position of the prostate, integrity of the rectal wall, and to check for evidence of internal bleeding.

7 Pass a large-bore nasogastric tube, or orogastric tube if a basal skull or mid-face fracture is present (see p. 380).

8 Splint major limb fractures, cover compound injuries with sterile dressings and check the peripheral pulses.

9 Administer increments of morphine 2.5–5 mg i.v. titrated to analgesic response.

The above procedures will save life during the resuscitation phase, and allow a decision on priorities in proceeding to definitive care.

Table 5.2 Mnemonic for components of the history in multiple trauma

A	**A**llergies
M	**M**edications
P	**P**ast history, including alcohol and cigarette use; **P**regnancy
L	**L**ast meal
E	**E**vents/**E**nvironment relating to the injury, including time, speed of impact, initial vital signs, and any change in condition

Obtain as full a history as possible from ambulance crew, witnesses or relatives, as well as the patient. A useful mnemonic for remembering the components in the history is AMPLE (see Table 5.2).

Make sure an ongoing record is kept of all vital signs, clinical findings, and investigation results, and keep re-examining the patient regularly.

FURTHER DIAGNOSIS AND MANAGEMENT OF MULTIPLE INJURIES: DEFINITIVE CARE

This is considered under the following headings:
- Head and facial injuries.
- Neck injuries.
- Chest injuries.
- Abdominal and pelvic trauma.
- Additional orthopaedic injuries.

HEAD AND FACIAL INJURIES

DIAGNOSIS AND MANAGEMENT

1 Scalp
   (i) Look for lacerations, haematomas, penetrating wounds and foreign bodies.
   (ii) Palpate for evidence of deformity and fracture.
   (iii) Assess the level of consciousness if a major head injury is suspected, and manage as described on p. 29.

2 Face
   (i) Check the integrity of the airway again, and remember the possibility of an unrecognized neck injury.
   (ii) Look for bruising, swelling or deformity suggesting orbital, nasal, malar or mandibular fractures (see p. 377).

(iii) Look for parotid and facial nerve damage in injuries to the face in the area in front of the ear.

(iv) Clean and evaluate all facial lacerations. They will require meticulous debridement and formal closure when the patient's condition is stable, and all serious injuries have been dealt with.

3 Eyes

(i) Inspect the eyes for evidence of penetrating or blunt injury. Look for specific conditions such as iris prolapse, hyphaema, lens dislocation and traumatic mydriasis (see p. 350).

(ii) Assess the pupil size and reactions, and look for an afferent pupillary defect (Marcus Gunn pupil – see page 356) as evidence of vitreous or retinal haemorrhage and/or a large retinal detachment.

(iii) Check the visual acuity and eye movements.

4 Nose

(i) Examine for evidence of blood or cerebrospinal fluid (CSF) leakage suggesting a basal skull fracture (see p. 31).

(ii) Palpate for deformity and nasal bone fracture (see p. 367).

(iii) Look specifically for a septal haematoma, which, if large, will require incision and drainage to reduce the risk of subsequent cartilage necrosis (see p. 367).

5 Mouth

(i) Examine for broken or missing teeth. They may have been inhaled (see p. 376).

(ii) Check for dental malocclusion, suggesting maxillary or mandibular fracture (see p. 377).

(iii) Assess for nasopharyngeal bleeding, which may be profuse and associated with a basal skull fracture. Look for any tongue lacerations, although they rarely need repairing (see p. 376).

6 Ears

(i) Examine for skin and cartilage damage, which will require drainage and suture later.

(ii) Consider perforation of the eardrum, although if frank bleeding is seen, do not examine with a speculum to avoid introducing infection

(a) this bleeding may be associated with either a temporal bone fracture or damage to the external ear canal (see p. 363).

NECK INJURIES

CERVICAL SPINE INJURY

This should be considered in all patients with localized neck pain or pain on palpation following trauma. It should also be *assumed* in any unconscious head injury, multiply injured patient, a patient under the influence of alcohol or drugs, and a patient with a locally distracting injury above the clavicles.

DIAGNOSIS

1 Ask about local pain or tenderness on midline palpation if the patient is conscious, and about any associated limb weakness or sensory deficit noticed.

2 Check the vital signs. A cervical or high thoracic spinal cord lesion will cause respiratory difficulty, tachypnoea and abdominal breathing.

   (i) Loss of sympathetic tone will also cause bradycardia, hypotension and hypothermia from vasodilation if the ambient temperature is low (neurogenic shock).

3 Palpate for areas of tenderness, swelling or deformity in the neck. Assess for limb tone, weakness, reflex loss and sensory deficit, including loss of perineal sensation and anal tone.

4 Describe any motor weakness found by the myotome and reflex abnormalities:

   (i) Myotomes in the upper limb. Nerve roots C5 to T1 supply the muscles of the upper limb (see Table 5.3).

   (ii) Use the Medical Research Council scale to grade muscle weakness, so that the same terminology is used by each doctor examining the patient (see Table 5.4).

   (iii) Reflexes in the upper limb: assess for the biceps, triceps and supinator upper limb reflexes, which indicate normal or other functioning of certain motor roots (see Table 5.5 for motor roots of the reflexes)

      (a) use reinforcement (Jendrassik's manoeuvre) before concluding that a reflex is absent, e.g. ask the patient to clench the teeth hard or hold the knees together when testing a reflex.

Table 5.3 Myotomes in the upper limb and their associated actions

Root	Action
C5	Shoulder abduction
C6, C7	Shoulder adduction
C5, C6	Elbow flexion
C7	Elbow extension
C6	Pronation and supination
(C6), C7	Wrist flexion
C6, (C7)	Wrist extension
C8	Finger flexion
C7	Finger extension
T1	Intrinsic hand muscles

Table 5.4 Medical Research Council (MRC) scale used to grade muscle weakness

Recorded grade	Physical finding
Grade 0	Complete paralysis
Grade 1	A flicker of contraction only
Grade 2	Movement possible only if gravity is eliminated
Grade 3	Movement against gravity
Grade 4	Movement against gravity and resistance
Grade 5	Normal power

Table 5.5 Reflexes in the upper limb

Reflex	Root
Biceps	C5, (C6)
Supinator	(C5), C6
Triceps	(C6), C7, C8

Table 5.6 Dermatomes supplying the upper limb

Root	Dermatomal distribution
C5	Outer upper arm
C6	Outer forearm
C7	Middle finger
C8	Inner forearm
T1	Inner upper arm

5 Describe sensory deficit by dermatomes:
- (i) Assess sensation by testing pain fibres using pinprick (spinothalamic tracts), and examine fine touch or joint position sense (posterior columns).
- (ii) Dermatomes C5–T1 supply the upper limb (see Table 5.6).
- (iii) Dermatomes C4 and T2 are adjacent on the front of the chest at the level of the first and second ribs.

6 The myotomes, reflexes and dermatomes in the leg are described on p. 280.

7 Cervical spine imaging
- (i) *Lateral cervical spine X-ray:*
  - (a) make sure an adequate view is obtained and that all seven cervical vertebrae and the C7/T1 junction are visualized. A swimmer's view may be required
  - (b) look for appropriate alignment of the cervical spine longitudinal lines. Anterior displacement of >3 mm implies ligament disruption and cervical spine instability (see Fig. 5.1)

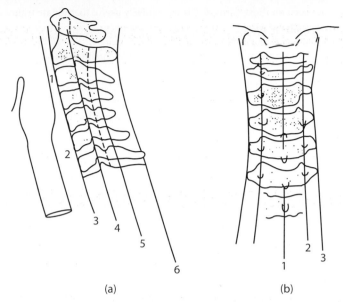

Figure 5.1 Cervical spine x-ray in the adult.
(a) Lateral view: (1) retropharyngeal space (<5 mm), (2) retrotracheal space (less than the width of one vertebral body), (3) anterior longitudinal ligament line, (4) posterior longitudinal ligament line, (5) spinolaminar line, (6) posterior spinal line. Lines 3, 4, 5 and 6 should all be parallel, following the normal gentle lordotic curve of the cervical spine. The spinal cord runs between lines 4 and 5.
(b) Anteroposterior view: (1) interspinous line, (2) foramen transversarium line, (3) transverse processes line. Lines 1, 2 and 3 should be straight in the normal neck.

    (c) observe the bony vertebrae for signs of fractures such as wedge and teardrop. Examine the soft-tissue shadows in front of the vertebral bodies (see Fig. 5.1)
      – the retropharyngeal space should be <5 mm between C1 and C4/C5
      – the retrotracheal space should be less than the width of one vertebral body in adults between C4/C5 and T1.
  (ii) *Open-mouth odontoid view*: examine the odontoid peg and dens of C2, and the lateral masses of C1 for evidence of fracture.
 (iii) *Anteroposterior cervical spine X-ray*: look for rotation of the vertebrae, loss of joint space and transverse process fracture.
 (iv) *Cervical spine CT scan*: Perform this following plain cervical spine X-rays if bony injury is still suspected clinically, or to further define any cervical fracture and vertebral subluxation

seen on those films. CT is particularly useful to evaluate trauma patients with:

(a) abnormal plain films

(b) suspicious, inadequate or incomplete plain films

(c) neurological deficit

(d) suspected vascular, airway, oesophageal or other soft-tissue injury

(e) head injury requiring CT head scan, particularly if intubated.

(v) MRI is more sensitive than CT and plain X-ray for identifying soft-tissue damage such as ligamentous injuries, disc herniation or a haemorrhage causing compression of the spinal cord or cervical nerve roots

(a) it is rarely available in the acute situation, but may be arranged subsequently particularly in the presence of focal neurological signs.

MANAGEMENT

1 Always apply a semi-rigid collar, minimize head movements in any suspected neck injury, and use laterally placed sandbags taped to the forehead to prevent head rotation.

2 Arrange urgent airway control with orotracheal intubation for the unconscious patient or for respiratory distress.

(i) Only an airway-skilled doctor should perform this, usually by a rapid sequence induction (RSI) intubation technique (see p. 467) with in-line manual immobilization to protect the neck from any movement.

3 Restore the circulatory volume if the patient is hypotensive.

(i) First look for sources of blood loss **before** diagnosing neurogenic shock.

(ii) Neurogenic shock causes hypotension in a patient with a cervical cord injury due to loss of sympathetic tone with vasodilation and bradycardia.

(iii) Place a urinary catheter to monitor urinary output.

4 Severe ligamentous damage with cervical spine instability can occur, with an apparently normal X-ray.

(i) This is more likely in young children with serious spinal injuries, 20–30% of whom have normal X-rays and/or CT scan (SCIWORA – spinal cord injury without radiological abnormality).

(ii) Neck hyperextension may cause predominant weakness of the arms in elderly patients with cervical spondylosis, often without any associated fracture or dislocation, known as the central cord syndrome.

(iii) Arrange an MRI in these circumstances.

5   Refer all suspected cervical spine injuries to the orthopaedic or surgical team and begin pressure-area nursing.

6   The value of high-dose methylprednisolone to improve neurological outcome in patients with complete or incomplete spinal cord damage is unconvincing, controversial and may cause harm. It has now been abandoned in most centres.

   (i)   Start treatment within 8 h of injury, guided by the advice of the regional spinal injuries unit.

   (ii) Infuse methylprednisolone 30 mg/kg over 15 min, followed 45 min later by 5.4 mg/kg per hour for 23 h.

AIRWAY INJURY

DIAGNOSIS

1   Airway injuries may be penetrating or blunt, isolated, or associated with multiple injuries.

2   Patients may present with a hoarse voice, pain, stridor, cough and/or haemoptysis.

3   Examine for local swelling, subcutaneous emphysema, respiratory distress, pneumothorax or haemothorax.

4   Perform anteroposterior and lateral cervical spine X-rays and a CXR, only if the patient is considered stable.

MANAGEMENT

1   Call for urgent senior ED staff to help. Do not leave the patient unattended at any stage.

2   Perform endotracheal intubation or cricothyrotomy, or insert an endotracheal tube directly into a gaping wound in the trachea to maintain patency of the airway.

3   Refer the patient immediately to the surgical team for admission.

   (i)   Arrange a CT scan once the airway has been protected by an endotracheal tube.

VASCULAR INJURY IN THE NECK

DIAGNOSIS AND MANAGEMENT

1   Vascular injury causes obvious external haemorrhage, or internal bleeding with rapid haematoma formation, which may compromise the airway.

2   *Never* attempt to probe or explore any penetrating wound in the ED. Leave all penetrating objects *in situ*.

3   The patient will require angiography and panendoscopy after urgent surgical referral to arrange formal wound exploration in theatre.

NERVE INJURY IN THE NECK

DIAGNOSIS AND MANAGEMENT

1   Damage to the following nerves causes specific signs and symptoms:
- (i) *Recurrent laryngeal branch of the vagus*: hoarseness and vocal cord paralysis.
- (ii) *Accessory nerve*: loss of function of trapezius and sternomastoid.
- (iii) *Phrenic nerve*: loss of diaphragmatic movement.
- (iv) *Hypoglossal nerve*: deviation of the tongue to the affected side.
- (v) *Cervical sympathetic cord*: Horner's syndrome, with partial ptosis, a constricted pupil, and decreased sweating on the same side of the face.

2   Refer any of these injuries to the surgical team.

OESOPHAGEAL INJURY

DIAGNOSIS AND MANAGEMENT

1   Oesophageal injury in the neck causes dysphagia, drooling and localized pain, with the development of surgical emphysema.

2   Refer this rare condition to the surgical team for immediate admission.
- (i) Arrange a CT scan providing the airway is protected by an endotracheal tube as necessary.

NECK SPRAIN

DIAGNOSIS

1   Neck sprain is most commonly associated with hyperextension injuries resulting from sudden deceleration in a motor vehicle collision.
- (i) The lay term for this mechanism of injury is 'whiplash'. In practice, neck sprain occurs with other directions of impact, including hyperflexion.

2   The resultant neck pain and stiffness often go unnoticed at the time of injury. Patients typically present 12–24 h later, often with symptoms of headache.

3   The pain may radiate to the shoulders and arms, causing paraesthesiae, but neurological examination does not show any objective deficit. Neck movements are restricted by pain.

4   Cervical spine X-ray may show loss of the normal anterior curvature due to muscle spasm.

MANAGEMENT

1   Treat the patient with a non-steroidal anti-inflammatory analgesic drug (NSAID), such as ibuprofen 200–400 mg orally t.d.s. or naproxen 250 mg orally t.d.s., and encourage early mobilization.

2 Refer the patient to the physiotherapy team if the pain fails to settle, for heat treatment and motion exercises.

3 Unfortunately, symptoms may continue for months, and may be exacerbated by further minor injuries.

CHEST INJURIES

PNEUMOTHORAX

DIAGNOSIS

1 *Tension pneumothorax*
- (i)   This causes extreme respiratory distress, tachypnoea and hypotension. There is tracheal deviation away from the affected side, distended neck veins, loss of chest expansion on the affected side, a hyper-resonant percussion note, and diminished or absent breath sounds.
- (ii) Perform immediate decompression. Use a large-bore i.v. cannula inserted into the second intercostal space in the mid-clavicular line, followed by placement of an intercostal drain (see p. 473).

2 *Simple pneumothorax*
- (i)   This is caused by blunt or penetrating chest trauma, and penetrating abdominal trauma breaching the diaphragm.
- (ii) It is surprisingly easy to miss. Examine for subcutaneous emphysema, decreased chest expansion, and quiet breath sounds.
- (iii) Confirm the diagnosis with an erect CXR to highlight a small apical pneumothorax, provided there is no possibility of spinal injury
  - (a) the supine CXR may appear normal and miss a small pneumothorax lying anteriorly
  - (b) however, a CT scan of the chest will show the pneumothorax.

MANAGEMENT

1 Most cases of traumatic pneumothorax require chest-drain insertion to avoid the subsequent development of tension, particularly if positive-pressure ventilation is necessary, or transport by air.
- (i)   Insert an intercostal drain into the fifth or sixth intercostal space in the mid-axillary line (see p. 473).

2 A small asymptomatic pneumothorax may be closely observed.

3 Refer all of these injuries to the surgical team.

HAEMOTHORAX

DIAGNOSIS

1 This results from chest wall damage, penetrating or blunt lung injury and great vessel damage.

2 It causes hypotension, respiratory difficulty with reduced chest expansion, quiet breath sounds and a dull percussion note at the base of the affected lung.

3 Request an erect or semi-erect CXR to identify a fluid level, provided there is no possibility of spinal injury.

4 Look for diffuse ground-glass haziness over one hemithorax if the CXR is taken supine, which is easy to miss.

5 Alternatively, take a lateral decubitus CXR, although the diagnosis is usually made on CT chest scan.

MANAGEMENT

1 Give high-dose oxygen and commence i.v. fluid, including blood.

2 Insert a large-bore 32- or 36-French gauge intercostal drain in the fifth or sixth intercostal space in the mid-axillary line, using blunt dissection down to and through the pleura (see p. 473).

3 A thoracotomy may be required if bleeding is significant i.e. >1500 mL or persists (see p. 187).

RIB AND STERNUM FRACTURES

DIAGNOSIS

1 These injuries are associated with direct trauma, including from a seat belt. They cause localized pain and tenderness, worse on breathing or springing the chest wall.

2 Associated injury may occur with fractures in the following areas:
   (i) *Clavicle, first and second ribs*: damage to the subclavian vessels, aorta, trachea, main bronchus, and spinal cord or brachial plexus.
   (ii) *Sternum*: damage to the myocardium, great vessels and upper thoracic spine.
   (iii) *Right lower ribs*: damage to the liver and right kidney.
   (iv) *Left lower ribs*: damage to the spleen and left kidney.

3 A flail segment with paradoxical chest wall movement from multiple rib fractures in two sites causes hypoxia, mainly from the underlying pulmonary contusion.

4 Perform an ECG to exclude myocardial contusion (see below).

5 Request a CXR to look for the associated complications of pneumothorax, haemothorax and a widened mediastinum, not simply to visualize the fractures.
   (i) A lateral sternal X-ray is indicated for a suspected sternal fracture.

MANAGEMENT

1 Give the patient high-flow oxygen by face mask and aim for an oxygen saturation of 94%.

2 Commence i.v. resuscitation as required, insert an intercostal drain if indicated, and administer adequate analgesia such as increments of morphine 2.5–5 mg i.v.

3 Refer the following patients to the surgical team for admission:
    (i) Pneumothorax, haemothorax.
    (ii) Fractured sternum with severe pain or ECG abnormalities.
    (iii) Injury to other thoracic or abdominal organs.
    (iv) Pre-existing lung disease with poor respiratory reserve.
    (v) Rib fractures with significant pain. These patients may require a thoracic epidural.

4 Positive-pressure ventilation may be required for deteriorating respiratory function, although an intercostal drain must be inserted first for any pneumothorax, however small.

5 Discharge remaining patients with uncomplicated rib fractures or an isolated sternal fracture with a normal ECG and CXR.

6 Provide an analgesic such as paracetamol 500 mg and codeine phosphate 8 mg two tablets orally q.d.s.
    (i) Recommend regular deep-breathing exercises to prevent atelectasis.
    (ii) Contact the general practitioner (GP) by fax or letter.

MYOCARDIAL CONTUSION

DIAGNOSIS

1 This is due to blunt deceleration injury and is associated with rib fractures, sternal fracture and chest wall contusion. It is difficult to diagnose as there is no agreed gold standard.

2 It may be asymptomatic, but can cause chest pain, arrhythmias or rarely cause transient right ventricular dysfunction with distended neck veins, tachycardia and hypotension.

3 Gain i.v. access and send blood for full blood count (FBC), U&Es, cardiac biomarkers and group and save (G&S).
    (i) Troponins are a reliable indicator of cardiac myocyte damage, but do not quantify the potential risk
        (a) in addition they may diagnose antecedent myocardial infarction, if raised.

4 Perform an ECG.
    (i) Myocardial contusion may result in ventricular conduction abnormalities and arrhythmias.

(ii) ECG abnormalities range from sinus tachycardia, atrial fibrillation, bundle branch block and ventricular extrasystoles to non-specific ST and T wave abnormalities or ST elevation.

5 Request a CXR.

6 Organize an echocardiogram if hypotensive, which may show wall motion abnormalities but is most useful to exclude cardiac tamponade or acute valvular rupture.

MANAGEMENT

1 Give the patient high-dose oxygen and administer a cautious fluid challenge if hypotensive.

2 Give morphine 2.5–5 mg i.v. with an antiemetic such as metoclopramide 10 mg i.v. for pain.

3 Admit all patients with arrhythmias and haemodynamic instability to the intensive care unit (ICU).

4 Refer a stable patient with ECG abnormalities, age >50 years or pre-existing cardiac disease to a coronary care unit (CCU) for cardiac monitoring if there is evidence of significant blunt myocardial trauma with a raised troponin.

5 Discharge home patients <50 years with normal ECG findings, and without a history of cardiac disease with oral analgesia.

AORTIC RUPTURE

DIAGNOSIS

1 This occurs following high-speed deceleration injury, when the aorta is torn just distal to the left subclavian artery.

(i) It is increasingly being recognized in lower-speed injuries including side-impact.

2 Always consider this diagnosis in any deceleration injury >60 k.p.h. (45 m.p.h.) or following a fall from >5 m (15 ft).

3 Only 10–15% of patients with rupture of the thoracic aorta survive to reach hospital.

4 Clinical signs of aortic rupture are subtle or absent and so diagnosis is suspected largely based on the mechanism of injury, or from a history of chest or interscapular pain, unequal blood pressures in each arm, or different femoral and brachial pulse volume, and the initial CXR.

5 Insert two large-bore i.v. cannulae and cross-match 4–6 units of blood.

6 Perform a CXR and look for the following signs of aortic rupture:

(i) Widened mediastinum (≥8 cm on a 1 m supine anteroposterior X-ray):

(a) 10% of these patients will have a contained aortic rupture confirmed

       (b) other causes of a widened mediastinum include a mediastinal haematoma from sternal fracture, lower cervical or thoracic spine fracture, oesophageal injury, local venous oozing and projection artefact.

   (ii) Blurred aortic outline with obliteration of the aortic knuckle.

   (iii) Left apical cap of fluid in the pleural space and a left haemothorax.

   (iv) Depressed left main stem bronchus.

   (v) Displacement of the trachea to the right.

   (vi) Displacement of a nasogastric tube in the oesophagus to the right.

7 Look for a cervical, thoracic or sternal fracture clinically and on X-ray, although exclusion of aortic rupture remains necessary irrespective of the other clinical findings when the CXR is suggestive.

8 Perform a high-speed helical CT angiogram scan of the chest to look for blood contiguous with the aorta, or an abnormal aortic wall indicative of rupture.

MANAGEMENT

1 Administer fluid cautiously.

   (i) Initial hypotension responds to modest fluid replacement in contained aortic rupture.

   (ii) Take care to avoid over-transfusion or hypertension from poorly controlled pain, etc.

2 Refer the patient urgently to the surgical or vascular team for further evaluation, if the patient has a high-risk mechanism of injury and positive radiographic findings.

   (i) Urgent thoracotomy and repair are indicated when these show a rupture, or endovascular stenting if the expertise is available locally.

DIAPHRAGM RUPTURE

DIAGNOSIS

1 This may occur from blunt or penetrating chest or abdominal trauma, including crush fracture of the pelvis. Left-sided lesions are more common and allow eventration of the stomach or intestine into the chest.

2 75% of patients with ruptured diaphragm have associated intra-abdominal injuries.

3 It causes difficulty in breathing, and occasionally bowel sounds are audible in the chest.

4 Perform a CXR and look for the following signs seen in diaphragm rupture:

   (i) Haemothorax, pneumothorax, elevated hemidiaphragm and coils of bowel or a nasogastric tube curled up in the left lower chest.

   (ii) The diagnosis is often missed, as the CXR appears normal in up to 25% of cases.

5 Arrange a CT scan of the chest and abdomen to define the injury.

MANAGEMENT

1   Decompress the stomach with a nasogastric tube.

2   Carefully insert an intercostal drain for an associated haemothorax or pneumothorax, using blunt dissection down to and through the parietal pleura (see p. 473).

   (i)   **Never** use the trocar introducer to insert the drain.

3   Refer the patient to the surgical team following resuscitation.

OESOPHAGEAL RUPTURE

DIAGNOSIS

1   This rare injury is most commonly associated with penetrating trauma or following blunt trauma to the upper abdomen.

   (i)   Other causes include instrumentation, swallowing a sharp object, and spontaneous rupture from vomiting (Boerhaave's syndrome).

2   The patient complains of retrosternal pain, difficulty in swallowing and occasionally haematemesis. Look for cervical subcutaneous emphysema.

3   Establish venous access with a large-bore i.v. cannula.

4   Request a CXR to look for a widened mediastinum or mediastinal air (pneumomediastinum), a left pneumothorax, pleural effusion or haemothorax. These findings in the absence of rib fracture should suggest the possibility of rupture.

5   Request a CT scan to better define air in the mediastinum or perioesophageal fluid collections.

MANAGEMENT

1   Administer oxygen and replace fluids. Give morphine 2.5–5 mg i.v. for pain with an antiemetic.

2   Commence broad-spectrum antibiotics if rupture is considered likely, such as gentamicin 5 mg/kg i.v., ampicillin 1 g i.v., and metronidazole 500 mg i.v.

3   Carefully insert an intercostal drain if there is a pleural effusion.

4   Refer the patient to the surgical team for a Gastrografin swallow and/or oesophagoscopy, followed by surgical repair if feasible.

PENETRATING CHEST INJURY

DIAGNOSIS

1   Penetrating chest injury may be predicted by wounds:

   (i)   Medial to the nipple line anteriorly or tips of the scapulae posteriorly – high risk of heart or great vessel injury.

    (ii)   Above the umbilicus – injury to the lungs, heart or great vessels.

    (iii) Below the fourth intercostal space – injury to the abdominal contents as well.

2   Patients usually present with pain and dyspnoea. However, some patients are deceptively undistressed.

3   The patient may become hypotensive due to blood loss from a haemothorax, or the development of cardiac tamponade or tension pneumothorax.

4   Gain i.v. access and send bloods.

5   Request a CXR to look for any of the above complications.

6   Arrange an urgent focused bedside ultrasound if cardiac tamponade is suspected, particularly in the presence of a raised JVP.

MANAGEMENT

1   Assess and secure the airway, give high-flow oxygen, and perform needle thoracocentesis if required. Commence fluid resuscitation.

2   80% of penetrating chest injuries are managed conservatively with the insertion of an intercostal drain (see p. 473).

3   Injuries involving the heart and great vessels require a thoracotomy, either in the ED or urgently in theatre.

4   *Emergency department thoracotomy*
    Patients in cardiac arrest secondary to trauma require an immediate thoracotomy in the resuscitation room:

    (i)   Optimum survival rates are found in patients with:
       (a) palpable pulse and spontaneous respirations at the scene of the incident
       (b) elapsed time since cardiac arrest of <10 min
       (c) penetrating trauma secondary to stab wound or low-velocity bullet.

    (ii) Conversely traumatic cardiac arrest is nearly always fatal in patients with:
       (a) blunt chest trauma or a high-velocity bullet wound
       (b) absence of palpable pulse or respiratory effort at the scene of the incident
       (c) elapsed time without signs of life >15 min.

5   *Operating room thoracotomy*
    Transfer patients with the following injuries *immediately* to the operating theatre for an urgent thoracotomy:

    (i)   Penetrating cardiac injury.
    (ii) Massive haemothorax with >1500 mL initial drainage or >200 mL/h for 2–4 h.
    (iii) Persistent large air leak suggesting tracheobronchial injury.
    (iv) Cardiac tamponade following trauma.

ABDOMINAL AND PELVIC TRAUMA

BLUNT ABDOMINAL TRAUMA

DIAGNOSIS

1 This should be suspected in the following:
- (i) Road traffic crash or a fall from a height, particularly if there is evidence of chest, pelvic or long-bone injury (e.g. injuries on either side of the abdomen).
- (ii) Trauma victims with unexplained hypotension in the absence of obvious external bleeding or a thoracic injury.

2 Ask about referred shoulder-tip pain or localized pain suggesting lower rib, pelvic or thoracolumbar spine injury.

3 Look for the imprint of clothing or tyre marks as indicators of potential intra-abdominal injury.
- (i) Bruising from a lap seat belt may be associated with duodenal, pancreatic or small bowel injury, and/or fracture-dislocation of the lumbar spine.

4 Examine the chest, as well as the abdomen, pelvic area and perineum including genitalia. Consider a vaginal examination when there are signs of local injury.

5 Log-roll the patient to examine the thoracolumbar spine. Inspect the buttock area and perform a rectal examination.

6 Insert two large-bore i.v. cannulae and send blood for FBC, U&Es, LFTs, blood sugar, lipase/amylase, and cross-match at least 4 units of blood.

7 Request initial radiology including chest, pelvis and thoracolumbar spine X-rays.
- (i) Erect CXR: this may demonstrate a thoracic injury or free gas under the diaphragm. Look particularly for lower rib fractures that may be associated with liver, splenic and renal injury.
- (ii) Pelvis X-ray: a fractured pelvis may be associated with major intra-abdominal or retroperitoneal injuries.

MANAGEMENT

1 Give high-flow oxygen. Assess response to initial crystalloid such as normal saline or Hartmann's (compound sodium lactate), and commence blood for continuing shock.

2 Pass a nasogastric tube to drain the stomach.

3 Insert a urethral catheter to measure the urine output and to look for haematuria.
- (i) Omit this if a urethral injury is suspected from blood at the meatus, a scrotal haematoma or a high-riding prostate on rectal examination.

4   Consider the need for an immediate laparotomy, call the surgeon if not present and alert theatre. Indications include:

    (i)   Persistent shock.

    (ii) Evisceration or penetrating object in situ.

    (iii) Radiological evidence of free gas or ruptured diaphragm.

5   Commonly there are no immediate indications for laparotomy and further investigation is needed:

    (i)   *Ultrasound*

        (a) focused assessment by sonography for trauma (FAST) ultrasound is ideal for unstable patients unable to be transferred for CT evaluation

        (b) it is rapid, repeatable at the bedside, non-invasive and highly sensitive for free intraperitoneal fluid, i.e. blood from a haemoperitoneum. It can also demonstrate cardiac tamponade

        (c) however, it is operator dependent, and may miss hollow viscus, diaphragmatic and retroperitoneal injuries.

    (ii) *CT scan*

        (a) patients *must* be stable enough to be transported out of the resuscitation room

        (b) CT provides anatomical information on the intra-abdominal organs injured allowing non-operative management

        (c) CT also visualizes the retroperitoneum, pelvis and lower chest, although it can still miss hollow viscus and diaphragmatic injuries.

    (iii) *Diagnostic peritoneal lavage (DPL)*

        (a) has largely been entirely superseded by FAST and CT scans

        (b) whilst highly sensitive for intraperitoneal bleeding it provides no indication about its source or volume, and misses retroperitoneal injury to the duodenum, pancreas, kidney and pelvis, or a diaphragm rupture.

6   Involve the admitting surgical team at all stages of investigation, as the decision on emergency laparotomy is theirs.

PENETRATING ABDOMINAL TRAUMA

DIAGNOSIS

1   Penetrating abdominal injury may occur in stab wounds, industrial incidents, road traffic crashes, explosions and gunshot wounds.

2   Gunshot wounds may be divided into three types:

    (i)   *High-velocity wound*

        (a) the muzzle velocity of a bullet from a high-velocity rifle is >1000 m/s

        (b) a small entry wound is associated with gross internal tissue damage from cavitation and a large exit wound.

(ii) *Low-velocity wound*
- (a) the muzzle velocity from a hand gun reaches 250 m/s
- (b) the bullet causes local internal damage by perforation and laceration, often passing through several structures and deflecting to end up in a different body area.

(iii) *Shotgun wound*
- (a) usually fatal from a range of <3 m (10 ft), and causes massive superficial internal damage from close range (<7 m)
- (b) there is scattering of shot if the shotgun is fired from >7 m, perforating structures within the abdomen.

3   An entry wound may be obvious, with evisceration of bowel, or may be difficult to find especially if hidden by a gluteal fold or in the perineum.

4   The most important signs to look for are hypotension and shock.

5   Abdominal examination is unreliable as abdominal tenderness on examination is absent in up to 50% of patients with acute haemoperitoneum.
- (i) Positive examination findings include local rigidity and guarding with reduced bowel sounds.

6   Remember that an associated chest injury can occur with any wound above the umbilicus.

7   Insert a large-bore i.v. cannula and send blood for FBC, U&Es, lipase/amylase and cross-match.

8   Request a CXR to look for associated thoracic injury, and an abdominal X-ray (AXR) to assess for metallic foreign bodies.

9   Arrange a CT scan with i.v. contrast particularly if non-operative management is considered.

MANAGEMENT

1   Cover any exposed bowel with saline-soaked pads.

2   Give oxygen, and replace fluid cautiously with normal saline aiming for SBP 80–100 mmHg. Titrate analgesic requirements by administering 2.5–5.0 mg morphine i.v.

3   Commence broad-spectrum antibiotics, e.g. gentamicin 5 mg/kg i.v., ampicillin 1 g i.v. and metronidazole 500 mg i.v. Give tetanus prophylaxis.

4   Refer all patients to the surgical team for urgent admission and laparotomy for all gunshot wounds and the vast majority of stab wounds.

PELVIC INJURY

The major complication of a pelvic fracture is massive blood loss, with up to 3 L or more of concealed haemorrhage, which may continue despite resuscitation.

DIAGNOSIS

1   Pelvic injuries usually result from high-energy blunt trauma in road traffic crashes, crush injuries and from falls.

2   Associated bladder, urethral, rectal and vaginal injuries occur, which account for further morbidity. A ruptured diaphragm must also be excluded.

3   There is local pain, tenderness and bruising. Persistent hypotension associated with pelvic haemorrhage is an ominous sign.

4   Rectal examination is indicated to identify rectal or urethral injury.

5   Insert two large-bore i.v. cannulae and send blood for FBC, U&Es, lipase/amylase, coagulation profile, blood sugar, lactate and cross-match 4–6 units of blood.

6   Request a pelvic X-ray in **all** multi-trauma patients, especially if there is unexplained hypotension.

7   Pelvic fractures associated with the greatest risk of haemorrhage include:
     (i)   Quadripartite 'butterfly' fracture of all four pubic rami.
     (ii)   Open-book fracture with diastasis of the symphysis pubis over 2.5 cm.
     (iii) Vertical shear fracture with hemipelvic disruption, such as the Malgaigne fracture.

8   Arrange a CT scan with i.v. contrast providing the patient is not haemodynamically unstable.

MANAGEMENT

1   Give high-flow oxygen. Commence i.v. fluid resuscitation, and change to blood and blood products early.

2   Do not attempt to catheterize the bladder if urethral rupture is suspected, but await assistance from an experienced ED doctor, or the surgical team.

3   Fashion a pelvic sling from a sheet secured tightly around the front of the pelvis, or preferably use one of the radiolucent, commercially available pelvic binders applied at the level of the greater trochanters.

4   Exclude intraperitoneal bleeding with an early bedside ultrasound (FAST), or CT scan with i.v. contrast when stable enough to image to define the extent of the injuries.

5   Call the surgical, orthopaedic and interventional radiology team immediately.
     (i)   Control of haemorrhage secondary to pelvic trauma may require external fixation, arterial embolization and/or laparotomy with pelvic packing, followed by admission to ICU.

BLUNT RENAL INJURY

DIAGNOSIS

1   This may be associated with injury to the vertebral column, lower ribs, ureters, aorta, inferior vena cava and intra-abdominal contents.

2   Blunt renal trauma causes haematuria, loin pain and tenderness, and rarely a flank mass may be felt.

3 Hypotension is due to retroperitoneal bleeding or sometimes an associated paralytic ileus.

4 Insert a large-bore i.v. cannula and send blood for FBC, U&Es and cross-match 2–4 units of blood.

5 Request a thoracolumbar spine X-ray to exclude skeletal trauma.

6 Proceed to radiological imaging of the kidney and ureters. Indications include:
  (i) Significant deceleration injury with the risk of renal pedicle injury.
  (ii) Local physical signs such as pain or ecchymoses.
  (iii) Macroscopic haematuria.
  (iv) Microscopic haematuria with shock (systolic blood pressure ≤90 mmHg) at any time.
  (v) Penetrating proximity trauma.

7 Request a CT scan with i.v. contrast to evaluate suspected renal injury in the presence of any of the above.

MANAGEMENT

1 Resuscitate the patient with i.v. fluids and exclude associated intra-abdominal injuries with ultrasound (FAST) or CT.

2 Refer the patient to the surgical team for admission and observation. Over 85% of blunt renal injuries settle on conservative management with bed rest and analgesia.

PENETRATING RENAL INJURY

DIAGNOSIS

1 These are rare and usually involve injury to the abdominal contents, ureter or vertebral column. They may be multiple or associated with penetrating anterior truncal injury.

2 There is usually haematuria, localized pain, and tenderness, although significant renal or ureteric injury may be present without haematuria.

3 Ureteric colic can occur from the passage of blood clots.

4 Insert a large-bore i.v. cannula and send blood for FBC, U&Es, and cross-match 2–4 units.

5 Perform special imaging with a CT scan with i.v. contrast (or an IVP if that is all that is available).
  (i) These demonstrate the nature of the renal injury and also confirm the presence and normal function of the other kidney.
  (ii) CT scan gives essential additional information on intra- or retroperitoneal injury.

MANAGEMENT

1   Resuscitate the patient with i.v. fluids, commence antibiotics such as gentamicin 5 mg/kg i.v. and ampicillin 1 g i.v. and give tetanus prophylaxis as indicated.

2   Refer the patient to the surgical team for admission.

BLADDER AND URETHRAL INJURIES

DIAGNOSIS

1   These injuries are more commonly associated with direct blunt trauma to the lower abdomen and with major pelvic fractures.

2   *Bladder rupture*
    This may be intraperitoneal or extraperitoneal.
    (i)   Intraperitoneal is associated with shock and peritonism.
    (ii)   Extraperitoneal:
           (a) causes signs of urine extravasation and local bruising
           (b) >95% have macroscopic haematuria.

3   *Urethral rupture*
    This may occur to the membranous or bulbous urethra.
    (i)   Membranous urethra:
           (a) associated with difficulty voiding urine and urethral bleeding, which mimics extraperitoneal rupture of the bladder
           (b) rectal examination reveals a high-riding prostate, often with an underlying boggy haematoma.
    (ii)   Bulbous urethra:
           (a) caused by a straddle injury (falling astride an object)
           (b) results in local perineal bruising, pain and meatal bleeding.

MANAGEMENT

1   Call for a senior ED doctor and attempt to gently catheterize the bladder, but stop if any resistance at all is encountered.

2   Treat the patient for pain and blood loss, and give antibiotics such as gentamicin 5 mg/kg i.v. and ampicillin 1 g i.v.

3   Refer to the surgical team for an ascending urethrogram or cystogram, **before** a CT scan of the abdomen with i.v. contrast is performed.

ADDITIONAL ORTHOPAEDIC INJURIES IN MULTIPLE TRAUMA

Early orthopaedic team involvement is common for pelvic trauma particularly if associated with haemorrhage, as well as for thoracic and lumbosacral spine injury, and major limb injury.

THORACIC AND LUMBOSACRAL SPINE INJURY

DIAGNOSIS

1 This type of injury is caused by blunt trauma from a fall, a direct blow or following a traffic crash. A fractured sternum may accompany a hyperflexion wedge fracture of the upper thoracic spine.

2 Always examine the back in multi-trauma patients. Maintain spinal precautions and carefully log-roll all patients with a suspected spinal injury.

3 Look for bruising, deformity and evidence of penetrating injury.

4 Palpate for localized tenderness and swelling around the vertebral column or for an abnormal gap between the spinous processes suggesting a fracture, or overlying the renal areas suggesting a kidney injury (see p. 191).

5 Perform a careful neurological examination, assessing for sensory deficit and a sensory level, loss of perianal sensation, and for motor and reflex loss in the legs (see p. 280 for the dermatomes, myotomes and reflex roots in the legs).

   (i)   The spinal cord ends at the level of the first lumbar vertebra, so any injury distal to this involves the cauda equina only, causing lower motor neuron weakness.

6 Send blood for FBC, U&Es, blood sugar and G&S.

7 Request thoracolumbar spine X-rays or spinal reformatting on CT scans of the chest and abdomen in all the following high-risk patients:

   (i)   Fall from 3 m (10 ft).
   (ii)   High-speed motor vehicle crash at over 80 k.p.h. (50 m.p.h.).
   (iii)   Ejection from motor vehicle or motor cycle.
   (iv)   GCS score of ≤8.
   (v)   Neurological deficit.
   (vi)   Back pain or tenderness (may be absent).

8 X-rays may show vertebral body fractures, e.g. a distraction 'Chance' fracture or a wedge fracture, transverse process fracture, or a dislocation (particularly between T12/L1, and L4/L5).

9 Request a CT scan for all suspicious areas on plain films or potentially unstable fractures.

MANAGEMENT

1 Treat associated thoracic and abdominal injuries as a priority. Maintain spinal precautions, log-roll the patient and minimize unnecessary movements, as thoracolumbar fractures are commonly unstable.

2 Commence i.v. fluid if there is hypotension from local or retroperitoneal bleeding, or from loss of sympathetic tone in a high thoracic cord injury.

3 Refer the patient to the orthopaedic team.

   (i)   Methylprednisolone i.v. for spinal cord damage within 8 h of injury is rarely, if ever, used now, and then only after consultation with the regional Spinal Injuries unit (see p. 179).

LIMB INJURY

The management of limb injuries in the multi-trauma patient does not take precedence over head, thoracic, abdominal or pelvic injuries, even though they may appear more dramatic and attract instant attention.

Limb injuries are covered in detail in Section VI, Orthopaedic Emergencies.

DIAGNOSIS

1 Look for obvious deformity, swelling, tenderness, abnormal movement or crepitus (if the patient is unconscious).

2 Check the distal pulses, particularly in a supracondylar humeral fracture or a dislocated knee.

3 Remember that closed fractures bleed extensively with little external evidence, and open fractures bleed even more. See Table 5.7 for the amounts of concealed blood loss expected with pelvic and limb injuries in multiple trauma.

4 Note any neurological deficit, e.g. sciatic nerve damage in posterior hip dislocation, or radial nerve damage in humeral shaft fracture.

MANAGEMENT

1 Restore any deformity to a normal anatomical alignment. This will reduce the risk of neurovascular compromise and maintain skin integrity, reducing long-term complications. Examples include:
    (i) Posteriorly dislocated hip, to prevent sciatic nerve damage.
    (ii) Dislocated knee, to maintain vascular circulation to the distal extremity.
    (iii) Dislocated ankle, to prevent ischaemic pressure necrosis of the skin overlying the malleolus (see p. 259).

2 Give increments of morphine 2.5–5 mg i.v. for pain with an antiemetic such as metoclopramide 10 mg i.v.

3 Cover compound fractures with a saline-soaked sterile dressing. Give flucloxacillin 2 g i.v. or cephazolin 2 g i.v. and tetanus prophylaxis.

4 Immobilize the fracture using a plaster of Paris backslab, or commercially designed traction splint for femoral shaft or tibial fractures.
    (i) Splinting reduces pain, making handling easier; it also reduces blood loss and the risk of neurovascular injury.

Table 5.7 Expected concealed blood loss from orthopaedic injuries in multiple trauma

Site of closed fracture	Predicted blood loss
Pelvic ring	Up to 6 units or more
Femoral shaft	2–4 units
Tibial shaft	1–3 units

5 Obtain urgent vascular and orthopaedic consults if distal ischaemia is present. Otherwise refer the patient when the other major injuries have been stabilized.

6 *Traumatic amputation of a limb or digit*
  (i) Control haemorrhage by direct pressure and elevation of the stump.
  (ii) Consider the possibility of replantation, especially in a clean, sliced wound without crushing
      (a) preserve the amputated part by wrapping in a saline-soaked sterile dressing
      (b) seal the wrapped part in a sterile dry plastic bag, and immerse in a container of crushed ice and water
      (c) give i.v. antibiotics and tetanus prophylaxis as for a compound fracture
      (d) X-ray the limb and severed part
      (e) refer the patient to the orthopaedic or plastic surgery team for consideration of microvascular surgery ideally performed within 6 h of injury.

HEAD INJURY

The diagnosis and management of head injuries is best considered in two groups:
- Severe head injury – see page 29, Section I, Critical Care.
- Conscious head injury.

CONSCIOUS HEAD INJURY
The aim is to differentiate patients requiring admission from those who may be allowed home.

DIAGNOSIS

1 *History*
  Enquire about:
      (i) The nature and speed of impact.
      (ii) Subsequent loss of consciousness, drowsiness, vomiting or seizures.
      (iii) The length of post-traumatic amnesia (PTA) from the time of injury to the time of the return of memory for consecutive events. This is often underestimated
          (a) >10 min PTA is significant.
      (iv) Associated alcohol or drug intoxication.
      (v) Relevant medical conditions and drug therapy, including warfarin or NOAC.

2   Examination
   (i)   Record the temperature, pulse, blood pressure and respirations.
   (ii) Assess higher mental functions, including the level of consciousness, using the GCS score (see p. 30).
   (iii) Check the pupil size and reactions, eye movements, cranial nerves and the limbs for lateralizing neurological signs.
   (iv) Examine the scalp for bruising, lacerations or palpable fractures and haematomas.
   (v)   Exclude associated neck or other injuries.

3   Radiological imaging
   (i)   Request three-view cervical spine X-rays, if there is any suggestion of an associated neck injury
         (a) lateral cervical spine view, with an anteroposterior and open-mouth odontoid view
         (b) make sure C1–C7/T1 are visualized, if necessary by traction on the shoulders (see p. 177).
   (ii) CT head scan.
         Request a CT scan of the head as the investigation of choice for the detection of acute, clinically important brain injuries.
   (iii) Indications for a CT head in the conscious GCS 15 head injury patient following *any* loss of consciousness or significant anterograde amnesia (PTA) include:
         (a) drug or alcohol intoxication at time of trauma or evaluation
         (b) headache or repeated vomiting >2 episodes
         (c) age >65
         (d) warfarin, NOAC or other bleeding tendency, e.g. chronic liver disease
         (e) dangerous mechanism, such as high-speed injury, injury from a sharp or heavy object
         (f) deep scalp laceration, large haematoma, or skull fracture suspected on palpation
         (g) seizure or focal neurological sign
         (h) suspected open skull fracture
         (i) signs of a basal skull fracture such as cerebrospinal fluid or blood loss from the nose or ear.
   (iv) Skull X-rays. These now only have a limited role, if any, for instance detection of non-accidental injury in children, or when CT scanning services are unavailable, in conjunction with inpatient observation.

MANAGEMENT

1   Clean scalp lacerations thoroughly, trim the edges and remove any foreign bodies. Then suture in layers using a monofilament synthetic non- absorbable material such as nylon or polypropylene.

2   Give tetanus prophylaxis according to the patient's immune status.

3   *Admission*

(i)   Admit patients following a minor head injury with any of the following features under the surgical team for neurological observation:

(a)   confusion or decreased level of consciousness regardless of imaging result

(b)   neurological symptoms or signs; persistent headache or vomiting

(c)   abnormal CT head scan

(d)   skull fracture

(e)   difficulty assessing, e.g. alcohol, drugs, epilepsy

(f)   other medical condition, e.g. warfarin or NOAC, coagulation defect

(g)   significant associated injuries requiring inpatient care.

(ii)   Make certain all of the above have had radiological imaging with a CT head scan. Some will be discussed with the neurosurgery team.

4   *Discharge*

(i)   Send the following patients with a minor head injury home, provided there is someone with them and home circumstances are suitable:

(a)   fully conscious and oriented

(b)   normal CT head scan (normal skull X-ray when CT unavailable)

(c)   no other significant injuries

(d)   no seizures or focal neurological signs

(e)   no persistent headache or vomiting.

(ii)   Give each patient a standard head injury advice card

(a)   these cards advise patients to return if complications such as confusion, drowsiness, seizure, visual disturbance, vomiting or persistent headache occur in the 24 h after discharge.

(iii)   This still leaves some patients with a minor head injury yet to be dealt with. Admit the following patients to the ED short-stay ward for observation:

(a)   no one to accompany them

(b)   poor home circumstances

(c)   an unreliable history, particularly if they were under the influence of alcohol or drugs

(d)   other painful injuries, e.g. to the face or nose, etc.

5   *Remember*

(i)   Look for the cause of any preceding fall in the elderly, such as postural hypotension, Stokes–Adams attack or other syncopal episode

(a)   these require diagnosis and management in their own right, in addition to the resultant head injury.

(ii) A head injury in a child may be due to non-accidental injury (see p. 319).

(iii) Cervical spine injuries are associated with head injuries and appropriate examination and investigation is performed based on clinical grounds.

BURNS

These are considered in the following categories:

- Major burns.
- Minor burns and scalds.
- Minor burns of the hand.
- Minor burns of the face.

MAJOR BURNS

DIAGNOSIS

1 Determine the nature of the fire, how it started, whether there was any explosion, the time of the incident and delay in reaching hospital.

2 Ask if the patient was in an enclosed place and, if so, for how long. Ascertain whether smoke or fumes, which predispose to carbon monoxide and cyanide poisoning, were present and the duration of exposure.

3 Examine for signs of a respiratory burn.

(i) Look for burns around the face and neck, burnt nasal hairs, and soot particles in the nose and mouth.

(ii) Look for signs of tachypnoea, hoarseness, stridor or wheezing.

(iii) Assess for headache and confusion suggesting carbon monoxide poisoning.

4 Consider the possibility of cyanide poisoning from burning plastics and fabrics, especially in patients with:

(i) Tachypnoea, respiratory failure, cardiac arrhythmias, hypotension, convulsions and coma.

(ii) Severe, persistent, raised anion gap metabolic acidosis with a venous lactate level of >10 mmol/L despite fluid resuscitation (see p. 412).

5 Check for associated injuries, particularly if burns occurred from an explosion, blast injury or high-voltage electrocution.

6 Determine the extent of the burn.

(i) Use Wallace's *Rule of Nines* in adults, ignoring areas of mere erythema (see Fig. 5.2).

(ii) Use comparison with the size of the child's palm, equal to 1% of

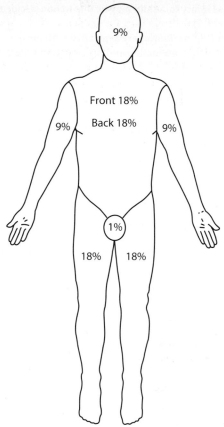

Figure 5.2 Wallace's Rule of Nines in adults, for estimating the percentage of body surface area burned.

body surface area (BSA), when estimating the extent of a burn in children. A child's head is relatively larger than an adult's (12–14%) and the legs are relatively smaller (14%).

    (iii) Or use a body map such as a Lund and Browder chart.

7   Determine the depth of the burn.

      (i) *Full-thickness*: the skin is white or brown, dry, leathery, and anaesthetic with no capillary refill. This will require skin grafting.

      (ii) *Partial-thickness*

        (a) deep dermal – the skin is pink or white, feels thickened, does not blanch, and has reduced sensation. This should heal over in about 3 weeks, but some areas may require grafting to avoid leaving a scar

    (b) superficial – the skin is red, moist and blistered, blanches and is painful. This should heal spontaneously in 10–14 days.

    (iii) *Superficial*: erythema, blanching and pain occur, followed by peeling as in sunburn. This should heal rapidly in 5–7 days.

8 Insert two large-bore i.v. cannulae and send blood for FBC, U&Es, CK, blood sugar, lactate, G&S and a drug screen if there is suspected alcohol or drug abuse.

    (i) The cannula may be placed through burned skin if absolutely necessary, or use a cut-down technique if no vein is found.

    (ii) Avoid central line insertion as there is a high risk of sepsis from this procedure.

9 Check ABGs or VBGs. An elevated carboxyhaemoglobin level will confirm exposure to carbon monoxide (see p. 411).

10 Monitor the ECG and attach a pulse oximeter to the patient.

11 Request a CXR.

MANAGEMENT

1 Confirm the adequacy of the airway and give 100% oxygen by tight-fitting mask with reservoir bag.

2 Give salbutamol 5 mg nebulized for wheeze.

3 Organize for an airway-skilled person to perform urgent endotracheal intubation using an RSI technique with an uncut endotracheal tube in patients with:

    (i) Significant burns involving the face, lips and pharynx.

    (ii) Stridor, hoarseness, respiratory distress or a deteriorating level of consciousness.

    (iii) Carbon monoxide or cyanide toxicity with coma from smoke and fume inhalation.

4 Commence i.v. fluids in any burn >10% BSA in a child or 15% BSA in an adult, or for associated injuries causing hypovolaemia.

5 Determine the rate of fluid administration using the Parkland formula:

    (i) Give fluid at 4 mL/kg per percentage of BSA burned

        (a) administer the first 50% in the initial 8 h, and the remaining 50% in the subsequent 16 h.

    (ii) More rapid fluid replacement may be required to catch up if there has been a delay in reaching hospital.

    (iii) Give additional maintenance fluid at 1.0–1.5 mL/kg per hour of normal saline.

    (iv) The Parkland formula and other fluid resuscitation formulae such as the Muir and Barclay are a guide only. Aim for at least 0.5 mL/kg/h urine output.

6 The quantity of fluid is more important than the type.

    (i)   Consider albumin initially in extensive, deep (e.g. electrical) burns, or when resuscitation is delayed.

    (ii)   Otherwise, use a crystalloid solution alone, such as Hartmann's (compound sodium lactate).

7 Insert a urinary catheter to assess the adequacy of resuscitation, aiming for a urine output of 0.5 mL/kg/h in adults, or 1 mL/kg per hour in children <30 kg.

8 Pass a nasogastric tube in patients with burns >20%, who may develop gastric stasis.

9 Give morphine 0.1 mg/kg i.v. with an antiemetic such as metoclopramide 10 mg i.v. Remember that under-transfusion or hypoxia are more common causes of restlessness than pain.

10 Give tetanus prophylaxis to all burn patients (see p. 269).

11 Leave any adherent clothing alone and do not break blisters in the burnt area. Remove constricting articles such as rings, bracelets and watches.

    (i)   Cover the burn with a non-adherent, paraffin-impregnated gauze dressing or plastic cling wrap. Beware of hypothermia in children if wet soaks were left on.

    (ii)   Avoid silver sulfadiazine cream at this stage until the patient has been assessed by the surgical or burns unit team.

12 Consider the need for escharotomy in the following:

    (i)   Circumferential, leathery, full-thickness burns that may cause distal ischaemia in limbs or digits by restricting blood flow, and respiratory compromise by constricting chest wall movements.

    (ii)   Ask the surgical or burns unit team to perform relieving incisions through the burn area.

13 All full-thickness burns of >1–2% BSA require hospital admission by the surgical team. Refer patients on to a specialist burns unit with:

    (i)   Burns >10% in children and 15% in adults.

    (ii)   Burns of important functional areas, such as the face, hands, feet, perineum and genitalia.

    (iii)   Respiratory burns.

    (iv)   Chemical burns and electrical burns, including lightning injury.

14 Assess all serious burns with care and resuscitate fully before departure, similar to the precautions taken when transferring serious head injuries to a neurosurgical unit.

    (i)   Remember the risk of sudden respiratory obstruction during transit.

    (ii)   Make sure a senior doctor has assessed the need for endotracheal intubation in any significant respiratory burn, prior to departure.

Tip: burn injuries are frightening and unexpected, and relatives (particularly parents of children) may feel guilty and angry. Early counselling and reassurance from the outset aid coming to terms with the injuries and allay anxiety, to facilitate optimal support for the victim.

MINOR BURNS AND SCALDS

These include full-thickness burns <1% or partial-thickness burns <15% BSA in adults and <10% in children. The aim is to manage them as outpatients, as distinct from patients with major burns, who require admission (see above).

INITIAL MANAGEMENT

1   Irrigate the wound immediately with copious running cool water until the pain is relieved.

2   Assess the extent and depth of the burn (see p. 200). Superficial partial-thickness burns heal spontaneously, deep dermal partial-thickness burns heal slowly with scar formation; and full-thickness burns do not heal at all, unless <1–2 cm in diameter, when epithelium will cover the area from the edges. Otherwise grafting is required.

3   Clean with sterile saline or an antiseptic such as chlorhexidine.

4   Give adequate analgesia such as paracetamol 500 mg with codeine 8 mg two tablets orally q.d.s. and/or ibuprofen 200–400 mg orally t.d.s. Give children 15 mg/kg of paracetamol elixir.

5   De-roof large blisters that have broken, or aspirate the fluid if the blister is tense. Otherwise leave blisters intact to protect the healing epithelium.

6   Apply silver sulfadiazine cream and cover the burn with a non-adherent paraffin-impregnated gauze dressing.

7   Then apply gauze and an absorbent layer consisting of a cotton-wool and gauze combine pad, overlapping the paraffin-impregnated gauze dressing by 3 cm at either end.

8   Finally, keep the absorbent layer in place with a firm crêpe bandage, again overlapping each end by 3 cm, and seal with adhesive tape.

9   Always elevate the limb using a high-arm sling for arm and hand burns.

10   Give tetanus prophylaxis and oral analgesics such as paracetamol 500 mg and codeine phosphate 8 mg two tablets q.d.s. to take home.

11   Remember that burns of the perineum, feet or hands in children may be due to non-accidental injury.
  (i)   Suspect this when there has been a delay in seeking treatment and the explanation is tenuous, or there is absence of any evidence of splashing.
  (ii) Refer the child to the paediatric team for admission if non-accidental injury is possible, however trivial the burn (see p. 319).

FOLLOW-UP MANAGEMENT

1 Review the patient after 24–48 h to clean the affected site, reassess the condition of the burn, and to ensure that no evidence of secondary infection is present. Re-dress the site, but omit the silver sulfadiazine.

2 Thereafter, change the dressing every 5 days, unless the wound becomes painful, or smells, or the bandage becomes soaked ('strike through'), when the dressing should be renewed immediately.

    (i) Leave the paraffin-impregnated gauze in place when changing the dressing, if it has become adherent to the skin, to avoid destroying the delicate new epithelium forming underneath.

3 When the wound is healing and has become epithelialized, leave it exposed or cover it with a dry, non-adherent dressing.

4 Refer burns that have not healed in 10–12 days to a plastic surgery unit for review and consideration for skin grafting.

5 Warn the patient that healed burns will initially be both hypersensitive and photosensitive, will have dry scaly skin, and that there may be depigmentation in dark-skinned races.

MINOR BURNS OF THE HAND

DIAGNOSIS AND MANAGEMENT

These are difficult to dress.

1 Cover the hand with silver sulfadiazine cream and place the hand inside a sterile polythene bag, bandaged over a gauze ring as a seal at the wrist.

2 Elevate the hand and encourage the patient to move the fingers regularly.

3 Give tetanus prophylaxis and analgesia.

4 Replace the silver sulfadiazine cream and bag daily, as turbid fluid collects in the bag.

MINOR BURNS OF THE FACE

DIAGNOSIS AND MANAGEMENT

1 Leave these alone and exposed to heal in 10 days. A proprietary moisturizing lotion may be used.

2 Exclude corneal damage by staining with fluorescein.

3 Warn the patient that facial swelling may develop the following day.

ACUTE ABDOMEN

The aims are to resuscitate critically ill patients; differentiate those requiring referral to the surgical, gynaecological, urological, vascular or medical team; and to determine who can be allowed home.

SERIOUSLY ILL PATIENT

DIAGNOSIS AND MANAGEMENT

1 Clear the airway, give oxygen, and attach a cardiac monitor and pulse oximeter to the patient. Check the temperature, pulse, blood pressure, respiratory rate and blood sugar level.

2 Obtain a brief history of the onset, duration, nature and character of the pain, prior episodes of pain, relevant previous operations and illnesses, present medication and known drug allergies.

3 Examine the chest and heart, and then lay the patient flat to examine the abdomen, including the femoral pulses.

4 Look for a ruptured abdominal aortic aneurysm (AAA), pancreatitis, inferior myocardial infarction, mesenteric infarction or a ruptured ectopic pregnancy in any shocked patient presenting with *sudden* acute abdominal pain.

5 Perform a rectal examination to look for blood.

6 Insert one or two large-bore i.v. cannulae and send blood for FBC, U&Es, LFTs, blood sugar, lipase/amylase and a lactate. Cross-match blood if haemorrhage is suspected. Send blood cultures if pyrexial. Check an arterial or venous blood gas.

7 Commence an i.v. infusion with normal saline.

8 Catheterize the bladder. Test the urine for sugar, blood, protein, bile and urobilinogen, and send for microscopy and culture.
- (i) Perform a urinary β-human chorionic gonadotrophin (hCG) pregnancy test in females of reproductive age.

9 Perform an ECG.

10 Arrange a focused bedside ultrasound for a suspected AAA or ectopic pregnancy.

11 Request urgent radiology:
- (i) Erect CXR or lateral decubitus abdominal film if the patient is unable to sit upright, to look for free gas in suspected perforation.
- (ii) AXR for possible bowel obstruction, volvulus or for abnormal air such as the 'double-wall sign' in a perforation.
- (iii) CT abdomen scan providing the patient is not too unstable.

12 Insert a nasogastric tube if there is evidence of intestinal obstruction, ileus or peritonitis.

13 Commence broad-spectrum antibiotics such as gentamicin 5 mg/kg, ampicillin 1 g i.v. and metronidazole 500 mg i.v. for generalized peritonitis.

14 Refer the patient early to the surgical team.

STABLE PATIENT WITH AN ACUTE ABDOMEN

DIAGNOSIS AND MANAGEMENT

1   Determine the onset and nature of pain:
   (i)   *Explosive and excruciating pain*: consider myocardial infarction, ruptured aortic aneurysm, perforated viscus, and biliary or renal colic.
   (ii) *Rapid, severe and constant pain*: consider pancreatitis, strangulated bowel, mesenteric infarction and ectopic pregnancy.
   (iii) *Gradual, steady pain*: consider cholecystitis, appendicitis, diverticulitis, hepatitis and pelvic inflammatory disease (salpingitis).
   (iv) *Intermittent pain with crescendos*: consider mechanical obstruction.

2   Ask about the location and radiation of pain:
   (i)   Central abdominal pain radiating to the back suggests an aortic aneurysm or pancreatitis.
   (ii) Flank pain radiating to the genitalia suggests ureteric colic, or rarely ruptured aortic aneurysm.
   (iii) Otherwise pain tends to localize over the organ affected, provided there is peritoneal involvement, with radiation to a shoulder tip if the diaphragm is irritated, e.g. by cholecystitis or a ruptured spleen.

3   Look for associated features such as:
   (i)   Nausea and vomiting:
      (a) pain tends to precede the nausea and vomiting in the surgical acute abdomen
      (b) a medical condition such as gastroenteritis or gastritis is more likely if the nausea and vomiting precede the pain.
   (ii) Fever and rigors:
      (a) a low-grade pyrexia is usual in appendicitis or diverticulitis
      (b) a high fever and rigors suggest cholecystitis, cholangitis, diffuse peritonitis, pyelonephritis or acute pelvic inflammatory disease (salpingitis).

4   Check the temperature, pulse, blood pressure and respiratory rate.

5   Inspect for visible peristalsis and distension, palpate for local tenderness, guarding and masses, percuss for free gas, and listen for increased or absent bowel sounds. Examine the hernial orifices, particularly in cases of intestinal obstruction.

6   Perform a rectal examination, external genitalia examination in male patients, and consider a vaginal examination in female patients.

7   Insert an i.v. cannula and send blood for FBC, U&Es, LFTs, blood sugar and lipase/amylase.
   (i)   Their true discriminatory value in differentiating between the various conditions is limited, apart from the lipase/amylase.

8 Test the urine for sugar, blood, protein, bile and urobilinogen, and send for microscopy and culture in suspected UTI.

   (i) Perform a β-hCG pregnancy test in females with abdominal pain.

9 Record an ECG.

10 Plain and special radiology.

Request radiologic investigation for the following specific indications:

   (i) Erect CXR – to look for evidence of basal pulmonary disease, a secondary pleural reaction from intra-abdominal disease and free gas under the diaphragm indicating a perforation.

   (ii) Erect and supine abdomen films – to look at the gas pattern for obstruction or volvulus, splenic shadow, renal outlines and psoas shadows, and for calcification and opacities.

   (iii) Upper abdominal ultrasound to confirm biliary colic or cholecystitis.

   (iv) Lower abdominal ultrasound to confirm an AAA or ureteric colic.

   (v) Pelvic ultrasound – to look for a gynaecological cause (remember to do the β-hCG first).

   (vi) CT abdomen scan

      (a) with i.v. contrast for a suspected aortic aneurysm, provided the patient is haemodynamically stable

      (b) with i.v. plus or minus oral contrast for difficult diagnoses particularly in the older patient, such as suspected bowel cancer or other complex masses, diverticulitis, appendicitis

      (c) without contrast to confirm ureteric colic.

11 Give all patients i.v. analgesia as required, such as morphine 2.5–5 mg i.v. with metoclopramide 10 mg i.v. This will *not* interfere with the surgical diagnosis, which may even be facilitated.

12 Refer all cases to the surgical team if an acute surgical condition is suspected or cannot be excluded.

CAUSES OF ACUTE ABDOMINAL PAIN

Disorders causing acute abdominal pain may be categorized as intestinal, biliary, vascular, pancreatic, urinary, peritoneal and retroperitoneal, gynaecological and medical. See Table 5.8 for a complete list.

ACUTE APPENDICITIS

DIAGNOSIS

1 Acute appendicitis causes poorly localized central abdominal pain, worse on coughing or moving, which classically shifts to the right iliac fossa. There is associated anorexia, nausea, vomiting, and diarrhoea or constipation.

2 Low-grade pyrexia, localized abdominal tenderness, rebound and guarding are found.

3 Always perform a urinalysis to look for glycosuria, white cells, and a β-hCG pregnancy test. Even if positive, none of these rules out appendicitis.

Table 5.8 Causes of acute abdominal pain

Intestinal disorders	Acute appendicitis
	Intestinal obstruction
	Intussusception
	Perforation of a viscus
	Diverticulitis
	Inflammatory bowel disease
Biliary disorders	Biliary colic
	Acute cholecystitis
	Ascending cholangitis
Vascular disorders	Ruptured aortic aneurysm
	Ischaemic colitis
	Mesenteric infarction
	Ruptured spleen
Pancreatic disorder	Acute pancreatitis
Urinary disorders	Renal and ureteric colic
	Pyelonephritis
	Acute urinary retention
	Acute epididymo-orchitis
	Acute testicular torsion
Peritoneal/retroperitoneal disorders	Primary peritonitis
	Retroperitoneal haemorrhage
Gynaecological disorders	
Medical disorders	

4 Gain i.v. access.
    (i) FBC is frequently performed, but rarely influences decision making alone.
5 Request an ultrasound in females to rule out pelvic pathology, or a CT scan in equivocal cases particularly in older patients.
6 Diagnosis is most difficult in very young, elderly or pregnant patients.

MANAGEMENT

1 Commence a normal saline infusion and administer i.v. analgesia.
2 Keep the patient nil by mouth. Give gentamicin 5 mg/kg i.v., ampicillin 2 g i.v. q.d.s. and metronidazole 500 mg i.v. t.d.s. if rupture is suspected with peritonitis.

3   Admit all patients under the surgical team, whether the diagnosis appears clear or is just suspected in an atypical case, such as:

  (i)   Confused elderly patient, infant with diarrhoea, or older child off his or her food, any of whom could have appendicitis.

INTESTINAL OBSTRUCTION

DIAGNOSIS

1   The causes are many, including adhesions, an obstructed hernia, carcinoma, diverticulitis, volvulus, intussusception, mesenteric infarction, and Crohn's disease.

2   Intermittent colicky abdominal pain occurs with abdominal distension and vomiting in high obstruction, and constipation with failure to pass flatus in low obstruction.

3   Visible peristalsis may be seen, associated with tinkling bowel sounds and signs of dehydration.

4   The pain becomes more continuous and generalized if strangulation occurs (most common with a femoral hernia), associated with tachycardia and signs of shock.

5   Always examine the hernial orifices and perform a rectal examination.

6   Gain i.v. access and send blood for FBC, U&Es, lipase/amylase and blood sugar.

7   Request erect and supine abdominal X-rays and look for the following features:

  (i)   Small bowel obstruction:

    (a) X-rays show dilated loops of small bowel and a colon devoid of air

    (b) small bowel is usually central in distribution with regular transverse bands (*valvulae conniventes*) extending across the entire diameter of the bowel

    (c) fluid levels, with over five considered significant. Note fluid levels also occur in gastroenteritis.

  (ii)   Large bowel obstruction:

    (a) X-rays show dilated large bowel, with a peripheral distribution, irregular haustral folds and faecal mass content.

8   Request a CT abdomen scan to determine the level and cause of the obstruction.

MANAGEMENT

1   Commence an infusion of normal saline to correct dehydration from vomiting and fluid loss into the bowel.

2   Pass a nasogastric tube, administer analgesia, and refer the patient to the surgical team.

INTUSSUSCEPTION

DIAGNOSIS

1 This is caused by telescoping or prolapse of one portion of bowel into an immediately adjacent segment. It usually occurs in children aged 3–18 months and is characterized by intermittent abdominal pain with sudden screaming and pallor, followed by vomiting.

2 Abdominal distension and a mass may be felt, with blood-stained mucus ('redcurrant jelly') passed per rectum.

3 Send blood for FBC, U&Es and blood sugar if the child is unwell.

4 Request erect and supine AXRs, which may be normal in the early stages, or reveal signs of intestinal obstruction.
   (i) Look for evidence of a soft-tissue mass surrounded by a crescent of air ('doughnut sign') or free air from perforation of a viscus.

5 Arrange an abdominal ultrasound, or a contrast or air enema.
   (i) Both have high degrees of sensitivity, with an enema resulting in therapeutic reduction in 75% of cases.

MANAGEMENT

1 Insert an i.v. cannula and commence careful i.v. rehydration with analgesia.

2 Refer immediately to the surgical team.

PERFORATION OF A VISCUS

DIAGNOSIS

1 Perforation may occur anywhere in the gastrointestinal tract. Common sites are a peptic ulcer, the appendix, or a colonic diverticulum.
   (i) There may be an antecedent history of alcohol or NSAID ingestion, dyspepsia, or lower abdominal pain, or
   (ii) Perforation can occur *de novo*.

2 It presents with severe pain and signs of generalized peritonitis with board-like rigidity. Shock soon supervenes.

3 Gain i.v. access and send blood for FBC, U&Es, blood sugar and lipase/amylase.

4 Request an erect CXR to look for gas under the diaphragm, seen in >70% of cases.

5 Arrange a CT scan of the abdomen with i.v. and oral contrast.

MANAGEMENT

1 Treat shock with i.v. normal saline, administer i.v. analgesia with morphine in 2.5–5 mg increments and pass a nasogastric tube.

2   Commence broad-spectrum antibiotics such as gentamicin 5 mg/kg once daily, ampicillin 2 g i.v. q.d.s. and metronidazole 500 mg i.v. t.d.s.

3   Refer the patient immediately to the surgical team.

DIVERTICULITIS

DIAGNOSIS

1   This follows inflammation of one or more colonic diverticulae.

2   It causes lower abdominal pain radiating to the left iliac fossa, and altered bowel habit sometimes with blood and diarrhoea.

3   Look for a low-grade fever, abdominal tenderness, and guarding on the left with a palpable mass.

4   Complications of perforation, severe bleeding, fistula formation and bowel obstruction may occur.

5   Gain i.v. access and send blood for FBC, U&Es, blood sugar and G&S.

6   Perform an ECG and request an erect CXR if perforation is suspected.

7   Organise a CT scan of the abdomen with i.v. contrast.

MANAGEMENT

1   Commence an i.v. infusion to treat dehydration or shock.

2   Refer the patient to the surgical team for analgesia and antibiotics such as gentamicin 5 mg/kg once daily, ampicillin 2 g i.v. q.d.s. and metronidazole 500 mg i.v. t.d.s., or for surgery if bowel obstruction or a pelvic abscess is suspected.

INFLAMMATORY BOWEL DISEASE

DIAGNOSIS

1   Ulcerative colitis associated with bouts of diarrhoea with blood-stained mucus may present as a fulminating attack with fever, tachycardia and hypotension.

2   Crohn's disease, associated with recurrent abdominal pain, diarrhoea, malaise and perianal fistulae or abscesses, may present acutely with obstruction, perforation or right iliac fossa pain. This can mimic acute appendicitis.

3   Gain i.v. access and send blood for FBC, U&Es, blood sugar, lipase/amylase and blood cultures.

   (i)   Send a faecal sample for *Clostridium difficile* toxin, as well as ova, cysts and parasites.

4   Request a plain AXR to look particularly for the following:

   (i)   Ulcerative colitis: extensive mucosal ulceration may leave normal mucosal islands (pseudopolyps) visible on plain film. Dilation of the transverse colon >6 cm indicates the presence of a megacolon. Perforation is a major risk.

(ii) Crohn's disease: free air associated with perforation may be seen. Stenotic regions of small bowel are best visualized with barium follow-through studies, or on colonoscopy.

5 Organize a CT scan of the abdomen with i.v. contrast.

MANAGEMENT

1 Commence an i.v. infusion and treat pain with i.v. analgesia, but avoid excessive doses in severe disease.

2 Refer all cases with shock, fever, peritonitis, severe bleeding or an obstructed bowel immediately to the surgical team.

3 Organize urgent gastroenterology advice for a toxic megacolon with fever, tachycardia and hypotension.

(i) Start hydrocortisone 200 mg i.v. 6-hourly, and broad-spectrum antibiotics such as gentamicin 5 mg/kg once daily, ampicillin 2 g i.v. q.d.s. and metronidazole 500 mg i.v. t.d.s.

BILIARY COLIC

DIAGNOSIS

1 This presents with discrete episodes of colicky pain in the right hypochondrium, referred to the scapula.

2 Look for right upper quadrant tenderness on examination. The patient may be jaundiced if the common bile duct is obstructed, with yellow sclera, and bilirubin in the urine.

3 Gain i.v. access and send blood for FBC, U&Es, LFTs and lipase/amylase.

4 Request an upper abdominal ultrasound.

MANAGEMENT

1 Treat pain with i.v. analgesia such as morphine 0.1 mg/kg i.v. with an antiemetic such as metoclopramide 10 mg i.v.

2 Refer the patient to the surgical team if the pain is severe or acute cholecystitis is suspected.

3 Otherwise, advise the patient to eat a diet low in saturated fats and refer them to the GP or surgical outpatients for follow-up.

ACUTE CHOLECYSTITIS

DIAGNOSIS

1 This causes acute, constant right upper quadrant pain referred to the scapula, with anorexia, nausea and vomiting.

2 Look for localized tenderness, with involuntary guarding and rebound tenderness. Painful splinting of respiration on deep inspiration and right upper quadrant palpation is frequent (Murphy's sign). Fever is common.

3 Occasionally a gall bladder may be palpable in association with jaundice, although more commonly the gall bladder is not felt as it is shrunken and contracted.

4 Gain i.v. access and send blood for FBC, U&Es, blood sugar, LFTs, lipase/ amylase, and blood cultures.

5 Request an upper abdominal ultrasound.

MANAGEMENT

1 Give analgesia such as morphine 0.1 mg/kg i.v. with an antiemetic such as metoclopramide 10 mg i.v., and commence an i.v. infusion of normal saline.

2 Give gentamicin 5 mg/kg i.v., and ampicillin 2 g i.v. q.d.s.

3 Refer the patient to the surgical team for bed rest, analgesia, antibiotics and cholecystectomy.

ASCENDING CHOLANGITIS

DIAGNOSIS

1 This causes fever, rigors, upper abdominal pain and jaundice. Confusion and shock occur in severe cases.

2 It is associated with biliary obstruction from gall stones, duct stricture and malignancy.

3 Look for fever, jaundice and right upper quadrant tenderness. Tachycardia, hypotension and confusion are seen from septic shock.

4 Gain i.v. access and send blood for FBC, U&Es, blood sugar, LFTs, lipase/ amylase, lactate and blood cultures.

5 Request an urgent upper abdominal ultrasound, or CT scan if well enough.

MANAGEMENT

1 Commence an i.v. infusion of normal saline.

2 Give gentamicin 5 mg/kg i.v., and ampicillin 2 g i.v. q.d.s.

3 Refer the patient to the surgical team or ICU, although an urgent drainage procedure such as ERCP is needed in severe cases.

RUPTURED ABDOMINAL AORTIC ANEURYSM

DIAGNOSIS

1 This classically presents with sudden abdominal pain radiating to the back or groin, syncope, collapse or unexplained shock. Tachycardia and hypotension occur in 50% of cases.

2 Feel for a tender mass with expansile pulsation on examination, or a vague fullness with discomfort to the left of the umbilicus.

3   Always consider this diagnosis in men >45 years in particular, even when only one feature of the 'classic triad' of abdominal or back pain, shock, and a pulsatile or tender abdominal mass is present.

  (i)   Also consider a ruptured AAA first in the older patient with apparent 'ureteric colic'.

4   Gain large-bore i.v. access in both arms and send blood for FBC, U&Es, blood sugar, lipase/amylase and cross-match 4–6 units of blood.

5   Catheterize the bladder.

6   Record the ECG because ischaemic heart disease is usually associated with or exacerbated by the hypotension.

7   Request a CXR if there is time.

8   Perform a rapid bedside ultrasound scan to confirm the presence of an abdominal aneurysm if the patient is haemodynamically unstable and the diagnosis is uncertain.

9   Or proceed directly to theatre if the patient is moribund.

10   Only request a CT scan if the patient is haemodynamically stable. Remember to modify the dose of i.v. contrast depending on the renal function.

MANAGEMENT

1   Give the patient high-flow oxygen by face mask and commence a slow i.v. infusion.

  (i)   Only give minimal amounts of normal saline or Hartmann's (compound sodium lactate), aiming for a systolic blood pressure of no more than 90–100 mmHg (i.e. minimal volume or hypotense resuscitation).

  (ii)   **Avoid** giving large fluid volumes, as this leads to coagulopathy, hypothermia, increases the bleeding and causes a higher mortality.

2   Refer the patient urgently to the vascular surgical team for immediate laparotomy.

  (i)   Contact the duty anaesthetist, alert theatre, and inform ICU.

ISCHAEMIC COLITIS

DIAGNOSIS

1   This usually occurs in an elderly patient with recurrent abdominal pain, progressing to episodes of bloody diarrhoea or intestinal obstruction from stricture formation.

2   Gain i.v. access and send blood for FBC, coagulation profile, electrolyte and liver function tests (ELFTs), blood sugar, lipase/amylase, lactate and G&S.

3   Record an ECG.

4   Request a plain AXR that may reveal 'thumb-printing' of the colonic wall, or proximal colon dilation, intramural gas, and the most ominous sign of gas within the portal vein.

5 Arrange a CT scan with i.v. contrast that may show free fluid and colonic-wall oedema or air, although many of the features are non-specific.

   (i)   Request CT angiography to best define the extent.

MANAGEMENT

1 Commence an i.v. infusion of normal saline.

2 Give analgesia and keep the patient nil by mouth.

3 Refer the patient to the surgical team.

MESENTERIC INFARCTION

DIAGNOSIS

1 This may be due to embolism from atrial fibrillation or a myocardial infarction, or due to arterial or venous thrombosis, or arterial occlusion such as following an aortic dissection.

2 There is sudden onset of severe, diffuse abdominal pain, usually in an elderly patient, associated with vomiting and bloody diarrhoea.

3 Abdominal examination reveals distension, generalized tenderness, absent bowel sounds and fresh rectal blood.

4 Gain i.v. access and send blood for FBC, U&Es, LFTs, lipase/amylase, blood sugar and cross-match 2–4 units of blood. Send a lactate as a marker of severity in late stage disease, but it may not be elevated early.

5 Record the ECG.

6 Arrange a CT abdomen scan with angiography, if the patient is haemodynamically stable enough.

MANAGEMENT

1 Commence an i.v. infusion of normal saline or Hartmann's (compound sodium lactate) to treat shock.

2 Refer the patient to the surgical team, who will determine the need for urgent surgery. However, the prognosis is poor.

RUPTURED SPLEEN

DIAGNOSIS

1 Left lower rib injuries following blunt trauma are associated with splenic damage in up to 20% of cases. Occasionally, trivial injury to an already enlarged spleen from glandular fever, malaria or leukaemia can cause rupture.

2 Presentation of the splenic rupture may be:

   (i)   *Acute*: causing tachycardia, hypotension and abdominal tenderness with pain referred to the left shoulder.

   (ii) *Delayed*: occurring up to 2 weeks or more after an episode of trauma. Initial localized discomfort and referred shoulder-tip pain give way to signs of intra-abdominal haemorrhage.

3 Gain large-bore i.v. access and send blood for a FBC and cross-match 2–4 units of blood for an acutely ruptured spleen.

4 Request a CXR to look for fractured left lower ribs and a basal pleural effusion, especially in delayed splenic rupture.

5 Arrange an urgent abdominal ultrasound if the patient is unstable, or a CT scan with i.v. contrast if the patient is stable.

MANAGEMENT

1 Commence an infusion of normal saline and refer the patient immediately to the surgical team.

ACUTE PANCREATITIS

DIAGNOSIS

1 Predisposing factors include alcohol abuse, gallstones, viruses such as mumps, hepatitis B and cytomegalovirus, trauma, ischaemia or vasculitis, and following endoscopic retrograde cholangiopancreatography (ERCP).

2 Acute pancreatitis presents with sudden, severe abdominal pain radiating to the back, that is eased by sitting forward, associated with repeated vomiting or retching.

3 Vital signs may reveal a low-grade fever and tachycardia with hypotension.

4 Look for epigastric tenderness, guarding and decreased or absent bowel sounds on abdominal examination.

5 Insert a large-bore i.v. cannula and send blood for FBC, U&Es, LFTs, blood sugar, calcium, lipase/amylase and G&S. Check an arterial or venous blood gas.

6 Record the ECG, which may show diffuse T wave inversion, in the absence of myocardial ischaemia.

7 Request an erect CXR to exclude viscus perforation or lobar pneumonia as a cause of the pain.

8 Perform an upper abdominal ultrasound to rule out associated gall stone disease.

9 Perform a CT scan of the abdomen in severe cases that provides both diagnostic and prognostic information.

MANAGEMENT

1 Commence an i.v. infusion of normal saline and pass a nasogastric tube. Give morphine 5–10 mg i.v. with an antiemetic such as metoclopramide 10 mg i.v.

2 Refer the patient to the surgical team.

3 Admit patients with hypoxia, shock, metabolic acidosis, hypocalcaemia or renal impairment to ICU.

RENAL AND URETERIC COLIC

DIAGNOSIS

1   Renal and ureteric calculi may cause pain, haematuria, hydronephrosis or infection.

2   Symptoms are caused by obstruction of one or more calyces, the renal pelvis or ureter.

3   Characteristically these include sudden, severe colicky pain radiating from the loin to the genitalia, restlessness, vomiting and sweating. There may also be urinary frequency and haematuria.

4   Look for loin tenderness in the costovertebral angle.
   (i)   Remember to consider a possible ruptured abdominal aortic aneurysm in men >45 years, especially with an apparent first episode of renal colic, and/or if haematuria is absent (see p. 214).

5   Gain i.v. access and send blood for FBC, U&Es, LFTs, lipase/amylase, calcium and uric acid.

6   Perform a bedside urinalysis for macroscopic or microscopic haematuria, which occurs in 90%.
   (i)   Send a formal midstream urine (MSU) for microscopy and culture.

7   Request a non-contrast abdominal CT scan of the renal tract in patients with acute flank pain, to also rule out other retroperitoneal pathology at the same time.
   (i)   CT can determine the presence of calculi, their size, degree of ureteric obstruction and exclude other important differential diagnoses, particularly an AAA.

8   Alternatively request a renal ultrasound, particularly in the younger patient or for recurrent colic.

9   An IVP is best reserved for post complex urological surgery only.

10 Request a plain AXR KUB (kidneys, ureters, bladder) when subsequently tracking the course of a calculus, as most renal calculi are radio-opaque.

MANAGEMENT

1   Start analgesia:
   (i)   Give morphine 0.1 mg/kg i.v. with an antiemetic such as metoclopramide 10 mg i.v. particularly if the pain is intense and incapacitating.
   (ii) Alternatively, use diclofenac 75 mg i.m. or indomethacin (indometacin) 100 mg p.r.

2   Admit patients with resistant pain, a stone >6 mm in diameter with an obstructed kidney (these are unlikely to pass spontaneously), or any evidence of infection.
   (i)   An infected obstructed kidney is a urological emergency needing immediate drainage.
   (ii) Call the urology team urgently for percutaneous nephrostomy insertion.

3 Discharge the remainder to their GP or urology outpatients for follow-up, and recommend a reduced sodium and low-protein diet that decreases the likelihood of recurrent calcium-based stones.

PYELONEPHRITIS

DIAGNOSIS

1 Typically symptom onset is rapid and characterized by frequency, dysuria, malaise, nausea, vomiting and sometimes rigors.

2 Raised temperature, renal-angle tenderness, and vague low abdominal pain are found.

3 Dipstick urinalysis shows blood, protein and nitrites.

4 Insert an i.v. cannula and send blood for FBC, U&Es, blood sugar and blood cultures in any patient who is significantly ill.

5 Send an MSU to look for bacteria, leucocytes and red blood cells on microscopy and for culture.

MANAGEMENT

1 Significantly ill patients.
   (i)   Include those with vomiting or prostration; pregnant, very young or old; urinary tract abnormalities, e.g. a duplex system, horseshoe kidney or renal/ureteric stones; diabetes or immunosuppression.
   (ii) Commence i.v. fluids. Give gentamicin 5 mg/kg i.v. and ampicillin 2 g i.v. q.d.s.
   (iii) Refer these patients to the medical or urology team for admission, and arrange a renal ultrasound scan.

2 Otherwise, if the symptoms are mild, commence an oral antibiotic depending on local prescribing policy, such as cephalexin 500 mg q.d.s, or amoxicillin 875 mg with clavulanic acid 125 mg one tablet b.d., or trimethoprim 300 mg once daily, all for 10 days.

3 Return the patient to the GP with a letter requesting the GP to organize a repeat urine culture after the completion of a full antibiotic course, to ensure that the infection has been eradicated.

4 Arrange a renal ultrasound in any male with a proven urinary tract infection and refer to urology outpatients for follow-up.

ACUTE URINARY RETENTION

DIAGNOSIS

1 Predisposing factors include prostatic hypertrophy, urethral stricture, pelvic neoplasm, anticholinergic drugs, pregnancy, local painful condition such as genital herpes and faecal loading in the elderly.

2   Occasionally, retention is due to a neurogenic cause such as multiple sclerosis or cauda equina syndrome.

3   The enlarged bladder is easily palpable, dull to percussion and is usually painful, although in the semiconscious patient it may manifest as restlessness.

4   Always perform a rectal examination, and assess perineal sensation and leg reflexes in every patient.

5   Send blood for FBC, ELFTs and blood sugar.

MANAGEMENT

1   Carefully pass a urethral catheter as a strict aseptic procedure, and send a specimen of urine for microscopy and culture (see p. 484).

2   Refer the patient to the surgical team or gynaecology as appropriate.

ACUTE EPIDIDYMO-ORCHITIS

DIAGNOSIS

1   This occurs in sexually active men with a preceding history of urethritis, or non-sexually following urinary tract infection or instrumentation including catheterization.

2   Pain begins gradually and is usually localized to the epididymis or testis, associated with a low-grade fever.

3   Send a FBC to look for a neutrophilia. Request a urine microscopy to look for leucocytes and to culture.

   (i)   Arrange a first-void urine for PCR if sexually acquired to test for Chlamydia and gonorrhoea.

MANAGEMENT

1   **Never** diagnose epididymo-orchitis in a patient <25 years old without considering testicular torsion first (see below).

2   Give the patient a scrotal support if torsion has been excluded, analgesics such as paracetamol 500 mg and codeine phosphate 8 mg two tablets q.d.s., and an antibiotic.

3   The choice of antibiotic depends on the suspected aetiology:

   (i)   *Sexually acquired epididymo-orchitis*
         Give ceftriaxone 500 mg i.v., plus azithromycin 1 g orally once, plus either another 1 g orally 1 week later or doxycycline 100 mg orally b.d. for 14 days
         (a) arrange follow-up in a genitourinary medicine clinic or by the GP, and partner treatment.

   (ii) *Bacterial cystitis with epididymo-orchitis*
         Give cephalexin 500 mg b.d., or amoxicillin 875 mg with clavulanic acid 125 mg one tablet b.d., or trimethoprim 300 mg once daily, all for 7–14 days and refer to the urology clinic.

ACUTE TESTICULAR TORSION

DIAGNOSIS

1 Suspect this diagnosis in any male under 25 years with sudden pain in a testicle, which may radiate to the lower abdomen. There may be associated nausea and vomiting.

2 The testicle lies horizontally and high in the scrotum, and is very tender. There may be a small hydrocoele.

3 Urinalysis is typically negative and the blood white cell count normal.

MANAGEMENT

1 Always refer every suspected case urgently to the urology team, as the testicle becomes non-viable after 6 h of torsion.
    (i) Still refer the patient for surgery even if >6 h have elapsed, as orchidopexy is required on the other side to prevent subsequent torsion there.

2 Only arrange scrotal ultrasound if the diagnosis is in doubt or the history is prolonged, to assess blood supply and to look for an alternative diagnosis. This must **never** delay urgent urological assessment.

PRIMARY PERITONITIS

DIAGNOSIS AND MANAGEMENT

1 Primary bacterial peritonitis occurs almost exclusively in patients with ascites, particularly due to cirrhosis or the nephrotic syndrome.

2 Look for fever, abdominal pain with tenderness and sometimes confusion.

3 Send blood for FBC, U&Es, LFTs, blood sugar and blood cultures. Check a urinalysis.

4 Refer the patient to the medical team for a diagnostic peritoneal tap and culture, and give ceftriaxone 2 g i.v.

RETROPERITONEAL HAEMORRHAGE

DIAGNOSIS

1 This may occur following trauma to the pelvis, kidney or back, or from aortic aneurysm rupture, or from trivial trauma – even spontaneously in those with a bleeding tendency, on anticoagulants or haemodialysis.

2 It presents with hypovolaemic shock following trauma, in the absence of an obvious external or internal thoracic or abdominal source for haemorrhage. A paralytic ileus may develop.

3 Insert a wide-bore i.v. cannula and send blood for FBC, coagulation profile, ELFTs, blood sugar, lipase/amylase and cross-match blood according to the degree of shock.
    (i) Check the urine for blood.

4 Request a CT scan of the abdomen with i.v. contrast to localize the bleeding.

MANAGEMENT

1 Commence an infusion of normal saline with correction of any coagulopathy.

2 Refer to the surgical team for admission.

GYNAECOLOGICAL CAUSES

The following causes are discussed in Section IX, Obstetric and Gynaecological Emergencies.

- Ruptured ectopic pregnancy (see p. 327).
- Pelvic inflammatory disease (acute salpingitis) (see p. 325).
- Ruptured ovarian cyst (see p. 326).
- Torsion of an ovarian tumour (see p. 326).
- Endometriosis (see p. 326).

MEDICAL DISORDERS PRESENTING WITH ACUTE ABDOMINAL PAIN

It is uncommon for non-surgical disorders causing acute abdominal pain to present without other symptoms or signs suggesting their true medical origin.

Always remember diabetic ketoacidosis (DKA), and perform a urinalysis in *every* patient with abdominal pain. DKA is suggested by finding glycosuria and ketonuria (see p. 79).

DIAGNOSIS

Medical disorders presenting with acute abdominal pain include:

1 *Thoracic origin*
  - (i) Myocardial infarction, pericarditis.
  - (ii) Pulmonary embolus, pleurisy, pneumonia.
  - (iii) Aortic dissection.

2 *Abdominal origin*
  - (i) Hepatic congestion from hepatitis or right heart failure.
  - (ii) Infection, including gastroenteritis, pyelonephritis and primary peritonitis.
  - (iii) Intestinal ischaemia from atheroma or sickle cell disease, vasculitis and Henoch–Schönlein purpura.
  - (iv) Irritable bowel syndrome.

> **Warning:** constipation, particularly in the elderly, should be regarded as a *symptom* and not a diagnosis. Other significant underlying conditions such as a bowel obstruction, diverticulitis, urinary or other sepsis, colon cancer, hypercalcaemia or neurological disease must be actively excluded.

3 *Endocrine and metabolic origin*
  - (i) Diabetic ketoacidosis.
  - (ii) Hypercalcaemia – 'stones, bones and abdominal groans'.
  - (iii) Addison's disease.
  - (iv) Lead poisoning, paracetamol or iron poisoning.
  - (v) Porphyria (acute intermittent).

4   Neurogenic origin
   (i)   Herpes zoster.
   (ii) Radiculitis from spinal cord degeneration or malignancy.
   (iii) Tabes dorsalis.

5   Thoracolumbar spine origin
   Collapsed vertebra due to osteoporosis, neoplasm or infection (see p. 281).

6   Psychiatric
   Münchausen's syndrome or 'hospital hopper':
   (i)   Be suspicious of a patient presenting with acute abdominal pain
         or renal colic, who usually does not live locally, and with no GP,
         who may have multiple abdominal scars from operations 'at
         another hospital'.
   (ii) Their aim is to gain narcotic analgesia or hospital admission by
         feigning illness.
   (iii) Ask for a previous hospital number or admission details, so you
         can 'go and verify their story'.
   (iv) Seek advice from the senior ED doctor.

7   Take a careful history in all patients, do a thorough examination, and send
        blood for FBC, U&Es, LFTs, blood sugar and lipase/amylase.

8   Request a urinalysis, perform an ECG and request a CXR to avoid missing
        the more serious diagnoses.

MANAGEMENT

1   Discuss the case with the senior ED doctor. Admit the patient as appropriate
        according to the suspected underlying diagnosis.

FURTHER READING

National Health and Medical Research Council (Australia). http://www.nhmrc.
   gov.au/guidelines/search

National Institute for Health and Care Excellence, NHS UK. http://www.nice.org.
   uk/guidance/published

Scottish Intercollegiate Guidelines Network. http://www.sign.ac.uk/

Spahn D, Bouillon B, Cerny V et al. (2013) Management of bleeding and coagulopathy following major trauma: an updated European guideline. *Crit Care*
   17:R76.

Trauma.org http://www.trauma.org/ (trauma education and management).

ORTHOPAEDIC EMERGENCIES

INJURIES TO THE SHOULDER AND UPPER ARM

FRACTURES OF THE CLAVICLE

DIAGNOSIS

1 These fractures are usually due to direct violence or to transmitted force from a fall onto the outstretched hand.

2 A fracture between the middle and outer thirds is common in adults. A greenstick fracture occurs in children.

3 The patient experiences pain on movement of the shoulder and examination reveals tenderness over the clavicle associated with local deformity.

4 An anteroposterior X-ray of the shoulder usually shows the fracture clearly.

MANAGEMENT

1 Support the weight of the arm in a triangular sling, and give an analgesic such as paracetamol 500 mg and codeine phosphate 8 mg two tablets q.d.s.

2 Rarely, comminuted fractures or fractures causing compression of underlying nerves or vessels are treated operatively.
    (i)   Refer these immediately to the orthopaedic team.

3 Otherwise, refer the patient to the next fracture clinic.

ACROMIOCLAVICULAR DISLOCATION

DIAGNOSIS

1 Acromioclavicular injuries usually occur following a fall on to the apex of the shoulder with the arm held in adduction.

2 A fall on to the shoulder that tears the acromioclavicular ligament results in subluxation.
    (i)   Dislocation occurs if the strong coracoclavicular ligaments are torn as well, with the clavicle losing all connection with the scapula.

3 Subluxation causes local tenderness to palpation with minimal deformity.
    (i)   Full dislocation causes a prominent outer end of the clavicle and drooping of the shoulder, with pain on movement.

4 Assess the clavicle and scapula for associated fractures.

5 X-ray the acromioclavicular joint with the patient standing to show the displacement of the clavicle. This can be highlighted by comparing the shoulders, with the patient holding a weight in each hand.

MANAGEMENT

1 Treat minor subluxations with ice, oral analgesics, sling immobilization, daily range of motion exercises, and refer to the next fracture clinic.

2 Start the same supportive treatment for a full dislocation, but discuss with the orthopaedic team for consideration of operative intervention.

    (i) Sling immobilization may be required for 4–6 weeks.

STERNOCLAVICULAR DISLOCATION

DIAGNOSIS

1 This dislocation is rare and is caused by either:

    (i) A direct blow to the anteromedial aspect of the clavicle forcing the clavicle backwards resulting in a posterior dislocation, or

    (ii) Transmission of indirect forces from the anterolateral or posterolateral shoulder, displacing the clavicle either forwards or backwards.

2 Patients complain of chest and shoulder pain exacerbated by arm movements, particularly when supine.

3 Anterior displacement results in local tenderness and asymmetry of the medial ends of the clavicles.

4 Posterior displacement can impinge on the trachea or great vessels and present with dyspnoea, dysphagia and arm paraesthesiae.

5 The diagnosis is largely clinical. On examination the affected shoulder appears thrust forward, and the medial aspect of the sternoclavicular joint is painful to palpate.

6 Plain X-rays are not easy to interpret, although anteroposterior and oblique views should be requested.

7 A computed tomography (CT) scan is required, particularly in posterior displacements.

MANAGEMENT

1 Treat subluxations with a triangular sling, oral analgesics and refer to the next fracture clinic.

2 Refer posterior dislocations with pressure symptoms immediately to the orthopaedic team.

3 Discuss full anterior dislocations with the orthopaedic team.

    (i) As with acromioclavicular dislocations, once reduced they are difficult to hold in place.

    (ii) Following reduction, provide sling immobilization for 4–6 weeks.

FRACTURES OF THE SCAPULA

DIAGNOSIS

1 These can be divided into fractures of the neck, body, spine, acromion and coracoid. They are usually due to direct trauma.

2   Their importance is that they 'flag' that considerable force has been applied to the area. Check for an associated rib, chest, vertebral column and shoulder injury.

3   Request an anteroposterior shoulder view and lateral scapula view to adequately visualize the majority of scapula injuries.

    (i)   A CT scan is indicated to delineate associated glenoid and/or coracoid fractures.

MANAGEMENT

1   Treat the associated injuries as a priority.

2   Manage the majority of isolated undisplaced scapula fractures that do not involve the glenohumeral articular surface with ice, sling immobilization, oral analgesics, and early range of motion exercises. Refer to the next fracture clinic.

3   Displaced fractures of the glenoid and scapula neck are associated with significant shoulder soft-tissue trauma and may require surgical reduction. Refer these to the orthopaedic team.

ANTERIOR DISLOCATION OF THE SHOULDER

DIAGNOSIS

1   This dislocation is caused by forced abduction, elevation and external rotation of the shoulder relative to the trunk. It is most common in young adults from sports or traffic crashes, or in the elderly from a fall.

2   It tends to become recurrent, when dislocation may occur with a trivial injury, movement or even spontaneously in bed.

3   Patients have severe shoulder pain and a limited range of movement.

4   The arm is held slightly abducted and the shoulder appears 'square', due to loss of the deltoid contour and a prominent acromion.

5   Look for the following complications before any attempt is made at manipulation:

    (i)   *Axillary (circumflex) nerve damage*
        Assess for pinprick sensory loss over the 'regimental badge' area on the upper lateral aspect of the deltoid (testing for shoulder movement by the deltoid is too painful to be meaningful).

    (ii) *Posterior cord of the brachial plexus*
        Test wrist extension by the radial nerve. Rarely other parts of the brachial plexus are damaged.

    (iii) *Axillary artery damage*
        Palpate the radial pulse. Prompt reduction usually restores the circulation.

    (iv) *Fracture of the upper humerus*
        Look carefully for this on the X-rays.

6 Always X-ray the shoulder, even if you are sure of the diagnosis, to avoid missing an associated humeral neck or head fracture. Look for the following features:

    (i) The humeral neck or head is displaced medially and anteriorly with loss of contact with the glenoid fossa on the anteroposterior view.

    (ii) Look at the lateral 'Y' view in doubtful cases. The humeral head lies anterior to the 'Y' in anterior dislocation.

    (iii) *Upper humeral fracture*

        (a) fracture of the greater tuberosity does not influence the initial reduction

        (b) refer a fracture through the humeral head, neck or upper humerus directly to the orthopaedic team. **Do not** attempt reduction.

MANAGEMENT

1 Give the patient morphine 2.5–5 mg i.v. with an antiemetic such as metoclopramide 10 mg i.v. if there is severe pain (unusual in recurrent dislocations). Reduce the dose of morphine in elderly patients.

2 Perform the reduction in a monitored area such as a resuscitation bay using procedural sedation with diazepam 5–10 mg i.v. or midazolam 2.5–5 mg i.v.

    (i) Ensure a second doctor is present, comprehensive monitoring and resuscitation equipment are available, and dentures, rings, etc. have been removed.

3 There are many different methods of reduction:

    (i) *Modified Kocher's manoeuvre*

        (a) hold the arm in adduction with the elbow flexed

        (b) apply gentle if any traction and slowly externally rotate. Stop briefly if muscle resistance is felt, then continue

        (c) the shoulder may 'clunk' back during external rotation. If it does not, lift the externally rotated arm to 90°, flex the shoulder and then adduct the arm across the chest in external rotation, and finally internally rotate it across the chest.

    (ii) *Milch technique*

        (a) stabilize the position of the humeral head in the supine or prone patient with one hand

        (b) using the other hand abduct the affected limb to the overhead position

        (c) then externally rotate the affected limb with one hand and use the other to push the humeral head laterally to achieve reduction.

    (iii) *Spaso technique*

        (a) hold the affected arm by the wrist with the patient lying supine

        (b) while applying mild traction, slowly lift the affected limb vertically

        (c) achieve reduction by externally rotating the shoulder and maintaining vertical traction.

     (iv) *Scapular rotation*
         (a) with the patient seated or prone, manipulate the scapula by medially displacing the inferior tip of the scapula using thumb pressure
         (b) keep stabilizing the superior part of the scapular with the other hand.

4 Place the arm in a sling strapped to the body after reduction, or enclosed under the patient's clothes, to prevent external rotation and a recurrent dislocation. Repeat the shoulder X-ray to confirm the reduction.

5 Test again for neurovascular damage.

6 Give the patient an oral analgesic, instructions to keep the arm initially adducted and internally rotated, and refer to the next fracture clinic.
     (i) Recurrent dislocation occurs in at least 50%, up to 85% if aged <20 yr.
     (ii) Operative repair is increasingly recommended in the young, certainly for four or more dislocations.

POSTERIOR DISLOCATION OF THE SHOULDER

DIAGNOSIS

1 This dislocation is uncommon and can be bilateral. It occurs classically during electrocution or a seizure, or from a direct blow (e.g. in boxing), and is easily missed.

2 The arm is held adducted and internally rotated, and the greater tuberosity of the humerus feels prominent.
     (i) Any attempts at external rotation are severely limited and painful.

3 Include two X-ray views of the shoulder, as the anteroposterior view will appear 'normal'.
     (i) Look for the 'light bulb' sign on the anteroposterior view, due to the internally rotated humerus displaying a globular head, and for an irregular, reduced glenohumeral joint space.
     (ii) Look for the humeral head lying behind the glenoid on the lateral scapular 'Y' view.

MANAGEMENT

1 Give the patient morphine 2.5–5 mg i.v. with an antiemetic such as metoclopramide 10 mg i.v.

2 Perform the reduction using procedural sedation with diazepam 5–10 mg i.v. or midazolam 2.5–5 mg i.v., provided that a second doctor is present, and monitoring and resuscitation equipment are available.
     (i) Apply traction to the arm abducted to 90°.
     (ii) Gently externally rotate the arm.

3 Place the arm in a sling and repeat the shoulder X-ray to confirm reduction. Occasionally, the reduction may be unstable and immediate orthopaedic referral will be required.

4 Give the patient an analgesic and refer to the next fracture clinic.

FRACTURES OF THE UPPER HUMERUS

DIAGNOSIS

1 These fractures usually occur in elderly patients following a fall onto the outstretched hand and may involve the greater tuberosity, the lesser tuberosity, the anatomical neck or most commonly the surgical neck of the humerus.

2 There is localized pain and loss of movement, often with dramatic bruising gravitating down the arm.

3 Complications include:
    (i) Dislocation of the humeral head.
    (ii) Complete distraction of the humeral head off the shaft.
    (iii) Axillary (circumflex) nerve damage causing anaesthesia over the upper, lateral aspect of the upper arm and loss of deltoid movement.
    (iv) Axillary vessel damage with compromised vascular supply to the humeral head or distal arm.

4 Confirm proximal head fracture and associated humeral head distraction or comminution with plain X-rays of the shoulder.

MANAGEMENT

1 Immediately refer to the orthopaedic team patients with:
    (i) Gross angulation or total distraction of the humeral head.
    (ii) Fracture associated with a dislocation.
    (iii) Associated neurovascular damage.

2 Otherwise, use a collar and cuff to allow gravity to exert gentle traction. Give the patient an analgesic such as paracetamol 500 mg and codeine phosphate 8 mg two tablets q.d.s.

3 Remember that the elderly patient may now need social services support in the form of 'meals on wheels', a home help, and possibly a community nurse.
    (i) Inform the GP by email and letter so he or she may visit the patient.

4 Refer the patient to the fracture clinic for follow-up.

FRACTURES OF THE SHAFT OF THE HUMERUS

DIAGNOSIS

1 These fractures are caused by direct trauma or a fall onto the outstretched hand.

2   Upper-third fractures result in the proximal fragment being adducted by the pectoralis major, whereas in middle-third fractures the proximal fragment is abducted by the deltoid.

3   Clinically the diagnosis is usually evident, with obvious local deformity and loss of function of the arm. Examine the affected arm for neurovascular complications, which are common.

4   Complications are usually seen in middle-third fractures, including:
-   (i)   Compound injury.
-   (ii) Radial nerve damage in the spiral groove, causing weak wrist extension and sensory loss over the dorsum of the thumb.

5   Always include views of the shoulder and elbow, remembering the old adage to 'X-ray the joint above and the joint below any fracture'.

MANAGEMENT

1   Immediately refer to the orthopaedic team patients with:
-   (i)   Grossly angulated or comminuted fracture.
-   (ii) Compound fracture.
-   (iii) Radial nerve palsy.

2   Otherwise, support the arm for comfort in a U-slab plaster or hanging cast. This should not require analgesia to apply.
-   (i)   Pad the arm well with cotton-wool and apply a 10–15 cm wide plaster slab medially under the axilla, around the elbow, up over the lateral aspect of the upper arm and on to the shoulder.
-   (ii) Hold the slab in place with a crêpe bandage, and support the arm in a sling.

3   Give the patient analgesics and review in the next fracture clinic. Social services support is needed for the elderly, who may require admission if they are unable to cope.

INJURIES TO THE ELBOW AND FOREARM

SUPRACONDYLAR FRACTURE OF THE HUMERUS

DIAGNOSIS

1   This fracture occurs most commonly in children from a fall onto the outstretched hand, although it is also seen in adults following a direct blow to the elbow.

2   There is tenderness and swelling over the distal humerus, but the olecranon and two epicondyles remain in their usual 'equilateral triangle' relationship (which is lost in dislocation of the elbow).

3   Test for median nerve damage and look for any signs of arterial occlusion, such as pain, pallor, paralysis, paraesthesiae, and pulselessness.

4   Complications include:
   (i)   *Brachial artery damage* – compression, intimal damage or division may be caused by posterior displacement of the lower end of the proximal humeral fragment.
   (ii) *Median nerve damage* – associated with sensory loss over the radial three-and-a-half fingers and weakness of abductor pollicis.
   (iii) *Local tissue swelling* – tense and rapidly progressive swelling may cause vascular compromise to the distal forearm.
   (iv) *Volkmann's ischaemic contracture* – a late but devastating complication resulting from tissue necrosis secondary to distal forearm arterial compromise.

5   X-ray will show any displacement, although one-third of fractures are undisplaced, some merely greenstick.
   (i)   An occult, undisplaced fracture may be inferred by the presence of a haemarthrosis causing a posterior or anterior fat pad sign on X-ray (see p. 232).
   (ii) Request comparison views of the other normal elbow if there is difficulty in interpreting the radiographs, especially in children with epiphyseal growth plates.

MANAGEMENT

1   Refer the patient immediately to the orthopaedic team if arterial occlusion is suspected, for urgent manipulation under procedural sedation or preferably general anaesthesia.

2   Refer displaced, comminuted, or severely angulated fractures also to the orthopaedic team, even if there is no arterial damage.

3   Manage undisplaced and greenstick fractures conservatively with analgesia, and a collar and cuff with the forearm flexed to at least 80° or more from extension, allowing the triceps to help splint the fracture.
   (i)   Arrange review in the next fracture clinic.

CONDYLAR AND EPICONDYLAR FRACTURES OF THE HUMERUS

DIAGNOSIS

1   The lateral condyle is usually fractured in children, and the medial epicondyle at any age, due to direct violence or forced contraction of the forearm flexors that attach to it.

2   There is pain, swelling (which may be minimal) and loss of full elbow extension if the medial epicondyle is trapped in the joint, usually following dislocation of the elbow.

3   Test for ulnar nerve damage, causing sensory loss over the medial one-and-a-half digits and weakness of the finger adductors and abductors.

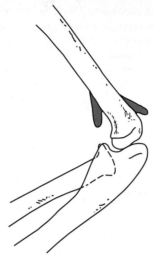

Figure 6.1 Line-drawing of a lateral elbow X-ray showing an anterior and posterior fat-pad sign (shaded areas are abnormal and indicate a joint effusion).

4   X-rays are often difficult to interpret in children, as many of the structures are still cartilaginous. Helpful clues to look for are:

    (i)   The posterior fat-pad sign (see Fig. 6.1). This indicates a joint effusion, and is indirect evidence of significant trauma. It is also typically seen with radial head fractures.

    (ii)   Comparison with the normal elbow placed in a similar anatomical position. Look for any differences between the two sides.

    (iii)   Suspect displacement from injury if an epiphysis that should be visible by age is missing

        (a)   the capitellum epiphysis is visible by age 1 year, the medial epicondyle epiphysis by age 6 years, and the lateral epicondyle epiphysis by age 11 years.

MANAGEMENT

1   Refer all these fractures to the orthopaedic team. The fractures are always more extensive than they appear on the X-ray, as the structures are mainly cartilaginous.

DISLOCATION OF THE ELBOW

DIAGNOSIS

1   This is caused by a fall on to the outstretched hand driving the olecranon posteriorly. Rarely anterior, medial or lateral displacement occurs.

2   The normal 'equilateral triangle' between the olecranon and two epicondyles is disrupted (unlike in a supracondylar fracture).

3 Look for the following complications:
   (i) Ulnar nerve damage, causing sensory loss over the medial one-and-a-half fingers and weakness of the finger adductors, with the fingers held straight.
   (ii) Median nerve damage, causing sensory loss over the radial three-and-a-half fingers and weakness of the abductor pollicis.
   (iii) Brachial artery damage, causing loss of the radial pulse with pain, pallor, paralysis, paraesthesiae and feeling cold in the forearm or hand.

4 Request an X-ray that usually shows the dislocation clearly.
   (i) Look for associated fractures of the coronoid process of the ulna or radial head in adults, and of the humeral epicondyles or lateral condyle in children.

MANAGEMENT

1 Support the elbow in a sling and give morphine 2.5–5 mg i.v. with an antiemetic such as metoclopramide 10 mg i.v.

2 Call a senior emergency department (ED) doctor to help perform the reduction under procedural sedation with diazepam 5–10 mg i.v. or midazolam 2.5–5 mg i.v., provided a second doctor is present, and full monitoring and resuscitation equipment are available.

3 Apply axial traction to the elbow in 30° of extension, and push the olecranon with the thumbs.

4 Apply a posterior plaster slab with the elbow in 90° of flexion, and forearm in neutral position (hand vertical).

5 Perform a post-reduction X-ray and refer all cases to the orthopaedic team for neurovascular observation.

6 Also refer complicated cases to the orthopaedic team, which include comminuted fracture of the radial head, humeral epicondyles or coronoid process, or those that were not able to be reduced.

PULLED ELBOW

DIAGNOSIS

1 This is common in children aged 2–6 years and usually follows axial traction applied to an extended arm, for example when pulling a child's hand to prevent a fall or to put on a sweater.
   (i) However, about half the cases report no history of trauma.

2 The radial head is subluxed out of the annular ligament, causing local pain and loss of use of the arm, particularly supination.

3 Examination reveals an anxious child protecting the affected arm, which is held by the side, with the elbow semi flexed and pronated. There is no neurovascular compromise and motor activity is normal.

4   X-rays are usually not necessary, but should be performed to exclude a fracture if there is extensive swelling over the elbow, or if reduction is not successful after two or three attempts.

MANAGEMENT

1   Fix the elbow and apply pressure to the region of the radial head with one hand. Applying axial compression at the wrist, supinate the forearm and gently flex the elbow with the other hand.

   (i)   The radial head is felt to click back in the majority of cases.

   (ii) If reduction fails, ensure the diagnosis is correct, then place in a broad arm sling and arrange fracture clinic follow up. Most cases resolve spontaneously within 48 h.

2   The child is often still reluctant to use the arm for the first 15–30 min following reduction, and so observe in the ED until adequate return of function has been demonstrated.

3   No immobilization is required unless reduction fails. Discharge the child with the parents following education to prevent a recurrence.

FRACTURES OF THE OLECRANON

DIAGNOSIS

1   These fractures follow a fall on to the point of the elbow or forced triceps contraction, which may then distract the olecranon, leaving a palpable subcutaneous gap.

2   Examine for local tenderness, swelling and loss of active elbow extension.

3   Request an X-ray to confirm the diagnosis and to delineate the degree of fracture displacement, angulation or comminution.

   (i)   Anterior dislocation of the elbow may accompany a displaced olecranon fracture.

MANAGEMENT

1   Give the patient analgesia and a sling, and refer immediately to the orthopaedic team for operative reduction if there is displacement of the olecranon, or an associated anterior dislocation of the elbow.

2   Treat an undisplaced hairline fracture with a long-arm plaster, with the elbow flexed, and review at the next fracture clinic.

FRACTURES OF THE RADIAL HEAD

DIAGNOSIS

1   These fractures are caused by direct violence or by indirect force, such as falling onto the outstretched hand, when the radius is driven proximally against the capitellum.

2   There is localized pain and tenderness over the radial head, discomfort on supination of the forearm and a loss of full elbow extension.

3 This injury is commonly missed, usually because it is not thought of or because it is not seen on X-ray.

4 Request an X-ray of the elbow.
  (i) It may be difficult or impossible to see the fracture, but look for corroborating evidence of a posterior fat-pad sign (see Fig. 6.1).
  (ii) If there is doubt, ask specifically for additional radial head views.

MANAGEMENT

1 Place a non-displaced fracture in a collar and cuff, and refer the patient to the next fracture clinic.

2 Use a plaster elbow backslab for comfort and protection if there is severe localized pain.

3 Refer the patient directly to the orthopaedic team if the radial head is severely comminuted or grossly displaced, for consideration of operative management.

FRACTURES OF THE RADIAL AND ULNAR SHAFTS

These two bones act as a unit, attached proximally at the radial head by the annular ligament, throughout their length by the interosseous membrane and distally by the radio-ulnar ligaments.

It is rare to fracture one bone in isolation and, as in humeral shaft fractures, it is essential to X-ray the joints above and below (here, the elbow and wrist).

DIAGNOSIS

1 Injury is caused by direct trauma or by falling onto an outstretched hand, usually with an element of rotation fracturing both bones.

2 There is localized tenderness, swelling and deformity. Compound injuries are more common with direct trauma.
  (i) Monitor for neurovascular compromise, compartment syndrome and musculotendinous injury.

3 X-ray will demonstrate the fractures. Look closely for an associated dislocation injury if one bone is fractured and angulated, but with no radiographic evidence of the other bone being broken.
  (i) *Monteggia fracture:* fracture of the proximal ulna with dislocation of the radial head. Dislocation is present if a line through the radius fails to bisect the capitellum in both X-ray views.
  (ii) *Galeazzi fracture:* fracture of the distal radius with dislocation of the inferior radio-ulnar joint at the wrist. Look for widening at the distal radio-ulnar joint space and dorsal displacement of the ulnar head on X-rays. An associated ulnar styloid fracture is common.

MANAGEMENT

1 Refer all these fractures to the orthopaedic team for open reduction and internal fixation.

2 Place the arm in a full-arm plaster cast from the metacarpal heads to the upper arm, with the elbow flexed at a right angle and the wrist in the mid-position, in the rare instance of an isolated, undisplaced, single forearm bone fracture.

    (i) Refer the patient to the next fracture clinic.

INJURIES TO THE WRIST AND HAND

COLLES' FRACTURE

DIAGNOSIS

1 This is a fracture of the distal radius usually within 2.5 cm of the wrist. It is most common in elderly women with osteoporosis and usually associated with a fall onto the outstretched hand.

2 The classical 'dinner fork' deformity is due to dorsal angulation and dorsal displacement of the distal radial fragment, which may also be impacted and radially displaced.

3 X-ray demonstrates the distal radial fracture, with an associated avulsion of the ulnar styloid process in up to 60% of cases.

4 Delayed complications of Colles' fracture include malunion, post-traumatic reflex sympathetic dystrophy (Sudeck's atrophy), acute carpal tunnel syndrome, reduced grip strength, shoulder stiffness or a 'frozen shoulder' and late rupture of the extensor pollicis longus.

MANAGEMENT

1 Treat undisplaced or minimally displaced fractures, particularly in the elderly, directly with a Colles' backslab, without manipulation.

2 Displaced, angulated fractures with radial deviation require reduction to promote optimal return of function and to reduce the delayed complications.

3 Options for reduction include procedural sedation, Bier's block, axillary nerve block, haematoma block or general anaesthesia, according to departmental policy.

4 *Bier's block technique of intravenous regional anaesthesia* (see p. 487).

    (i) Rest the patient for at least 2 h after completion while regular observations are made. Allow home with an accompanying adult if the plaster is comfortable and the patient feels well.

5 *Colles' reduction and immobilization*

    (i) Prepare a 20 cm width plaster slab measured from the metacarpal heads to the angle of the elbow. Cut a slot for the thumb and remove a triangle to accommodate the final ulnar deviation (see Fig. 6.2a, b).

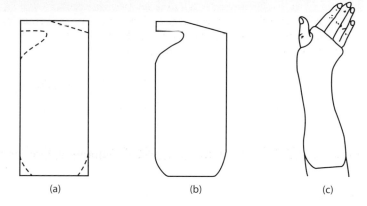

(a)   (b)   (c)

Figure 6.2 Colles' plaster of Paris backslab.
(a) and (b) the backslab is prepared by trimming to permit thumb movements, full elbow flexion and to allow for the final ulnar deviation of the wrist; (c) the backslab in position.

(ii) Disimpact the fracture by firm traction on the thumb and fingers, and by hyperextending the wrist in the direction of deformity. An assistant should provide countertraction to the upper arm, with the elbow kept flexed at 90°.

(iii) Next, extend the elbow and then use your thenar eminence to reduce the dorsal displacement and to rotate back the dorsal angulation, with the heel of your other hand acting as a fulcrum.

(iv) Alter your grip to push the distal fragment towards the ulna to correct radial displacement.

(v) Finally, hold the hand pronated in full ulnar deviation with the wrist slightly flexed. Pad the forearm with cotton-wool and apply the backslab to the radial side of the forearm (see Fig. 6.2c). Hold the backslab in place with a crêpe bandage.

(vi) Take a check X-ray to assess the adequacy of the reduction before terminating the anaesthetic:
  (a) reduction should be near perfect in a young person
  (b) up to 10° of residual dorsal angulation can be accepted, i.e. neutral position in an elderly person, and <5 mm radial shortening.

6   Give the patient a sling, with instructions to keep the shoulder and fingers moving, and review in the next fracture clinic.

7   Remember to check that an elderly patient will still be able to manage at home, particularly if they already rely on a walking frame. Social services help may be needed. Inform the GP by fax and letter.

SMITH'S FRACTURE

DIAGNOSIS

1 This fracture is caused by a fall on to the dorsum of the hand, a hyperflexion or a hypersupination injury. It results in a distal radial fracture with volar displacement. It is often termed a reversed Colles' fracture.

2 Examine for localized swelling and a classical 'garden spade' deformity. The patient is unable to extend the wrist and has pain on supination and pronation.

  (i) Assess for damage to the median nerve causing loss of sensation in the radial three-and-a-half digits and weakness of abductor pollicis.

MANAGEMENT

1 Reduce the fracture under procedural sedation, Bier's block, axillary block or general anaesthetic, according to departmental policy.

2 *Smith's reduction and immobilization*

  (i) Disimpact the fracture by firm traction to the forearm in supination, with an assistant providing countertraction to the upper arm.

  (ii) Apply pressure with the heel of the hand to reduce the distal fragment dorsally.

  (iii) Place a long-arm plaster to hold the reduced fracture in position

   (a) position the affected arm with the elbow in 90° flexion, the forearm in full supination, and the wrist dorsiflexed (extended)

   (b) mould an anterior slab around the radius with a slot cut for the thumb

   (c) extend the plaster above the elbow, kept at a right angle.

  (iv) Take a check X-ray to assess the adequacy of reduction before terminating the anaesthetic. If reduction fails, internal fixation may be necessary.

3 Give the patient a sling and analgesics, and review in the next fracture clinic.

  (i) As the fracture is often unstable, it is prone to slipping and the patient usually requires weekly X-ray follow-up to ensure continued fracture reduction.

BARTON'S FRACTURE–DISLOCATION

DIAGNOSIS

1 This is an intra-articular fracture of the distal radius with an associated subluxation of the carpus and wrist, which move in a volar or dorsal direction.

2 The volar Barton's fracture has a similar mechanism of injury to the Smith's fracture, and the intra-articular distal radius fracture is angulated in a palmar direction.

3 The dorsal Barton's fracture is caused by a fall onto the outstretched hand with the wrist extended and forearm pronated. The axial load causes the dorsal rim of the distal radius to fracture with anterior displacement.

MANAGEMENT

1 Refer the patient immediately to the orthopaedic team as this injury is unstable and open reduction with internal fixation is required.

RADIAL STYLOID FRACTURE

DIAGNOSIS

1 This is caused by a fall onto the outstretched hand causing an oblique intra-articular fracture of the radial styloid. It used to be termed the 'chauffeur's fracture' when caused by an engine starting-handle kickback.

2 There is pain over the lateral aspect of the distal radius.

3 Displacement is usually slight, but look for an associated scapholunate dissociation on X-ray.

MANAGEMENT

1 Apply a Colles'-type plaster backslab.

2 Give the patient a sling, with instructions to keep the shoulder and fingers moving, and review in the next fracture clinic.
  (i) Operative fixation may be necessary, and physiotherapy is required particularly if Sudeck's atrophy occurs.

DISTAL RADIAL FRACTURES IN CHILDREN

DIAGNOSIS

1 These represent the most common paediatric fractures.

2 They are associated with marked local tenderness, sometimes with deformity.

3 Request an X-ray to show the nature of the fracture:
  (i) *Plastic deformation:* most commonly associated with the ulna.
  (ii) *Greenstick fracture:* occurs when one side of a bone breaks as the opposite side is bent, usually where the force was directly applied.
  (iii) *Buckle or 'torus' fracture:* compressive forces cause one side of the bone to 'buckle' under pressure as the opposite side is bent.
  (iv) *Complete fracture:* involves the entire bone and both cortical surfaces.
  (v) *Epiphyseal fracture:* involves the growth plate and is classified using the Salter–Harris system. The radial epiphysis may displace dorsally, often in adolescents, to mimic a Colles' deformity.

MANAGEMENT

1 Refer all angulated fractures and displaced radial epiphyses to the orthopaedic team for reduction under general anaesthesia.

2 Otherwise, place the forearm in a Colles'-type plaster backslab for a minimally buckled cortex, which may be difficult to even see on an X-ray. Refer the patient to the next fracture clinic.

FRACTURES OF THE SCAPHOID

DIAGNOSIS

1   The scaphoid is the most commonly fractured carpal bone, usually caused by a fall onto the outstretched hand. Consider this in any patient presenting with a 'sprained wrist', particularly after a sporting injury.

2   There is pain on dorsiflexion or ulnar deviation of the wrist, as well as pain and weakness of pinch grip.

3   Look for localized pain and tenderness by:
    (i)   Compressive pressure along the thumb metacarpal.
    (ii) Palpating in the anatomical 'snuff box' between extensor pollicis longus and abductor pollicis longus.
    (iii) Palpating the scaphoid tubercle.

4   Ask specifically for scaphoid views as well as for anteroposterior and lateral wrist X-ray views. Unless the fracture is complete, it may be difficult to detect in the acute phase.
    (i)   Repeat X-ray in 10–14 days allows time for decalcification to occur at the fracture site and for the fracture to become visible.

5   Alternatively, request an immediate CT, bone scan or even magnetic resonance imaging (MRI) depending on availability, and local practice.

MANAGEMENT

1   Place the wrist in a removable splint or a double-elasticated stockinet bandage, if the X-rays are normal and pain or tenderness are minor. Provide a high-arm sling.
    (i)   Review every patient in either the ED or orthopaedic clinic within 10 days of injury depending on local policy.
    (ii) Repeat the X-ray if pain persists.

2   Otherwise, if a fracture is confirmed on X-ray, or if there is marked pain and tenderness particularly on moving the thumb or wrist, place the forearm in a scaphoid plaster.

3   *Scaphoid plaster* (see Fig. 6.3).
    (i)   The wrist should be fully pronated, radially deviated and partially dorsiflexed, and the thumb held in mid-abduction.
    (ii) Apply the plaster from the mid-shaft of the forearm to the metacarpal heads, to include the base of the thumb proximal to the interphalangeal joint.

4   Give the patient a high-arm sling and refer to the next fracture clinic.

5   The scaphoid has a critical role in the proximal carpal row and is important in maintaining radiocarpal stability.

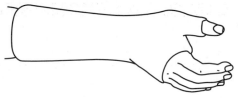

Figure 6.3 The scaphoid plaster. This extends from the angle of the elbow to the metacarpal heads, and around the base of the thumb to below (proximal to) the interphalangeal joint.

   (i)   Orthopaedic review is *essential* to reduce complications and potential loss of function, as well as to exclude a missed injury such as:
      (a) scapholunate dissociation with >4 mm space between these bones, radial styloid fracture, or even a Bennett's fracture of the base of the thumb metacarpal.
   (ii) Delayed complications of scaphoid fracture include avascular necrosis, non-union and osteoarthritis, which result in pain and loss of wrist function.

DISLOCATIONS OF THE CARPUS

DIAGNOSIS

1   Dislocations of the carpus are uncommon, and are caused by a fall on the outstretched hand. Two important types are seen:
   (i) *Dislocation of the lunate:* the distal carpal bones and hand maintain their normal alignment with the radius, but the lunate is squeezed out anteriorly, like a pip.
   (ii) *Perilunate dislocation of the carpus:* the lunate maintains its alignment with the radius, but the distal carpal bones and the hand are driven dorsally
      (a) a displaced fracture through the scaphoid is often present.

2   Test for median nerve compression in dislocation of the lunate, causing loss of sensation in the radial three-and-a-half digits and weakness of abductor pollicis.

3   Request X-rays that are easy to misinterpret as 'normal' in lunate dislocation, but look particularly for:
   (i) The normal curved joint space between the distal radius and the scaphoid and lunate is disrupted on the anteroposterior view, so the lunate looks triangular instead of quadrilateral.
   (ii) The dislocated lunate lies anteriorly on the lateral view, in the shape of the letter 'C'.

MANAGEMENT

1 Refer all cases immediately to the orthopaedic team, particularly if median nerve compression is found.

FRACTURES OF THE OTHER CARPAL BONES

DIAGNOSIS

1 These fractures are rare, and include fractures of the capitate, triquetral, hook of hamate and pisiform bones.

2 There is localized tenderness from direct trauma, sometimes with an associated ulnar nerve palsy affecting the deep branch that supplies most of the intrinsic hand muscles.

3 A common problem on X-ray is to remember the names of the eight carpal bones.

    (i) Try remembering that the 'trapezium is at the base of the thumb' and then use the mnemonic: '*Hamlet came to town shouting loudly to Polonius*', which refers to the hamate, capitate, trapezoid, trapezium, scaphoid, lunate, triquetral and pisiform bones (Fig. 6.4).

MANAGEMENT

1 Place all these fractures in a scaphoid plaster and refer to the next fracture clinic.

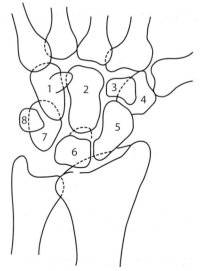

Figure 6.4 The two rows of carpal bones. **(1) hamate, (2) capitate, (3) trapezoid, (4) trapezium, (5) scaphoid, (6) lunate, (7) triquetral, (8) pisiform**.

FRACTURES OF THE THUMB METACARPAL

DIAGNOSIS

1 Injury usually results from forced thumb abduction, causing localized pain and tenderness.

2 Always X-ray to distinguish a stable from an unstable injury.
    (i) Stable injuries include transverse shaft and greenstick fractures.
    (ii) Unstable injuries include oblique shaft and comminuted fractures, and the fracture–dislocation of the base of the thumb (Bennett's fracture).
    (iii) *Bennett's fracture*
        (a) this is an oblique fracture through the base of the thumb metacarpal involving the joint with the trapezium, with subluxation of the rest of the thumb radially
        (b) look for swelling of the thenar eminence, sometimes with local palmar bruising
        (c) make sure the X-ray includes the base of the thumb to avoid missing this injury.

MANAGEMENT

1 Splint a stable fracture with a scaphoid plaster and refer the patient to the next fracture clinic.

2 Refer unstable fractures (including Bennett's) to the orthopaedic team for possible open reduction and internal fixation.

DISLOCATION OF THE THUMB METACARPAL

DIAGNOSIS

1 This may occur in motorcycle, skiing and football accidents, from forced thumb abduction or hyperextension.

2 Request an X-ray to exclude an associated fracture.

MANAGEMENT

1 Reduce under procedural sedation, a Bier's block or under general anaesthesia, according to departmental practice.
    (i) Apply traction to the thumb with pressure over the metacarpal head. After the manipulation, repeat the X-ray to confirm the reduction.
    (ii) Place the forearm in a scaphoid plaster with plenty of cotton-wool padding, and refer the patient to the next fracture clinic.

2 Refer the patient immediately to the orthopaedic team if the reduction fails.
    (i) The metacarpal head may have 'button-holed' through the joint capsule between tendons, and require open reduction.

RUPTURE OF THE ULNAR COLLATERAL LIGAMENT

DIAGNOSIS

1 This condition ('gamekeeper's thumb', which referred to a chronic lesion) is caused by forced thumb abduction, typically in motorcycling or skiing accidents.

2 It is often missed and must be suspected whenever pain and swelling are seen around the metacarpophalangeal (MCP) joint of the thumb, after an abduction injury.

3 Look for tenderness over the ulnar aspect of the MCP joint.

   (i) Test for laxity of the ulnar collateral ligament by applying a gentle abduction stress to the proximal phalanx, which reproduces the pain and demonstrates movement at the MCP joint.

   (ii) Pinch grip and power are lost.

4 X-ray may show an avulsion fracture of the proximal phalanx or a degree of MCP joint subluxation.

MANAGEMENT

1 Immobilize the thumb in a thumb spica cast or splint, and refer to the orthopaedic team, for consideration of operative repair.

2. Permanent disability may follow missed or untreated ruptures.

FRACTURES OF THE OTHER METACARPALS

DIAGNOSIS

1 These are caused by direct trauma and may be multiple. The classical, isolated, little-finger metacarpal neck fracture or 'boxer's fracture' is due to punching a hard object.

2 Examine all cases for any rotational deformity. On flexing the fingers into the palm, the fingertips should point to the scaphoid. If not, a rotational deformity of that finger exists.

3 Obtain anteroposterior, lateral and oblique X-rays of the hand.

MANAGEMENT

1 Refer multiple fractures, rotated fractures, compound fractures, and fractures associated with marked soft-tissue swelling from crushing to the orthopaedic team.

2 Otherwise, for an undisplaced, isolated fracture, give the patient a high-arm sling, an analgesic such as paracetamol 500 mg and codeine phosphate 8 mg and either a padded crêpe bandage, or a plaster of Paris volar slab with the hand in the 'position of safe splintage'.

3   **Position of safe splintage**
  (i)   Hold the wrist extended, the MCP joints flexed, the interphalangeal joints extended, and the thumb abducted with the volar slab, which is kept in place with a crêpe bandage.
  (ii) Pad well with cotton-wool, and extend the volar slab over the flexor aspect of the forearm, on to the palm of the hand to the fingertips.
  (iii) Instruct the patient to keep the hand elevated.
  (iv) Refer all patients to the next fracture clinic.

4   **Isolated, little-finger knuckle 'boxer's injury'**
  Many different methods of reduction and splintage have been tried.
  (i)   Simple 'buddy-strapping' of the little finger to the ring finger, a padded crêpe bandage, a sling and analgesia are as effective as any, particularly if angulation is less than 45°.
  (ii) Remember that if the knuckle struck a tooth and the skin has been broken, this is a potentially serious injury. It may involve underlying tendons or penetration of the joint capsule and there is high risk of infection
    (a) explore the wound in both the neutral position and with the fist clenched. If there is any suggestion of penetration into the joint space or tendon, refer the patient immediately to the orthopaedic team for surgical exploration and debridement. Give flucloxacillin 2 g i.v.
    (b) otherwise, take a wound swab for bacterial culture and irrigate the wound with normal saline. Give the patient amoxicillin 875 mg and clavulanic acid 125 mg, one tablet b.d. for 5 days and tetanus prophylaxis
    (c) review the wound within 24 h.

FRACTURES OF THE PROXIMAL AND MIDDLE PHALANGES

DIAGNOSIS

1   Similar mechanisms of injury and rules of management apply, as described previously for metacarpal fractures.

2   Examine all cases for rotational deformity. Check that on flexing the fingers into the palm, the tips all point to the scaphoid.

3   X-ray all injuries to look for fractures, dislocations, subluxations and radio-opaque foreign bodies.

MANAGEMENT

1   Refer all multiple, compound, angulated or rotated fractures, and those associated with marked soft-tissue damage or involving a joint surface, to the orthopaedic team.

2   Otherwise, buddy-strap the finger, give the patient a high-arm sling to prevent oedema, and give an analgesic such as paracetamol 500 mg and codeine phosphate 8 mg. Refer to the next fracture clinic.

FRACTURES OF THE DISTAL PHALANGES

DIAGNOSIS

1 These fractures are usually caused by a crushing injury resulting in a comminuted fracture of the bone.

2 The main problem is the associated soft-tissue injury to the nail and pulp space.

MANAGEMENT

1 Provide adequate protection by using a plastic mallet-finger splint, elevate the hand and give analgesics.

2 *Fingernail injuries*

  (i) Cover the exposed bed with soft paraffin gauze if the nail is avulsed, and give tetanus prophylaxis and flucloxacillin 500 mg orally q.d.s. for 5 days.

  (ii) If the nail is partially avulsed from the base:
  (a) administer a ring block (see p. 490)
  (b) remove the nail to exclude an underlying nailbed injury
  (c) debride and clean the area, then replace the nail as a splint to the nail matrix, and as a dressing to the nailbed
  (d) reposition the nail bed with one or two fine sutures inserted into the sides of the tip of the finger, **not** into the nailbed.

  (iii) Dress the area, give tetanus prophylaxis and antibiotics, and elevate the hand in a high-arm sling.

3 *Subungual haematoma*
Relieve this by trephining the nail with a red-hot paper clip to release the blood under tension. This is a painless procedure bringing instant relief.

DISLOCATION OF THE PHALANGES

DIAGNOSIS AND MANAGEMENT

1 Dislocations of the phalanges result from hyperextension injuries and must be X-rayed to exclude an associated fracture. They almost always displace dorsally or to one side.

2 Reduce under a ring block by traction applied to the finger, followed by a repeat X-ray to confirm adequate reduction (see p. 490).

3 Immobilize by buddy-strapping and encourage active finger movements. Refer the patient to the next fracture clinic.

4 Complications include:
  (i) Rupture of the middle slip of the extensor tendon following proximal interphalangeal joint dislocation.
  (ii) Avulsion of the volar plate.

(iii) Rupture of one or both collateral ligaments. An accompanying small avulsion flake fracture may be seen on X-ray.

(iv) Button-holing of the head of the phalanx through the volar plate, necessitating open operation for a failed reduction.

FLEXOR TENDON INJURIES IN THE HAND

DIAGNOSIS

1 These injuries occur from direct laceration or blunt injury.

2 Assess for a flexor tendon injury:

(i) *Flexor digitorum profundus* causes flexion at the distal interphalangeal joint.

(ii) *Flexor digitorum superficialis* causes flexion of the finger at the proximal interphalangeal joint, while the neighbouring fingers are held extended.

(iii) Suspect a partial tendon division from pain or reduced function against resistance.

MANAGEMENT

1 Refer every suspected flexor tendon injury directly to the orthopaedic team.

2 Give tetanus prophylaxis for a penetrating wound.

EXTENSOR TENDON INJURIES IN THE HAND

DIAGNOSIS

1 Injury can occur by:

(i) Direct laceration.

(ii) Avulsion of the middle slip of the extensor tendon that inserts onto the middle phalanx.

(iii) Avulsion of the distal slip of the extensor tendon that inserts onto the distal phalanx.

2 Assess for an extensor tendon injury:

(i) Avulsion of the distal insertion causes a 'mallet-finger' deformity. The patient is unable to extend the distal interphalangeal joint with the middle phalanx held.

(ii) Avulsion of the middle slip that inserts onto the middle phalanx may be missed

(a) initially, the proximal interphalangeal joint can be extended by the two lateral bands, but as they displace into a volar direction, they then begin to act as flexors

(b) finally, the proximal interphalangeal joint becomes flexed and the distal interphalangeal joint hyperextended, resulting in the *boutonnière* deformity.

3 Request an X-ray to show an associated flake fracture of avulsed bone.

MANAGEMENT

1 Refer a lacerated tendon or middle slip avulsion immediately to the orthopaedic team.

2 Also refer patients to the orthopaedic team for consideration of open reduction and internal fixation, if more than one-third of the articular surface of the distal phalanx has been avulsed.

3 Manage a mallet-finger deformity in a plastic mallet-finger extension splint for 6 weeks, and refer the patient to the fracture clinic.

DIGITAL NERVE INJURIES

DIAGNOSIS

1 It is mandatory to test for digital nerve function **before** using any local anaesthetic blocks.

2 Sensory loss, paraesthesiae or dryness of the skin from absent sweating, demonstrated along either side of a digit, indicate digital nerve injury.

MANAGEMENT

1 Refer immediately to the orthopaedic team nerve injuries that are:
   (i) Proximal to the proximal interphalangeal joint.
   (ii) Along the ulnar border of the little finger.
   (iii) Along the radial border of the index finger.
   (iv) Affecting the thumb.

2 Injuries distal to the proximal interphalangeal joint rarely justify repair unless local departmental policy differs.

FINGERTIP INJURIES

MANAGEMENT

1 Clean and debride injuries of the distal fingertip that are <1 cm in diameter and that do not involve fracture of the terminal phalanx, under a digital nerve block (see p. 490).

2 Leave to granulate under a soft paraffin gauze dressing changed after 2 days.

3 Give tetanus prophylaxis.

4 Refer injuries involving substantial soft-tissue loss, distal phalanx exposure or a degloving directly to the orthopaedic team.
   (i) Nerve injury distal to the distal interphalangeal joint does not warrant repair.

CERVICAL SPINE INJURIES

See page 174.

THORACIC AND LUMBAR SPINE INJURIES

See page 194.

PELVIC INJURIES

See page 190.

INJURIES TO THE HIP AND UPPER FEMUR

DISLOCATION OF THE HIP

DIAGNOSIS

1   Dislocation of the hip occurs in violent trauma such as a traffic crash, a fall from a height or sometimes a direct fall on to the hip.

2   The hip joint is inherently stable so always look for associated injuries, as considerable force is required to produce dislocation.

3   The most common direction to dislocate is posteriorly (85%), such as when the knee strikes the dashboard of a car.
   (i)   Other associated injuries from this particular incident are a fractured femoral shaft and a fractured patella.

4   Less common are the central dislocation, fracturing through the acetabulum, or the rare anterior dislocation.

5   Note on examining a posterior dislocation that the hip is held slightly flexed, adducted and internally rotated; whereas in an anterior dislocation the hip is abducted and externally rotated.

6   Check for sciatic nerve damage in posterior dislocation of the hip, particularly if an acetabular rim fracture is present.
   (i)   Assess dorsiflexion (L5) and plantar flexion (S1) of the ankle, and sensation over the medial side of the ankle (L5) and the lateral border of the foot (S1).

7   Gain i.v. access and send blood for full blood count (FBC), urea and electrolytes (U&Es), blood sugar and group and save (G&S).

8   X-ray the pelvis, hip and the shaft of the femur in all cases.

9   Complications are more common with a posterior dislocation and include:
   (i)   *Avascular necrosis of the head of the femur.*
      (a)   risk of avascular necrosis developing is related to the length of time the hip remains dislocated, and increases dramatically after 6 h.

      (ii)   *Sciatic nerve neurapraxia* occurs in 15% and is usually relieved by reduction.

      (iii) Missed knee injuries occur in up to 15% of cases.

MANAGEMENT

1   Commence an infusion of normal saline.

2   Give morphine 5–10 mg i.v. and an antiemetic such as metoclopramide 10 mg i.v.

3   Refer all cases to the orthopaedic team for immediate reduction under general anaesthesia.

FRACTURES OF THE NECK OF THE FEMUR

DIAGNOSIS

1   These fractures are most common in elderly women following a fall, and may be divided into two groups:

    (i)   *Intracapsular*
       (a) subcapital – may be displaced or non-displaced
       (b) femoral head – rare and normally associated with hip dislocation.

    (ii) *Extracapsular*
       (a) intertrochanteric
       (b) pertrochanteric
       (c) subtrochanteric.

2   Typically, after a fall the patient is unable to bear weight, and the leg is shortened and externally rotated.

3   Occasionally the patient may be able to limp if the fracture impacts, and examination reveals localized tenderness and pain on rotating the hip.

4   Gain i.v. access and send blood for FBC, U&Es, blood sugar and G&S.

5   Record an ECG.

6   Request X-rays and include the pelvis, as well as anteroposterior and lateral views of the hip.

    (i)   Request a chest radiograph (CXR) in addition as a pre-operative aid for the anaesthetist.

    (ii) Look carefully for a fractured pubic ramus on the pelvic X-ray if no femoral neck fracture is seen, as this also presents with hip pain and a limp.

MANAGEMENT

1   Commence i.v. fluid resuscitation, as a comminuted extracapsular neck of femur fracture may be associated with up to 1.5 L blood loss.

2   Give i.v. analgesia titrated to response.

3   Consider a femoral nerve block (see p. 488) for proximal neck of femur fractures, especially in the elderly when opiates must be given with caution.

4   Keep the patient fasted until consultation with the orthopaedic team.

FRACTURES OF THE SHAFT OF THE FEMUR

DIAGNOSIS

1 These fractures are due to considerable violence, as in a traffic crash, crushing injury or fall from a height.

2 They may be associated with a hip dislocation, pelvic fracture or fracture of the patella, and may cause concealed haemorrhage of 1–2 L in a closed injury (more if compound).

3 Rarely there is damage to the femoral vessels or sciatic nerve.

4 Gain large-bore i.v. access and send blood for FBC, U&Es, blood sugar and cross-match 4 units of blood.

5 X-ray the pelvis, hip and knee, as well as the shaft of femur, to avoid missing other injuries.

MANAGEMENT

1 Give high-flow oxygen by face mask.

2 Commence an infusion of normal saline or Hartmann's (compound sodium lactate).

3 Perform a femoral nerve block to help relieve the pain (see p. 488).

4 Supplement the femoral nerve block with morphine 5–10 mg i.v. and an antiemetic such as metoclopramide 10 mg i.v. if required.

5 Apply traction as quickly as possible to reduce the pain and blood loss, and to facilitate movement of the patient during X-ray, which should not be done until **after** the splint is in place.
  (i) Use a commercially available Donway™ or Hare™ traction splint, or alternatively use a traditional skin traction device such as the Thomas splint.
  (ii) Get help to apply the splint, which cannot easily be placed alone.

6 Reassess lower limb neurovascular status after the traction splint has been applied.

7 Refer the patient to the orthopaedic team.

INJURIES TO THE LOWER FEMUR, KNEE AND UPPER TIBIA

SUPRACONDYLAR AND CONDYLAR FRACTURES OF THE FEMUR

DIAGNOSIS AND MANAGEMENT

1 These injuries are caused by direct trauma or a fall in an elderly person with osteoporotic bones.

2 A condylar fracture often causes a tense haemarthrosis, and rarely the popliteal artery is damaged by a supracondylar fracture.

3 Give the patient analgesics and refer immediately to the orthopaedic team for aspiration of any tense haemarthrosis and operative fixation in certain cases.

FRACTURES OF THE PATELLA AND INJURY TO THE QUADRICEPS APPARATUS

DIAGNOSIS

1 Damage is caused by direct trauma as in a traffic crash or fall, or by indirect force from violent quadriceps contraction.

2 Patients typically present with acute knee pain, swelling, bruising and loss of function. There is inability to extend the knee in most cases, associated with the local pain.

3 Remember to always examine the shaft of femur and the hip at the same time.

4 There may be a palpable defect in the suprapatellar region if the quadriceps mechanism is torn, with a low-lying patella.

5 Request an X-ray to demonstrate the patella fracture.
   (i)   Confusion may arise from a congenital bipartite or tripartite patella, although these are often bilateral, unlike a fracture, so if in doubt X-ray the other knee.
   (ii) Look for a lipohaemarthrosis causing a horizontal line fluid level on the lateral X-ray view of the knee, which is a useful indicator of an intra-articular fracture.
   (iii) Request a 'skyline' X-ray view in subtle patellar fractures.
   (iv) Consider a CT scan when a suspected fracture is not visible on plain X-ray.

MANAGEMENT

1 Refer distracted or comminuted patella fractures, and patients with disruption of the knee extensor mechanism directly to the orthopaedic team.

2 Otherwise, place the leg in a padded plaster cylinder from the thigh to the ankle if there is a stable, undisplaced fracture of the patella, and refer the patient to the next fracture clinic.

3 Aspirate a tense haemarthrosis first, before applying the plaster cylinder (see p. 491).

DISLOCATION OF THE PATELLA

DIAGNOSIS

1 The patella usually dislocates laterally in teenage girls and may become recurrent. It is most commonly associated with a direct blow to the anterior or medial surface of the patella.

2 Patients complain of the knee suddenly giving way, and inability to weight-bear or extend the knee and are often in considerable pain.

3 Examine for an anterior defect, a laterally deviated patella, and swelling and medial joint line tenderness of the partly flexed knee.

4 Sometimes, spontaneous reduction occurs and the patient then presents with a tender knee, particularly along the medial border of the patella.

    (i) A careful history and a positive 'patella apprehension' test (moving the patella laterally causes pain) suggest the original injury.

MANAGEMENT

1 Reduce under nitrous oxide with oxygen (Entonox™) analgesia by pushing the patella medially with firm pressure, while extending the knee.

2 Request a skyline patellar X-ray after the reduction to exclude an associated osteochondral fracture.

3 Place the leg in a padded plaster cylinder and refer the patient to the next fracture clinic.

4 Use a pressure bandage instead of a plaster cylinder if the dislocation is recurrent.

SOFT-TISSUE INJURIES OF THE KNEE

A careful history of the mechanism of injury and the subsequent events is essential, as knee examination is often difficult or impossible immediately afterwards due to acute pain. Always lie the patient on an examination trolley properly undressed.

DIAGNOSIS

1 Rapid swelling of the knee suggests a haemarthrosis, usually due to an anterior cruciate tear, peripheral meniscal tear, or intra-articular fracture.

    (i) Delayed swelling, occurring after several hours, is more likely to be due to a serous effusion.

2 Injuries may be deduced from the direction of force.

    (i) Sideways stresses will rupture the collateral ligaments or joint capsule.

    (ii) A twisting injury will damage one of the menisci, usually the medial.

    (iii) Combinations may be seen. A severe, twisting lateral blow to the knee, e.g. from a car bumper, will rupture the medial collateral ligament, tear the medial meniscus, and rupture the anterior cruciate ligament (O'Donoghue's 'unhappy triad')

        (a) this may result in a tense haemarthrosis, in the absence of a fracture.

3 Always undress the patient and examine on a trolley. Include the hip and spine, as the pain may be referred particularly in children. Perform the following in every knee examination:

(i) Observe the size and extent of knee swelling and the location of bruising.

(ii) Look at the position of the knee

    (a) meniscal tears may result in 'locking' of the knee with inability to fully extend the knee.

(iii) Palpate the knee to elicit the area of maximum pain.

(iv) Assess the medial and lateral collateral ligaments by stressing each side, with the knee slightly flexed.

(v) Assess the cruciate ligaments

    (a) with the knee flexed, attempt to move the tibia backwards (posterior cruciate tear) or abnormally forwards (anterior cruciate tear)

    (b) a posterior cruciate tear allows the head of the tibia to slip backwards on posterior stressing, which then moves forwards into a correct anatomical position on anterior stressing

    (c) this forwards movement does not equate to an anterior cruciate tear, which is only indicated by an *abnormally* forwards position.

> **Warning:** passive and active movements of the knee are restricted by the pain and swelling in the setting of acute injury and are difficult to evaluate accurately. Reassessment after a few days is essential.

4 X-ray all patients and look for an associated fracture, such as:

(i) Tibial condyle fracture.

(ii) Avulsion fracture of the tibial spine in cruciate ligament tears.

(iii) Flake fracture of the lateral or medial femoral condyle in collateral ligament tears.

(iv) Vertical avulsion fracture off the lateral tibial condyle from the lateral capsular ligament attachment (Segond fracture)

    (a) this is associated with an ACL rupture, and/or medial meniscal tear from a varus twisting injury.

(v) Avulsion of the tibial tubercle (Osgood–Schlatter's disease) due to traction apophysitis, more common in young male teenagers.

MANAGEMENT

1 Refer the following to the orthopaedic team, having given adequate analgesics:

(i) A tense effusion, including all haemarthroses with a suspected associated fracture.

(ii) A 'locked' knee with sudden loss of ability to extend the knee fully.

(iii) A suspected torn cruciate ligament.

(iv) Any penetrating wound of the knee suggested by air or foreign material in the joint on X-ray (which may be absent).

2   Otherwise, if there is only moderate swelling, a good range of joint movement and no ligamentous laxity:

(i) Aspirate the knee to reduce pain and improve chances of early mobilization (see p. 491).

(ii) Apply a double-elasticated stockinet bandage to the knee or a proprietary Velcro™-fitted knee splint.

(iii) Give the patient anti-inflammatory analgesics such as ibuprofen 200–400 mg orally t.d.s. or naproxen 250 mg orally t.d.s.

(iv) Lend the patient crutches to use until the acute symptoms settle.

(v) Review the patient within 5 days.

DISLOCATION OF THE KNEE

DIAGNOSIS AND MANAGEMENT

1   This severe injury is an orthopaedic emergency.

2   It is associated with over 30% incidence of damage to the popliteal vessels and lateral popliteal nerve, so requires urgent reduction.

3   Insert an i.v. cannula, administer opiate analgesia, check the distal pulses, X-ray and refer immediately to the orthopaedic team.

FRACTURES OF THE TIBIAL CONDYLES

DIAGNOSIS

1   These fractures are caused by falls from a height, or severe lateral or medial stresses, which in addition may rupture the knee ligaments.

2   A tense haemarthrosis is usual and precludes further detailed examination of the knee due to pain.

3   Always check for vascular damage by palpating the foot pulses.

4   Check for a lateral popliteal nerve palsy by testing for active foot dorsiflexion and eversion, and sensation over the lateral aspect of the calf.

5   Request an X-ray to show the tibial condyle fracture either laterally or (rarely) on the medial side, although sometimes they are subtle and difficult to see.

(i) Look carefully for avulsion of the tibial spine and/or intercondylar eminence, which may indicate a significant ligamentous injury.

(ii) A horizontal line fluid level in the suprapatellar pouch on the lateral view indicates a lipohaemarthrosis with an intra-articular fracture.

6   Request a CT scan to best demonstrate the extent of these fractures.

MANAGEMENT

1 Give the patient analgesics and refer immediately to the orthopaedic team.

INJURIES TO THE LOWER TIBIA, ANKLE AND FOOT

FRACTURES OF THE SHAFT OF THE TIBIA

DIAGNOSIS

1 These injuries are often compound and associated with direct trauma.

2 Greenstick fractures in children and stress fractures in athletes are also seen.

3 X-rays should always include the knee and ankle, as well as the shaft of the tibia.

4 Gain i.v. access and send blood for FBC, U&Es and blood sugar, and cross-match 2 units of blood in a compound injury.

MANAGEMENT

1 *Compound injury*
  - (i) Commence an i.v. infusion of normal saline or Hartmann's (compound sodium lactate).
  - (ii) Give morphine 5–10 mg i.v. with an antiemetic such as metoclopramide 10 mg i.v.
  - (iii) Restore anatomical alignment.
  - (iv) Cover the exposed area with a sterile dressing.
  - (v) Give flucloxacillin 2 g or cephazolin 2 g i.v. and tetanus prophylaxis.
  - (vi) Apply a temporary plastic adjustable splint or a long-leg plaster of Paris backslab from thigh to foot, with the ankle placed at a right angle, especially when there are other injuries to the chest or abdomen requiring more urgent care.
  - (vii) Refer the patient immediately to the orthopaedic team.

2 Refer all other tibial shaft fractures to the orthopaedic team, after giving the patient analgesia and applying a long-leg plaster of Paris backslab with the knee slightly flexed, and the ankle at a right-angle.

ISOLATED FRACTURES OF THE FIBULA

DIAGNOSIS AND MANAGEMENT

1 Associated with a direct blow to the lateral aspect of the lower leg, typically when playing football.

2 Patients present with local pain, swelling and difficulty walking.

3   Perform a neurovascular assessment especially for an isolated proximal fracture to exclude damage to the common peroneal nerve causing foot drop.

4   Request full-length anteroposterior and lateral X-rays of the tibia and fibula, including the ankle and knee joints.

5   Provided there is definitely no injury to the ankle, and no tibial fracture at another level, apply:
   (i)   *Either* a firm crêpe bandage with cotton-wool padding.
   (ii) *Or* a below-knee walking plaster, which affords more protection.

6   Refer the patient to the next fracture clinic.

INVERSION ANKLE INJURIES

DIAGNOSIS

1   These injuries are common following sports or tripping on a staircase or on uneven ground.

2   The aim of clinical examination is to distinguish a ligament tear from bony injury, and to assess the stability of the ankle.

3   Immediate swelling and inability to weight-bear suggest a fracture or serious ligament tear.
   (i)   Examine the ankle for evidence of pain over the following specific sites:
       (a) distal fibula and lateral malleolus
       (b) distal tibia and medial malleolus
       (c) medial (deltoid) ligament and lateral ligament (anterior talofibular - most commonly injured, middle calcaneofibular and posterior talofibular portions) of the ankle
       (d) anterior tibiofibular ligament
       (e) base of the fifth metatarsal, navicular and calcaneus
       (f) proximal fibula head (for the uncommon but serious Maisonneuve fracture).

4   *Ottawa ankle rules*
   These prospectively validated clinical decision rules reduce the number of ankle X-rays requested, without missing clinically significant fractures.
   Request an anteroposterior and lateral X-ray of the ankle based on these Ottawa criteria, if there is pain in the malleolar area and any one of the following:
   (i)   Inability to bear weight (e.g. unable to take four steps without assistance, regardless of limping) both within the first hour of injury and in the ED.
   (ii) Bone tenderness over the posterior edge or tip of the distal 6 cm of the medial malleolus.
   (iii) Bone tenderness over the posterior edge or tip of the distal 6 cm of the lateral malleolus.

5 *Ottawa foot rules*

Request an additional foot X-ray only when there is pain in the mid-foot and any one of the following:

(i)   Inability to bear weight both immediately and in the ED.

(ii)   Bone tenderness over the base of the fifth metatarsal.

(iii) Bone tenderness over the navicular.

MANAGEMENT

1 Refer the following injuries immediately to the orthopaedic team, after giving analgesia and applying a below-knee plaster backslab (see below):

(i)   Compound ankle injury.

(ii)   Displaced lateral malleolar or medial malleolar fractures, with widening or diastasis of the ankle mortice.

(iii) Bimalleolar and trimalleolar ankle fractures.

2 Treat conservatively in a below-knee plaster a stable ankle fracture such as an undisplaced lateral malleolar fracture or a malleolar avulsion fracture.

(i)   *Below-knee plaster slab:*

(a) Apply this from the metatarsal heads to below the tibial tubercle, with the ankle at a right-angle (**not** in equinus)

(b) Repeat the ankle X-ray after application of the plaster

(c) Refer the patient to the next fracture clinic, with instructions to keep the leg elevated as much as possible.

3 Patients able to bear weight, with minimal swelling and with no fracture seen on X-ray:

(i)   Apply a double-elasticated stockinet bandage, give the patient crutches or a walking frame, and give an anti-inflammatory analgesic such as ibuprofen 200–400 mg orally t.d.s. or naproxen 250 mg orally t.d.s.

(ii)   Recommend initial elevation, no weight-bearing and a cold compress (e.g. a bag of frozen peas) at home, followed by gradual mobilization.

(iii) Warn patients that they will not be fully fit for active sports for at least 4–6 or more weeks, and recommend physiotherapy if available.

(iv)   Review the patient after 5–10 days and refer to physiotherapy when there is persisting disability, if not already attending.

OTHER ANKLE INJURIES

DIAGNOSIS

1 Eversion injuries damaging the medial malleolus and medial deltoid ligament, hyperflexion injuries or rotational injuries tend to cause more complicated damage.

2   Examine the ankle as before to localize the maximum area of tenderness.

      (i)   Palpate the upper fibula for pain suggesting a high, oblique fracture (Maisonneuve) in addition.

     (ii)   The Maisonneuve fracture is a rare, unstable ankle injury associated with a widened ankle mortice and tibiofibular diastasis from tearing of the syndesmosis.

3   X-ray all patients meeting the Ottawa criteria on page 257, and include the upper tibia and fibula if there is proximal bony tenderness.

MANAGEMENT

1   Refer all fractures, a widened ankle mortice, or patients who are totally unable to bear weight, to the orthopaedic team.

2   Otherwise treat as in point (3) on page 258.

DISLOCATION OF THE ANKLE

DIAGNOSIS AND MANAGEMENT

1   This dislocation is most commonly posterior and is clinically obvious.

2   Give morphine 5 mg i.v. and metoclopramide 10 mg i.v. and X-ray immediately.

3   Then use procedural sedation with a second doctor present in a monitored resuscitation area to reduce this urgently, to prevent ischaemic pressure necrosis of the skin stretched across the malleolus.

4   Reduce the ankle dislocation by steady traction on the heel, applying gentle dorsiflexion to the foot.

5   After the reduction, re-examine the neurovascular status, and support the lower leg in a plastic splint or padded plaster backslab, before sending the patient for post-reduction X-rays.

6   Refer the patient to the orthopaedic team.

FRACTURES AND DISLOCATION OF THE TALUS

DIAGNOSIS

1   The talus articulates in three joints: the ankle joint with the tibia and fibula, the subtalar joint with the calcaneus, and the mid-tarsal joint with the navicular (along with the calcaneus and cuboid).

2   Injuries result from falls from a height or sudden violence to the foot, as from the pedal of a car being forced upwards in a car crash.

3   There is pain and swelling. Request an X-ray to define the injuries.

      (i)   Perform a CT if suspicion is high and plain films appear normal.

4   Complications of talar injuries include avascular necrosis and persistent pain and disability from osteoarthrosis, particularly if the injury is missed.

MANAGEMENT

1 Refer all fractures including the osteochondral dome fracture immediately to the orthopaedic team.

2 The only exception is an avulsion flake fracture of the neck of the talus from a ligamentous or capsular insertion.

(i) Treat this in a below-knee plaster and refer to the next fracture clinic.

3 Occasionally, the talus dislocates completely and lies laterally in front of the ankle joint.

(i) Refer the patient for urgent manipulation to avoid overlying skin necrosis, similar to the dislocated ankle.

FRACTURES OF THE CALCANEUS

DIAGNOSIS AND MANAGEMENT

1 These are usually due to a fall from a height, and are bilateral in 20% of cases.

2 Falls from a height are associated with a typical constellation of injuries, which includes fractures to the:

(i) Calcaneus.

(ii) Ankle.

(iii) Tibial plateau.

(iv) Femoral head or hip.

(v) Thoracolumbar vertebrae.

(vi) Atlas and base of the skull.

3 Look specifically for each of these in turn, and X-ray any tender area found.

4 The heel tends to flatten following a calcaneal fracture, and is locally tender with bruising spreading to the sole and even up the calf.

5 Request an anteroposterior and lateral ankle X-ray with an additional tangential (axial) calcaneal view to avoid missing a vertical calcaneal fracture.

6 Arrange a CT scan in a complex fracture, particularly to demonstrate involvement of the subtalar joint.

7 Elevate the foot and give analgesia.

8 Refer all fractures to the orthopaedic team.

RUPTURE OF THE TENDO ACHILLES

DIAGNOSIS

1 This injury is most common in middle-aged men following abrupt muscular activity. There is pain and weakness of plantar flexion, although some is still possible by the long toe flexors. However, the patient is unable to walk on tiptoe.

2   Feel for a palpable gap in the tendon, although this rapidly fills with blood and may then disappear.

3   Perform the 'calf squeeze' test. This demonstrates reduced or absent foot plantar flexion compared with the uninjured side.

   (i)   It is best performed with the patient kneeling on a chair with both feet hanging free over the edge.

   (ii) Squeeze the unaffected calf just distal to its maximal girth, and compare the reduced flexion response in the injured leg with the normal plantar flexion response elicited in the uninjured leg.

MANAGEMENT

1   Apply a below-knee posterior plaster with the ankle in equinus (plantar flexed) in the first instance.

2   Give the patient analgesics and refer to the orthopaedic team for a decision on operative repair or conservative treatment.

MID-TARSAL DISLOCATIONS

DIAGNOSIS

1   These follow a twisting injury to the forefoot, causing pain and swelling around the talonavicular and calcaneocuboid mid-tarsal joint.

2   Request a foot X-ray to show disruption of the mid-tarsal joint, often associated with fractures of the navicular, cuboid, talus or calcaneus. These may merely be avulsion flake fractures.

3   Arrange a CT scan to evaluate these complex injuries further.

MANAGEMENT

1   Give the patient analgesics, elevate the foot and refer to the orthopaedic team.

METATARSAL INJURIES AND TARSOMETATARSAL DISLOCATIONS

DIAGNOSIS

1   These are caused by direct trauma, crushing or twisting.

2   A transverse or oblique avulsion fracture of the base of the fifth metatarsal often accompanies an ankle inversion injury, at the site of insertion of peroneus brevis.

3   A stress fracture may occur, usually in the neck of the second metatarsal, known as the 'march fracture' after repetitive use.

4   The Jones fracture is a more distal horizontal fifth metatarsal fracture that extends into the intermetatarsal joint with the fourth toe typically in athletes.

5   Tarsometatarsal fracture-dislocation (Lisfranc fracture) is uncommon and usually involves multiple bones, resulting in widening of the gap between the base of the hallux and the second metatarsal, with lateral shift of the remaining metatarsals.

(i)   It is easy to miss, as the significance of the foot swelling is not appreciated and interpretation of the X-ray is difficult.

(ii) Look carefully for any signs of circulatory impairment in the forefoot.

MANAGEMENT

1   Refer immediately to the orthopaedic team all compound, displaced or multiple fractures, fractures of the first metatarsal, tarsometatarsal fracture-dislocations, injuries associated with crushing or marked oedema and any signs of circulatory impairment.

2   Treat a 'march fracture', and an avulsion fracture of the base of the fifth metatarsal as for an ankle sprain in a support bandage, or rarely in a below-knee plaster if the pain is severe.

(i)   A Jones fracture requires a below-knee plaster and referral to the orthopaedic team for consideration of operative intervention, as non-union is common.

FRACTURES OF THE PHALANGES OF THE FOOT

DIAGNOSIS AND MANAGEMENT

1   These fractures are usually caused by direct trauma.

2   Clean all the wounds and release any subungual haematoma by trephining.

3   Otherwise, give an analgesic and a support bandage after buddy-strapping the damaged toe.

4   Apply a below-knee plaster with a toe platform extension if pain is severe, particularly with injury to the great toe.

5   Refer all patients to the next fracture clinic.

DISLOCATIONS OF THE PHALANGES OF THE FOOT

DIAGNOSIS AND MANAGEMENT

1   These occur by direct trauma, usually to bare or unprotected feet.

2   Insert a digital nerve ring block (see p. 490).

3   Request an X-ray, to exclude an associated fracture.

4   Reduce by restoring normal anatomical alignment, with axial traction.

5   Buddy-strap and refer to the next fracture clinic.

Emergency Medicine Clinics of North America (2015) Vol 3 (2) (orthopedic emergencies).

McRae R, Esser M (2008) *Practical Fracture Treatment*, 5th edn. Churchill Livingstone, Edinburgh.

Stiell IG, McKnight RD, Greenberg GH *et al.* (1994) Implementation of the Ottawa ankle rules. *Journal of the American Medical Association* **271**: 827–32.

MUSCULOSKELETAL AND SOFT-TISSUE EMERGENCIES

SOFT-TISSUE INJURIES

The so-called 'minor injury' is of major importance to the patient and may lead to serious problems if managed incorrectly. Therefore, adopt a consistent, careful approach to every patient presenting with a soft-tissue injury.

GENERAL MANAGEMENT OF A SOFT-TISSUE INJURY

1 Assessment
   (i)   Obtain a history of:
         (a) the nature of the injury, and when and where it was sustained
         (b) the possibility of a foreign body, wound contamination, and damage to deeper structures
         (c) any crushing injury
         (d) current medical conditions and drug therapy
         (e) antibiotic allergy and tetanus immunization status.
   (ii) Examine nerves and tendons for evidence of damage, before infiltrating with local anaesthetic.
   (iii) Send the patient for X-rays before exploring the wound, if a radio-opaque foreign body (metal or glass) is suspected. Inform the radiographer of the nature of the foreign body.

2 Wound preparation
   (i)   When assessing and preparing the wound:
         (a) always lie the patient down on a trolley
         (b) wash hands thoroughly before and after wound review
         (c) wear sterile gloves and prepare a sterile field.
   (ii) Remove all the dirt and debris from around the edges of the wound prior to anaesthetic infiltration, using normal saline or a disinfectant, e.g. chlorhexidine with gentle swabbing.
   (iii) Only trim adjacent hair for 1–2 mm if absolutely necessary, but **never** shave the eyebrows or eyelashes.

3 Local anaesthetic infiltration and toxicity
   (i)   Simple laceration. Infiltrate 1% lignocaine (lidocaine) along the edge of the wound using a 25-gauge orange needle.
   (ii) *Digital nerve ring block*
         Use 2% plain lignocaine (lidocaine) without adrenaline (epinephrine) to ring block wounds around the nail, fingertip, distal finger and toes (see p. 490).
   (iii) The maximum safe dose of lignocaine (lidocaine) is 3 mg/kg. As a 1% solution contains 10 mg/mL, the maximum safe amount allowed in a 67 kg patient is 200 mg contained in:
         (a) 20 mL of a 1% solution or
         (b) 10 mL of a 2% solution (both contain 200 mg lignocaine (lidocaine)).

(iv) Signs of lignocaine (lidocaine) or other local anaesthetic toxicity include:
   (a) perioral tingling, a metallic taste, restlessness, dizziness and slurred speech
   (b) confusion, seizures and coma
   (c) bradycardia, hypotension and circulatory collapse.
(v) Treat seizures with midazolam, diazepam or lorazepam i.v., and circulatory collapse with inotropes or by commencing cardiopulmonary resuscitation if needed (see p. 2)
   (a) intravenous 20% lipid emulsion 1.5 mL/kg bolus followed by 0.25 mL/kg/min continued for 10 min following recovery of vital signs is now recommended for refractory arrhythmias with cardiovascular collapse.

4 Exploration, irrigation, debridement and haemostasis

(i) Look carefully for evidence of foreign bodies, and severed tendons, vessels or nerves within the wound. Seek assistance from the senior emergency department (ED) doctor if any of these are found.
(ii) Irrigate the wound using a 20 mL syringe filled with saline and fitted with a 23-gauge blue needle to provide a high-pressure jet. Repeat this procedure until the wound is clear of debris
   (a) use protective eyewear to prevent eye splash contamination with body fluids.
(iii) Excise any dead or contaminated tissue and remove local dirt on the skin by swabbing briskly
   (a) make certain all ingrained gravel and grit is removed to avoid permanent tattooing of the skin. A general anaesthetic may be necessary.
(iv) Achieve haemostasis by local pressure. Avoid using mosquito forceps to clamp a bleeding area, as this may cause further local tissue damage.

5 Sutures

(i) The aim is to appose the edges of the wound without tension using interrupted sutures, starting in the middle of the wound and halving the remaining distance each time.
(ii) The choice of suture material depends on the type of tissue being repaired and local practice
   (a) use an absorbable suture such as polydioxanone or polyglactin when closing deep wounds, to first close the deep space, and bury the knot at the depth of the wound
   (b) although silk was traditionally most popular for skin closure, it is more likely to cause micro-abscess formation with scarring

       (c) use non-absorbable synthetic monofilament sutures such as nylon or polypropylene instead. Although harder to tie, requiring an initial double throw and multiple knots, they cause much less of a foreign-body reaction.

  (iii) Use the smallest practical suture size:

       (a) *limb laceration:* 4/0 synthetic monofilament sutures removed at 7–10 days

       (b) *scalp:* 2/0 or 3/0 synthetic monofilament sutures removed at 7 days

       (c) *face:* 5/0 or 6/0 synthetic monofilament sutures removed at 4 days.

  (iv) Cover the wound with a non-adherent dressing. There is no need to keep the area dry after the first 24 hours.

  (v) Arrange an appointment for removal of the sutures in the ED or with the general practitioner (GP).

  (vi) Make a record in the notes of the size and nature of the wound, the deep structures involved, and the number of sutures used to close it.

6 *Antibiotics*

Do not use antibiotics indiscriminately. They are secondary to thorough surgical toilet in preventing infection, and are best reserved for:

  (i) *Cellulitis*

       (a) this is usually due to a β-haemolytic *Streptococcus* or *Staphylococcus aureus* if associated with a wound. Send a swab first

       (b) give 1 week of phenoxymethylpenicillin (penicillin V) 500 mg orally q.d.s., or flucloxacillin 500 mg orally q.d.s. if staphylococcal infection is suspected.

  (ii) *Dirty, contaminated wound*

       (a) give flucloxacillin 2 g i.v., gentamicin 5 mg/kg i.v. and metronidazole 500 mg i.v.

  (iii) *Bites*

       (a) clean, debride and irrigate with copious normal saline. Do not suture, except on the face

       (b) give amoxicillin 875 mg and clavulanic acid 125 mg one tablet orally b.d. for 5 days, unless just a trivial scratch. If penicillin-allergic, use doxycycline 100 mg once daily orally and metronidazole 400 mg orally t.d.s. Use roxithromycin if pregnant or breastfeeding, and in children

       (c) give tetanus prophylaxis

       (d) consider rabies prophylaxis if the patient was bitten abroad by a dog, or by a bat in Australia. Discuss this with a local infectious diseases expert. See page 158.

  (iv) *Compound fracture*

       (a) give flucloxacillin 2 g i.v. or cephazolin 2 g i.v.

       (b) remember tetanus prophylaxis.

7   Tetanus prophylaxis
See below.

TETANUS PROPHYLAXIS

DIAGNOSIS

1   Routine tetanus immunization was progressively introduced into Australasia and the UK after the second world war, so elderly people are now the most likely to be non-immune.

2   Virtually any wound can become contaminated, however trivial.

3   Meticulous wound toilet is an essential part of tetanus prophylaxis, rather than simply relying on tetanus immunization or antibiotics.

4   Treat patients according to their immune status and the type of wound (see Table 7.1):

   (i)   *Tetanus-prone wound*
         Wounds at significant risk of developing tetanus include:
         (a) wounds or burns with extensive tissue damage

Table 7.1 Guide to tetanus prophylaxis in wound management

History of tetanus vaccination	Time since last dose	Type of wound	DTPa, DTPa-combinations, dT, dTpa, as appropriate	Tetanus immunoglobulin* (TIG)
≥3 doses	<5 years	All wounds	No	No
≥3 doses	5–10 years	Clean minor wounds	No	No
≥3 doses	5–10 years	All other wounds	Yes	No
≥3 doses	>10 years	All wounds	Yes	No
<3 doses or uncertain†		Clean minor wounds	Yes	No
<3 doses or uncertain†		All other wounds	Yes	Yes

* The recommended dose for TIG is 250 IU, given by i.m. injection using a 21-gauge needle, as soon as practicable after the injury. If more than 24 h has elapsed, 500 IU should be given.
† Individuals who have no documented history of a primary vaccination course (three doses) with a tetanus toxoid-containing vaccine should receive all missing doses.
DTPa, age <8 years child formulations of diphtheria, tetanus and acellular pertussis-containing vaccines.
dT/dTpa, adolescent/adult formulations (much less amounts of diphtheria toxoid and pertussis antigens).
Reproduced with permission from *The Australian Immunisation Handbook*, 10th edn, 2013.

      (b) deep penetrating wound

      (c) superficial wound obviously contaminated by soil, dust or horse manure (especially if topical disinfection is delayed more than 4 h)

      (d) wounds containing foreign bodies especially wood splinters

      (e) compound fracture

      (f) bite

      (g) wounds complicated by pyogenic infections

      (h) reimplantation of an avulsed tooth.

  (ii) *Clean minor wound*

      Any wound that is clean, incised or superficial, i.e. does not fulfil any of the criteria above of the tetanus-prone wound.

5 *Tetanus vaccines and immunoglobulin*

  (i) Adsorbed tetanus toxoid in Australia is combined with diphtheria (ADT) and is suitable for use age ≥8 years. Prior to this age, combinations with diphtheria and pertussis as well as other agents for protection against polio, hepatitis B and *Haemophilus influenzae* type b are recommended

      (a) administer by deep i.m. injection 0.5 mL into upper arm or anterolateral thigh

      (b) contraindications to tetanus vaccine include prior anaphylaxis to tetanus toxoid or any of its components (extremely rare).

  (ii) Active tetanus toxoid immunization in the UK is recommended given combined with diphtheria, pertussis, *Haemophilus influenzae* type B (HiB) and inactivated polio vaccines up to age 10 years, then combined with diphtheria and inactivated polio thereafter.

  (iii) Confer additional passive protection immediately by administering tetanus immunoglobulin (TIG) when indicated (see Table 7.1):

      (a) give 250 IU by deep i.m. injection, or 500 IU if the wound is >24 h old, at a site distant from the tetanus toxoid combined vaccines.

MANAGEMENT

1 Tetanus immunization schedule (see Table 7.1).

  (i) *Clean minor wound*

      (a) patients fully immunized and with boosters up to date require no immunization

      (b) give patients with an incomplete tetanus immunization schedule a tetanus toxoid combined-vaccine booster, and arrange completion of a full tetanus course with the GP

      (c) give non-immune patients an initial dose of tetanus toxoid combined-vaccine followed by a full course of the tetanus vaccine.

    (ii) *Tetanus-prone wound*
       (a) administer tetanus immunoglobulin to patients who are non-immune, have not completed a full tetanus immunization programme, or are uncertain
       (b) also give non-immune patients an initial dose of tetanus toxoid combined-vaccine followed by a full course of the tetanus vaccine.

2 Tetanus itself is rare, but worldwide it is an important cause of death in parts of Asia, Africa and South America.
    (i) The incubation time from injury to first symptoms ranges from 3 to 21 days (usually about 10 days).
    (ii) The most common symptoms are jaw stiffness (trismus), dysphagia, neck stiffness and abdominal and back pain. Hypertonia is found on examination.
    (iii) Localized or generalized painful spasms follow within 24–72 h, becoming more severe and prolonged from minimal stimuli.
    (iv) Death may occur from laryngospasm, respiratory failure or autonomic dysfunction.
    (v) There is no rapid diagnostic test to prove the diagnosis, therefore admit a suspected case immediately to the intensive care unit (ICU).

CRUSH INJURY AND COMPARTMENT SYNDROME

DIAGNOSIS

1 Crush injuries may be caused by a roller or wringer injury, a direct blow or, for instance, a vehicle wheel passing over a limb.

2 Even with severe soft-tissue injury there may be little to see initially.

3 Always test for tendon, nerve or vessel damage.
    (i) Loss of skin blanching on digital pressure indicates shearing of capillaries, which may subsequently lead to extensive soft-tissue necrosis.

4 *Compartment syndrome*
    (i) Tissue capillary perfusion pressure is compromised due to raised pressures locally within closed anatomic spaces or compartments:
       (a) this is most commonly associated with the lower leg, and forearm volar compartments.
    (ii) Causes include crush injury, external compression from a tight plaster, fractures (especially tibial), constricting burns, local haemorrhage including from a bleeding disorder or anticoagulation, vigorous exercise and prolonged immobilization, e.g. coma following acute poisoning.

(iii) Consider the possibility of a compartment syndrome if there is marked pain, particularly on passive stretching of muscles, associated with paraesthesiae and loss of motor and sensory nerve function.

(iv) The entire area within the closed fascial compartment feels tense.

(v) However, arterial pulses and even skin perfusion may remain deceptively normal.

5 Send blood for full blood count (FBC), electrolyte and liver function tests (ELFTs), creatine kinase (CK) and dipstick the urine for evidence of myoglobinuria (positive for blood, yet negative for red cells on microscopy).

6 Perform an electrocardiogram (ECG) particularly if hyperkalaemia is suspected.

7 Request X-rays to exclude an underlying fracture.

MANAGEMENT

1 Gain i.v. access and give normal saline 20–40 mL/kg i.v. to improve any hypoperfusion, and give morphine 0.1 mg/kg i.v. and metoclopramide 10 mg i.v.

2 Eliminate any external constricting factors such as a tight bandage or plaster by cutting, or bivalving a cast.

3 Place the affected limb at the level of the heart. Excessive elevation reduces arterial flow and may worsen the ischaemia.

4 Refer every severe crush injury involving a limb, hand or foot to the orthopaedic team, including patients suspected of having a compartment syndrome.

(i) Management will include consideration of compartment pressure monitoring, the use of vasodilator agents, mannitol and sodium bicarbonate, or operative fasciotomy.

5 Otherwise, clean and debride an isolated finger or toe injury without suturing, elevate the limb to the level of the heart, and give the patient analgesics.

(i) Review within 3 days for consideration of delayed primary suture.

NECROTISING FASCIITIS

DIAGNOSIS

1 This is a rare, rapidly progressive potentially lethal soft tissue infection that spreads along fascial planes.

(i) It may affect the previously healthy, or those with diabetes, immunosuppression or chronic alcoholism.

(ii) It can follow an apparently minor penetrating or crush injury, or some surgical procedures. No antecedent is seen in 20%.

2 Constant severe, disproportionate pain with cutaneous hyper- or anaesthesia is typical, associated with fever and malaise followed by rapid systemic deterioration, shock and delirium.

3   Initial skin changes of cellulitis and erythema progress to spreading bruising, bullae, oedema and a 'woody' firmness, sometimes with crepitation.

4   Send blood for full blood count (FBC), electrolyte and liver function tests (ELFTs), creatine kinase (CK), lactate and two sets of blood cultures.

MANAGEMENT

1   Gain i.v. access and give normal saline 20 mL/kg i.v. to improve any hypoperfusion, and morphine 0.1 mg/kg i.v. with metoclopramide 10 mg i.v.

2   Start empiric i.v. antibiotics such as meropenem 1 g t.d.s, vancomycin 1.5 g b.d. and clindamycin 600 mg t.d.s.

3   Call for immediate senior ED doctor help, and refer to the surgical team urgently. Refer on clinical suspicion alone.
     (i)   Surgical exploration with extensive debridement is essential to definitively establish and manage the condition.

4   Contact the duty anaesthetist, alert theatre and inform ICU.

PUNCTURE INJURIES

DIAGNOSIS

1   This type of injury is caused by treading on a nail or pin, by penetration of a sewing-machine needle, or through industrial accidents including nailguns or high-pressure guns for grease, paint, water or oil.

2   Needlestick and sharps incidents are covered on page 152.

MANAGEMENT

1   Refer all high-pressure gun injuries immediately to the orthopaedic team, even if no apparent damage is seen initially. They will require extensive surgical debridement.

2   Otherwise, clean the wound with antiseptic, give tetanus prophylaxis, and consider the need for antibiotics.

3   Treat a rusty nail injury to the foot by soaking with Betadine and give amoxicillin 875 mg and clavulanic acid 125 mg one tablet orally b.d. for 5 days.

4   Instruct the patient to return immediately if signs of infection or gross oedema supervene.

HAND INFECTIONS

DIAGNOSIS AND MANAGEMENT

1   *Paronychia*
     (i)   This is pus formation adjacent to the nail, with throbbing pain.
     (ii)   Make a longitudinal incision parallel to the nail edge across the nail fold to release the pus, under a ring- block anaesthetic (see p. 490). Mop out the cavity with pledgets of cotton-wool.

   (iii) Dress the finger with paraffin-impregnated gauze tucked into the cavity, and apply a plain viscose stockinet tubular bandage without tension. Use a high-arm sling for 24 h, and review the dressing after 2 days.

2   Pulp space infection
   (i)   This is pus formation in the distal fat pad of the finger, also known as a felon.
   (ii)   Make a central longitudinal incision using a ring block, over the middle of the abscess. Take care not to cross the flexion crease of the distal interphalangeal joint, and mop out the cavity of pus.
   (iii) Dress and review as for paronychia.
   (iv)   The flexor tendon sheath is in danger in more extensive infections when swelling approaches the distal interphalangeal joint. Refer the patient directly to the orthopaedic team, after an X-ray to exclude osteomyelitis.

3   Suppurative tenosynovitis of the flexor tendons
   (i)   The original wound may have been forgotten, but intense discomfort, swelling and tenderness develop along the line of the flexor tendon, with characteristically severe pain on all passive finger movements.
   (ii)   Refer the patient directly to the orthopaedic team for operative debridement and i.v. antibiotics.

4   Deep palmar and web space infections
   (i)   These cause pain, swelling and loss of function with localized tenderness and the development of a 'flipper' hand, from pronounced swelling on to the dorsum of the hand.
   (ii)   Refer the patient directly to the orthopaedic team.

PRE-TIBIAL LACERATION

DIAGNOSIS

1   These are most common in elderly patients, often from trivial trauma tearing a flap of skin.

MANAGEMENT

1   Clean the wound, remove blood clots, trim obviously necrotic tissue and unfurl the rolled edges of the wound to determine actual skin loss.

2   Refer the patient immediately to the surgical team if there is significant skin loss or marked skin retraction preventing alignment of the skin edges, for consideration of early skin grafting.

3   Otherwise, lay the flap back over the wound and hold it in place with adhesive skin-closure strips (Steristrip™). Cover the wound with a single layer of paraffin-impregnated gauze and a cotton-wool and gauze combine pad.

4 Then apply a firm crêpe bandage and instruct the patient to keep the leg elevated whenever possible.

5 Enquire about tetanus immunization status.

6 Review the patient after 5 days, removing the dressing but leaving the Steri-strips™ in place.

   (i) Refer the patient to the surgical team for skin grafting if the skin is now obviously non-viable.

   (ii) Otherwise, review the patient weekly if healing is taking place, or discharge to the care of the GP and community nurse.

NON-ARTICULAR RHEUMATISM

Joint pain, swelling and tenderness that mimic arthritis may be due to inflammation of periarticular structures. Most patients can be treated with non-steroidal anti-inflammatory analgesics such as ibuprofen 200–400 mg orally t.d.s. or naproxen 250 mg orally t.d.s. and then be referred to outpatients or back to their GP. Leave joint aspiration and steroid injection to the experts, as it can be tricky and complications such as septic arthritis and joint destruction do occur.

Conditions include:
- Torticollis (wry neck)
- Frozen shoulder
- Rotator cuff tear: supraspinatus rupture
- Supraspinatus tendonitis
- Subacromial bursitis
- Tennis and golfer's elbow
- Olecranon bursitis
- de Quervain's stenosing tenosynovitis
- Carpal tunnel syndrome
- Prepatellar bursitis.

TORTICOLLIS (WRY NECK)

DIAGNOSIS AND MANAGEMENT

1 Torticollis is abnormal involuntary contraction of the neck musculature lateralizing to one side, resulting in the neck being held in a twisted or bent position.

2 Ask the patient about recent trauma, particularly if elderly.

3 Direct the physical examination to identifying an underlying aetiology, as well as documenting the degree of neck movement.

4 Look specifically for local sepsis such as tonsillitis, quinsy and a submandibular abscess, or for sensory or motor signs suggesting a cervical disc prolapse.

5 Remember to exclude drug-induced dystonia such as an oculogyric crisis due to metoclopramide, phenothiazines or butyrophenones such as haloperidol.

    (i) Give benztropine (benzatropine) 1–2 mg i.v. followed by 2 mg orally once daily for up to 3 days if dystonia is likely.

6 Request a plain X-ray of the cervical spine if bony trauma or cervical pathology is suspected.

7 Manipulate the neck into the neutral position in the absence of any alternative causes suggested above, and immobilize in a soft collar. Try diazepam 2–5 mg orally if muscular spasm is severe.

8 Give an analgesic such as paracetamol 500 mg and codeine phosphate 8 mg two tablets orally q.d.s. and/or a non-steroidal anti-inflammatory analgesic such as ibuprofen 200–400 mg orally t.d.s. or naproxen 250 mg orally t.d.s.

9 Return the patient to the care of the GP.

FROZEN SHOULDER

DIAGNOSIS AND MANAGEMENT

1 This can occur spontaneously, following local trauma, or following disuse of the arm after a fracture, cerebrovascular accident, myocardial infarction or even shingles. It is more common in the elderly.

2 There is pain and loss of all movement from an adhesive capsulitis.

3 Encourage active shoulder movements following the conditions above to prevent the capsulitis in the first place.

4 Otherwise, prescribe an anti-inflammatory analgesic and return the patient to the care of the GP.

5 Physiotherapy may help, but although the pain subsides, the loss of movement tends to persist for months or even years.

ROTATOR CUFF TEAR: SUPRASPINATUS RUPTURE

DIAGNOSIS

1 Sudden traction on the arm may tear the muscles that make up the rotator cuff. The onset may be insidious, but a traumatic incident may complete a tear causing sudden severe pain and reduced shoulder function.

2 Evaluate full active and passive range of movement at the glenohumeral joint.

    (i) There is reduction of active shoulder motion with inability to initiate abduction and weakness of external rotation of the shoulder.

3 Tenderness is localized over the greater tuberosity and the subacromial bursa, particularly with supraspinatus rupture. Other muscles forming the rotator cuff may also tear but are difficult to differentiate clinically in the acute stage.

4   Perform a shoulder X-ray that may reveal a decrease in the space between the head of the humerus and the acromion.

5   Request an ultrasound, which is useful for characterizing the extent of full-thickness rotator cuff tears and biceps tendon dislocation. It is less sensitive for partial-thickness tears.

6   MRI is highly sensitive and specific for delineating size, location and characteristics of rotator cuff pathology, when available.

MANAGEMENT

1   Refer an acute tear in a young patient to the orthopaedic team for consideration of operative repair, to ensure an optimal return to a full range of movement and function.

2   Give the elderly patient analgesics, an immobilizing sling and refer to the physiotherapy department for a physical therapy rehabilitation programme.

SUPRASPINATUS TENDONITIS

DIAGNOSIS AND MANAGEMENT

1   This is one of the causes of the 'painful arc' with pain between 60° and 120° of shoulder abduction.

2   Request X-ray which may show calcification in the supraspinatus tendon.

3   Give an anti-inflammatory analgesic, and consider referral to the orthopaedic or rheumatology clinic for aspiration and local steroid injection.

SUBACROMIAL BURSITIS

DIAGNOSIS AND MANAGEMENT

1   This may follow rupture of calcific material into the subacromial bursa, again causing a 'painful arc', or a constant severe pain.

2   Treat as for supraspinatus tendonitis above.

TENNIS AND GOLFER'S ELBOW

DIAGNOSIS AND MANAGEMENT

1   Tennis elbow causes pain over the lateral epicondyle of the humerus from a partial tear of the extensor origin of the forearm muscles used in repetitive movements (e.g. using a screwdriver or playing tennis).

2   Advise the patient to avoid the activity causing the pain, and to rest the arm. Give an anti-inflammatory analgesic.

3   Refer for local steroid injection if the pain is persistent.

4   Golfer's elbow is a similar condition affecting the medial epicondyle and the flexor origin.

OLECRANON BURSITIS

DIAGNOSIS AND MANAGEMENT

1 Painful swelling of this bursa is due to trauma, gout or infection, usually with *Staphylococcus aureus*.

2 Aspirate under sterile conditions and send fluid for culture and polarizing light microscopy if the latter two conditions are likely.
    (i) Refer the patient for formal drainage of the bursa under anaesthesia if infection is confirmed.

3 Otherwise, give a non-steroidal anti-inflammatory analgesic and refer back to the GP.

DE QUERVAIN'S STENOSING TENOSYNOVITIS

DIAGNOSIS AND MANAGEMENT

1 This causes tenderness over the radial styloid, a palpable nodule from thickening of the fibrous sheaths of the abductor pollicis longus and extensor pollicis brevis tendons, and pain on moving the thumb.

2 Treat by resting the thumb in a splint and by using an anti-inflammatory analgesic.

3 This condition may require surgical release of the first dorsal compartment if local injection of steroid fails.

CARPAL TUNNEL SYNDROME

DIAGNOSIS AND MANAGEMENT

1 This is a compressive neuropathy of the median nerve at the wrist, most commonly affecting middle-aged females.

2 Secondary causes include rheumatoid arthritis, post-trauma such as a Colles' fracture, overuse, pregnancy, and rarely myxoedema, acromegaly and amyloidosis. Most cases though are idiopathic or related to minor trauma.

3 Patients complain of pain and paraesthesiae in the distribution of the median nerve in the hand, primarily the thumb, index, middle and lateral aspect of the ring finger. It is typically worse at night or following repetitive strain such as computer work.

4 Test for reduced sensation over the palmar aspect of the affected digits and weakness of thumb abduction. This is associated with thenar muscle wasting in more chronic cases.

5 Perform Phalen's test, by reproducing paraesthesiae in the distribution of the median nerve following 60-second wrist hyperflexion. Or look for Tinel's sign eliciting median nerve paraesthesiae by tapping on the volar aspect of the wrist over the median nerve.

6   Treat with an anti-inflammatory analgesic, and immobilize the wrist in a volar splint in the neutral position, particularly at night.

7   Refer resistant cases to the orthopaedic clinic for consideration of carpal tunnel decompression.

PREPATELLAR BURSITIS

DIAGNOSIS AND MANAGEMENT

1   Prepatellar bursitis or 'housemaid's knee' is due to friction or infection.

2   Treat by giving an anti-inflammatory analgesic, avoiding further trauma and, if necessary, by aspiration and steroid injection by the GP or outpatient clinic (orthopaedic or rheumatology).

3   Refer the patient to the orthopaedic team if bacterial infection is suspected, with fever, malaise and increasing pain.

BACK PAIN

This is a common problem that can be considered under four headings:
- Direct back trauma
- Indirect mechanical back trauma
- Severe or atypical, non-traumatic back pain
- Mild to moderate, non-traumatic back pain.

DIRECT BACK TRAUMA

Manage back pain that follows direct trauma according to the principles in the section on multiple injuries (see p. 194).

INDIRECT MECHANICAL BACK TRAUMA

DIAGNOSIS

1   Bending, lifting, straining, coughing or sneezing may precipitate acute, severe low back pain.

2   There is intense muscle spasm, or even complete immobility. The normal lumbar lordosis is lost, with development of a scoliosis.

3   Assess for any reduction in straight-leg raise (SLR), suggesting sciatic nerve-root irritation.

     (i)   Inability to leg raise more than 30° due to pain going down the leg is abnormal.

     (ii)   Remember that being able to sit up in bed with the legs out straight is equivalent to a SLR of 90° on both sides.

4   Examine for neurological signs of nerve-root irritation or compression from an acute prolapsed intervertebral disc.

  (i) Look for motor loss occurring in the following myotomes:
    (a) L1, L2 – hip flexion (iliopsoas)
    (b) S1 – hip extension (gluteus maximus)
    (c) L5 – knee flexion (hamstrings)
    (d) L3, L4 – knee extension (quadriceps)
    (e) L5 – ankle dorsiflexion (extensor hallucis longus)
    (f) S1 – ankle plantar flexion (calf muscles).
  (ii) Check for reduced or absent reflexes:
    (a) L3, L4 – knee jerk
    (b) L5, S1 – ankle jerk.
  (iii) Assess for sensory loss in the following dermatomes:
    (a) L3 – medial lower thigh and knee
    (b) L4 – medial side of calf
    (c) L5 – lateral side of calf
    (d) S1 – lateral border of the foot and sole.

5 **_Central disc prolapse with cauda equina compression_**

Always assess for any signs of a central disc prolapse causing cauda equina compression. Look for the following diagnostic features:

  (i) History of difficulty emptying the bladder or bowels.
  (ii) Saddle-area anaesthesia over dermatomes S2, S3, S4 and S5.
  (iii) Weakness in both legs with absent or reduced reflexes.
  (iv) Lax anal sphincter tone on p.r. examination.

MANAGEMENT

1 Refer any patient with features of a central disc prolapse causing any signs of cauda equina compression immediately to the orthopaedic team. It is an orthopaedic emergency.

  (i) Arrange urgent MRI to best demonstrate the cauda equina (or any spinal cord) compression.

2 Also refer a patient who has signs of nerve-root compression and/or is completely unable to move, or those who fail a trial of mobilization within the ED, particularly if living alone or elderly.

3 Discharge patients with moderate pain and with no nerve root signs.

  (i) Give the patient a non-steroidal anti-inflammatory analgesic such as ibuprofen 200–400 mg orally t.d.s. or naproxen 250 mg orally t.d.s.
  (ii) Encourage early return to ordinary activities within the limits of the pain. Bed rest should be kept to an absolute minimum.
  (iii) Request review and follow-up by a physiotherapist or the GP for back-care education including correct posture, safe lifting techniques and abdominal (transversus abdominis) and back exercises.

SEVERE OR ATYPICAL, NON-TRAUMATIC BACK PAIN

DIAGNOSIS

1 The aim in particular is to exclude a potentially serious underlying pathological cause.

2 Ask about any 'Red Flags' suggesting cancer, infection or fracture:
- (i) *Cancer:* unexplained weight loss, a history of cancer, age >50 yr, night pain, failure to improve after 4 weeks.
- (ii) *Vertebral infection:* fever/sweats, rest pain, intravenous drug use, immunocompromised including diabetes and use of steroids, recent infection e.g. UTI.
- (iii) *Fracture:* recent significant trauma; or recent mild trauma if older than 50 yr, on steroids or known osteoporosis.

3 Most likely cause according to the patient's age:
- (i) <30 years:
  - (a) ankylosing spondylitis
  - (b) rheumatoid arthritis
  - (c) osteomyelitis
  - (d) discitis
  - (e) extradural abscess.
- (ii) >30 years:
  - (a) bony metastases
  - (b) myeloma
  - (c) lymphoma
  - (d) renal or pancreatic disease
  - (e) aortic aneurysm.
- (iii) >60 years:
  - (a) as (ii) above
  - (b) osteoporosis
  - (c) Paget's disease
  - (d) osteoarthritis
  - (e) spinal stenosis.

4 Enquire specifically about previous back trouble, joint trouble, minor trauma and for associated abdominal, pelvic or urinary tract symptoms.

5 Check the vital signs and note any temperature or tachycardia. Perform a full examination including respiratory system, breasts, abdominal, rectal and neurological system.

6 Send blood for FBC, ELFTs, CRP and blood cultures when malignancy or infection is suspected.

7 X-ray the chest, and thoracic and lumbosacral spine if fracture is suspected.
- (i) Proceed to CT scan or MRI when malignancy or infection is suspected.

8 Perform a urinalysis.

MANAGEMENT

1 Refer the patient to the appropriate specialist team according to the most likely suspected aetiology.

MILD TO MODERATE, NON-TRAUMATIC BACK PAIN

DIAGNOSIS AND MANAGEMENT

1 This nebulous group with no red flags, and no abnormal physical signs, apyrexial with a normal urinalysis may be discharged.

2 Prescribe a non-steroidal anti-inflammatory analgesic such as ibuprofen 200–400 mg orally t.d.s. or naproxen 250 mg orally t.d.s.

3 Give patients a letter for their GP to follow them up and to arrange physiotherapy, an abdominal and back exercise regimen, and behaviour modification, including weight reduction and safe lifting techniques, as appropriate.

FURTHER READING

Australian Government Department of Health (2013) *The Australian Immunisation Handbook.* 10th edn. http://www.health.gov.au/internet/immunise/publishing.nsf/Content/Handbook10-home (tetanus).

Department of Health UK. Immunisation Against Infectious Disease 2013 'The Green Book'. https://www.gov.uk/government/collections/immunisation-against-infectious-disease-the-green-book#the-green-book (tetanus).

Section VIII

PAEDIATRIC EMERGENCIES

1   It is essential to be able to recognize the sick or seriously ill child, and to understand the key differences between children and adults.

2   Knowing what is abnormal and identifying the sick child is only possible if the doctor can first distinguish 'normal' paediatric physiological and developmental parameters (see Tables 8.1 and 8.2).

3   Most emergencies are frightening to children, causing distress to the child that adds to parental anxiety.

    (i)   Explain things as clearly as possible to both the child and the parent.

    (ii)   Use distraction techniques such as toys, picture books, DVDs and other electronic devices to placate the distressed child.

    (iii)   Allow the parent to stay with the child at all times.

4   Commence your assessment from the first moment you see the child, while the parent or child is giving the history or the child alone is talking.

    (i)   Even infants and children unable to converse will give important non-verbal cues about their illness or pain, such as facial expressions, posture and gait.

Table 8.1 Developmental milestones in early childhood

Age	Developmental milestones
Neonate	Symmetrical antigravity movement of four limbs Cries Looks at faces, responds to light Startles to loud noises
6 months	Sits erect with support Alert and interested Localizes sound
1 year	Crawls on all fours Walks holding onto furniture Understands simple commands Babbles Socially responsive
2 years	Runs, manages stairs Joins words: simple phrases Dry by day
3–4 years	Stands on one foot momentarily Speaks full (three-word) sentences Gives full name Dry by night
5 years	Skips/hops/stands on one foot Fluent speech Dresses self unaided

Table 8.2 Normal paediatric physiological parameters

Age	Weight (kg)		Height (cm)		Heart rate (beats/min)	Systolic BP (mmHg)	Circulating blood volume (mL)	Respiratory (breaths/min) rate
	Male	Female	Male	Female				
0–1 years	3.5–10.3	3.4–9.6	50–75	50–74	110–160	70–90	300–800	30–40
1–2 years	–	–	–	–	100–150	85–90	–	25–35
2–5 years	12.5–19	12–18.5	85–107	84–106	95–140	90–95	990–1390	25–30
5–12 years	19–38	18.5–40	107–147	106–149	80–120	100–105	1390–1700	20–25
12+ years	49–60	51–56	160–172	160–162	60–100	110–120	3500–4000	15–20
	For 1–10 years: weight (kg) = 2 ×(age in years + 4)				SBP = 80 + (2 × age in years) DBP = $\frac{2}{3}$ × SBP mmHg		80–85 mL/kg	Tidal volume = 5–7 mL/kg

DBP, diastolic blood pressure; SBP, systolic blood pressure.

5 A complete examination of every child is guided by the clinical history, but as a standard should include:

(i) Weight and head circumference measurements plotted on a percentile chart.

(ii) An oral or tympanic temperature and full vital signs.

(iii) Examination of the eardrums, mouth, throat (not if epiglottitis suspected), chest, abdomen and skin.

6 Children may present with non-specific symptoms and signs. A potentially serious illness should be suspected in any child who has:

(i) Respiratory distress, stridor, grunting or gasping respirations, nasal flaring or a silent chest.

(ii) Pallor, reduced peripheral circulation, poor capillary refill or cyanosis.

(iii) Altered level of consciousness, drowsiness and lethargy – particularly the 'floppy' infant.

(iv) Decreased fluid intake or urine output with reduced skin turgor and dry mucous membranes.

7 Early recognition and immediate management of impending respiratory, circulatory or neurological failure will reduce mortality and secondary morbidity.

CARDIOPULMONARY RESUSCITATION

DIAGNOSIS

1 Signs of cardiopulmonary arrest include:

(i) Unresponsiveness to pain (coma).

(ii) Apnoea or gasping respirations.

(iii) Absent circulation.

(iv) Pallor or deep cyanosis.

2 Cardiac arrest in children is usually secondary to respiratory or circulatory failure rather than ventricular fibrillation triggered by myocardial ischaemia, as in adults.

3 The outcome is poor and if hypoxia, hypovolaemia and acidosis are untreated, bradycardia progressing to asystole is inevitable.

4 Early recognition and treatment of impending respiratory or circulatory failure is therefore **essential** to avoid cardiopulmonary arrest occurring.

5 Look out for signs of respiratory failure:

(i) Increased effort of breathing:

(a) respiratory rate outside normal range for age (too fast or too slow)

     (b) tracheal tug, intercostal, subcostal or sternal recession, stridor and wheeze

     (c) grunting and gasping respiratory effort, head bobbing (signs of severe respiratory distress, especially in infants).

 Warning: decreased or minimal effort of breathing heralds pre-terminal respiratory failure as the child nears exhaustion.

  (ii) Efficacy of breathing:

     (a) reduced oxygen saturations measured by pulse oximetry

     (b) shallow breathing, decreased chest expansion with reduced, asymmetrical or abnormal breath sounds. Beware the silent chest.

  (iii) Effects of hypoxia:

     (a) initial tachycardia, followed by pre-terminal bradycardia if hypoxia is prolonged

     (b) initial skin pallor with vasoconstriction. Cyanosis is a pre-terminal sign

     (c) altered level of consciousness leading to coma.

6 Look out for signs of circulatory failure (shock):

  (i) Increased heart rate (bradycardia is an ominous sign of decompensation).

  (ii) Decreased systolic blood pressure.

  (iii) Decreased peripheral perfusion, poor (prolonged >2 s) capillary refill, cool, pale or mottled skin.

  (iv) Weak or absent pulses.

  (v) Decreased urine output and a metabolic acidosis.

MANAGEMENT

This is based on the International Liaison Committee on Resuscitation (ILCOR) 2015 International Consensus on CPR Science with Treatment Recommendations (CoSTR). Similar principles and practice apply to those for adult resuscitation (see p. 2).

1 Specific points relevant to paediatric resuscitation are outlined below. Figure 8.1 is the advanced life support (ALS) algorithm for children.

2 *Ventilation and oxygenation*

  (i) Give high-flow oxygen, open the airway with head tilt and chin lift, and look, listen and feel for normal breathing for no more than 10 s.

  (ii) Clear the airway, if breathing is not normal or absent:

     (a) ensure there is adequate head tilt and chin lift, but do not over-extend the neck

     (b) position the head in a neutral position in infants <1 year, as overextension may occlude their airway.

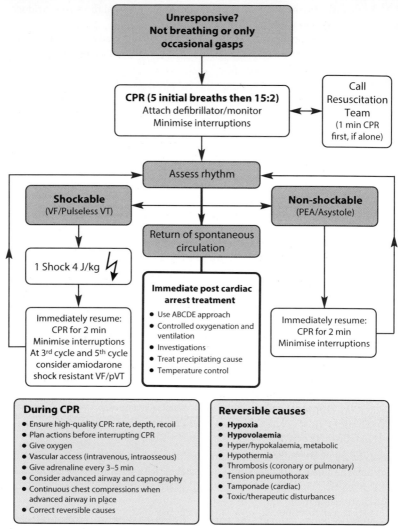

Figure 8.1 Paediatric advanced life support algorithm. ABCDE, airway/breathing/ circulation/disability/exposure; CPR, cardiopulmonary resuscitation; PEA, pulseless electrical activity; VF, ventricular fibrillation; pVT, pulseless ventricular tachycardia. Reproduced with kind permission from European Resuscitation Council (2015) European Resuscitation Council Guidelines for Resuscitation 2015. Section 1. Executive summary. *Resuscitation* **95**: 1–80.

(iii) Provide ventilatory assistance:
  (a) perform bag-mask ventilation – leave intubation to an airway-skilled doctor **only**:
    – use a face mask that fits closely over the nose and mouth. Soft circular plastic masks are ideal
    – attach a hand-ventilating device. Standard infant ventilating bags have a volume of 240 mL, require an oxygen flow rate of at least 4 L/min and are suitable for children up to 2 years
    – standard child ventilating bags have a volume of 500 mL and are suitable for children up to 10 years
  (b) insert an oropharyngeal airway under direct vision in the child who is unconscious with no gag reflex, and the tongue is occluding the airway
    – measure this airway from the centre of the incisors to the angle of the mandible
    – insert carefully avoiding damage to the soft palate
  (c) give five initial rescue breaths making certain the child's chest rises and falls with each breath, then give two rescue breaths after each 15 compressions.
(iv) If the airway is blocked by an inhaled foreign body:
  (a) hold the infant or small child head-down, prone and deliver up to five blows over the back with the heel of the hand, between the scapulae
  (b) follow with up to five chest thrusts in an infant, in the same position as for external cardiac compression one finger's breadth above the xiphisternum, but sharper and delivered at a slower rate
  (c) perform abdominal thrusts only in an older child, if back blows do not relieve the obstruction (see Heimlich's manoeuvre, p. 14).
(v) Have an endotracheal tube ready and both straight and curved-blade laryngoscopes for the airway-skilled doctor (see Table 8.3):
  (a) internal diameter of endotracheal tube (mm) = (age in years/4) + 4
  (b) oral endotracheal tube length uncuffed (cm) = (age in years/2) + 12
  (c) nasotracheal tube length uncuffed (cm) = (age in years/2) + 15.

3 *External cardiac massage*
  (i) Check the circulation for no more than 10 s, by looking for signs of life or palpate the carotid pulse (children) or femoral pulse (children and infants).

Table 8.3 Paediatric endotracheal tube sizes

Endotracheal tube (ET) size (formulae)		Age (years)									
		Birth	4/12	1	3	7	10	12	14	16	Adult
Internal diameter (mm): $\frac{age}{4} + 4$	Internal diameter (mm)	3.0	3.5	4.0	5.0	6.0	6.5	7.0	7.5	8.0	9.0
Oral length (cm): $\frac{age}{2} + 12$						(+ cuff)					
Nasal length (cm): $\frac{age}{2} + 15$	Oral length (cm)	9	10	12	13	16	17	18	21	22	23
Neonates: 3–3.5 mm ET tube											

(ii) Commence external cardiac massage if there are no signs of life, or if the pulse rate is <60/min:

(a) encircle the lower part of an infant's rib cage placing thumbs flat with tips pointing cranially, fingers supporting the back

(b) or if a lone rescuer in an infant, use two fingers over the lower half of the sternum in the centre of the chest

(c) use a single hand technique in a child, to compress the chest by one third of its depth or around 5 cm

(d) perform compressions at a rate of at least 100/min, but not exceeding 120/min.

4   Combine positive-pressure ventilation with chest compressions in the ratio of 15:2 effective breaths.

(i) Use a ratio of 30:2 if a lone rescuer, particularly if untrained or during basic life support.

(ii) Change to a ventilation rate of 10–12/min and compression rate of 100/min without interruption, once the airway is protected with an endotracheal tube

(a) use a ventilation rate of 12–20/min once the circulation is restored to achieve a normal $PaCO_2$.

5   *Vascular access*

(i) Vascular access will be difficult, but is needed to administer drugs and fluids and obtain blood samples. Request equipment for intraosseous (i.o.) access early in the resuscitation.

(ii) *Venous access*

(a) insert a 20- or 22-gauge cannula into a familiar site such as the antecubital fossa, the back of the hand, external jugular or internal jugular vein

    (b) perform i.o. (bone marrow) vascular access, if venous access is not gained within 60 s or is likely to take longer than this.

(iii) *Intraosseous access* (see p. 480).

    (a) i.o. access is rapid, safe and effective for administering drugs, fluids and blood products, and for drawing blood for cross-match, blood sugar and chemical analysis

    (b) use in children when i.v. access has failed or will take over 60 s to perform

    (c) insert the i.o. needle into the anteromedial surface of the proximal tibia, 1–2 cm distal to the tuberosity. Advance the needle with a gentle twisting or boring motion until it gives on entering the marrow cavity, and remove the stylet (see p. 480)

    (d) alternatively, use a semi-automatic, hand-held i.o. drill device

    (e) aspirate blood and marrow contents to confirm correct placement

    (f) flush each drug with a bolus of normal saline to ensure dispersal beyond the marrow cavity and to achieve faster central circulation distribution.

(iv) Connect an infusion of normal saline via a paediatric giving set slowed to a minimal rate to the vascular or venous access

    (a) give an initial fluid bolus of 20 mL/kg rapidly if systemic perfusion is inadequate with hypovolaemia.

6 Drug administration

(i) Recommended drug doses are shown in Table 8.4.

(ii) Give adrenaline 10 µg/kg i.v. or i.o. immediately in asystole or pulseless electrical activity (PEA), or after the third shock in ventricular fibrillation (VF)/pulseless ventricular tachycardia (pVT), then repeat every 3–5 min.

7 Defibrillation

See Figure 8.1 (p. 288).

(i) 'Time to defibrillation' is the main determinant of survival in the shockable rhythms VF or pulseless VT. They are uncommon in children, but increase with age.

(ii) Perform immediate defibrillation for VF and pulseless VT:

    (a) place defibrillator pads or paddles one below the right clavicle, and the other in the left axilla

    (b) administer defibrillation with 4 J/kg biphasic

    (c) resume cardiopulmonary resuscitation (CPR) immediately after each shock

    (d) review rhythm every 2 min

    (e) give further shocks at 4 J/kg if VF or pulseless VT persists.

Table 8.4 Paediatric emergency drugs

Drug		Dose and route of administration		
		Intravenous	Intraosseous	Intramuscular
Adrenaline (epinephrine)	1 in 10 000	Initial: 0.1 mL/kg (10 µg/kg)	Initial: 0.1 mL/kg (10 µg/kg)	–
	1 in 1000	–	–	0.01 mL/kg (10 µg/kg)
Atropine 0.6 mg/mL		i.v. or i.o. bolus over 1 min Birth–1 month: 15 µg/kg (0.025 mL/kg) 1 month–12 years: 20 µg/kg (0.033 mL/kg) (minimum 100 µg, maximum 600 µg)		–
Sodium bicarbonate 8.4%		i.v. or i.o. 1 mmol/kg or 1.0 mL/kg		–
Calcium chloride 10%		Central line or large i.v. 0.2 mmol/kg (0.2 mL/kg) to maximum 10 mL	–	–
Dextrose	10%	i.v. bolus 10%: 5 mL/kg	–	–
	25%	i.v. bolus 25%: 2 mL/kg	–	–
Lignocaine (lidocaine) 2% (100 mg/5 mL)		i.v. or i.o. 1 mg/kg (0.05 mL/kg), then i.v. infusion 15–50 µg/kg per minute		–
Lorazepam		i.v. or rectal or sublingual 0.1 mg/kg (maximum 4 mg) Give as a single dose (may be repeated once)	–	–

i.o., intraosseous; i.v., intravenous.

8   *Reversible causes*

Identify and treat any reversible causes of cardiopulmonary arrest, the 4 **Hs** and the 4 **Ts**, particularly hypoxia and hypovolaemia. Look for;

  (i)   **Hypoxia, Hypovolaemia, Hyper/hypokalaemia, Hypothermia.**
  (ii) **Tension pneumothorax, Toxins, Tamponade-cardiac, Thromboembolism.**

9   Heat loss

Remember sick infants and small children lose heat rapidly, so organize over-head heating, warming blankets or an incubator as appropriate.

(i)   However, once a child regains a spontaneous circulation but remains comatose after a period of CPR, he or she may benefit from targeted temperature management in particular avoiding hyperthermia >37.5°C for at least 24 h.

10   Parents in the resuscitation room

Invite and encourage parents to be present in the resuscitation room. A member of the team must stay with them and explain the resuscitation process with care and empathy:

(i)   Parents can then witness that everything possible is being done to help their child.

(ii)   They have the opportunity to say goodbye to their child, if death is inevitable:

(a) this facilitates the grieving process, and reduces parental anxiety and the risk of subsequent depression.

11   When to stop

The senior emergency department (ED) physician or paediatric doctor will decide at which point further resuscitation attempts are futile, usually after at least 20 min of failed resuscitation without ROSC.

(i)   He or she is also responsible for the distressing task of telling the parents, who may be present and watching.

12   Formal debrief

The resuscitation of a child is a highly emotional experience. Set aside time to allow any concerns to be aired, and for the resuscitation team to reflect on the clinical and psychological details in a supportive environment.

BREATHLESS CHILD

Disorders of the respiratory tract are common in childhood. Most respiratory illnesses are self-limiting minor infections, but a few present as potentially life-threatening emergencies. Important causes of a breathless child are:

• Asthma
• Bronchiolitis
• Pneumonia
• Anaphylaxis.

ASTHMA

DIAGNOSIS

1   This is an episodic, chronic inflammatory disorder characterised by reversible airways obstruction and bronchospasm.
    (i)   Exacerbations are most commonly precipitated by viral infection, or allergy, atopy, exercise and/or emotion.

2   It is one of the most common reasons for admission to hospital in childhood.

3   Asthma presents with dyspnoea, wheeze and cough. Obtain a history regarding trigger factors, current treatment and compliance, intercurrent illness and previous intensive care unit (ICU) admissions.

4   Assess the heart rate, respiratory rate, oxygen saturation and peak flow prior to treatment.

5   Look for tachycardia, tachypnoea with prolonged expiratory phase, nasal flaring, intercostal recession and expiratory wheeze on examination.
    (i)   Asymmetry on auscultation may be due to mucus plugging, but consider inhalation of a foreign body if the wheeze is of sudden onset (see p. 13).

6   Markers of severe asthma include any one of:
    (i)   Oxygen saturation <92% in air.
    (ii) Too breathless to talk or feed.
    (iii) Respiratory rate of ≥50 breaths/min if aged 2–5 years, or >30/min if >5 years.
    (iv) Tachycardia ≥130 beats/min if aged 2–5 years, or >120/min if >5 years.

7   Markers of a critical, life-threatening attack include any one of:
    (i)   Silent chest with absent wheeze on auscultation.
    (ii) Exhaustion.
    (iii) Altered level of consciousness.

8   Send blood for full blood count (FBC), urea and electrolytes (U&Es) and blood sugar levels *only* if the attack is severe, or an alternate diagnosis is considered.
    (i)   Hypokalaemia and hyperglycaemia are side effects of treatment.

9   Only perform a chest radiograph (CXR) if the diagnosis is in doubt, severe infection is suspected, or there is sudden deterioration suggesting a pneumothorax.
    (i)   Mucus plugging or collapse can be mistaken for pneumonia.

MANAGEMENT

1   Sit the child up and give oxygen, ideally with the parent in attendance to reassure the child. Attach a pulse oximeter, aiming for an oxygen saturation above 92%.

2   Give a bronchodilator such as salbutamol:
    (i)   Use a metered-dose inhaler with spacer device (MDI spacer). Administer 6 puffs if the child is <6 years of age and 12 puffs if >6 years, as a 'single dose'.
    (ii) Review the response after 10 min in a mild case.

    (iii) Administer a burst of three doses i.e. 20 min each over one hour in moderate to severe attacks and review.

    (iv) The severity of the attack will determine the frequency of administration thereafter.

3   Add ipratropium bromide (4 puffs if <6 years and 8 puffs if >6 years) to the MDI spacer every 20 min for the first hour of treatment in moderate to severe asthma, and/or if the response to salbutamol is ineffective.

4   Give prednisolone 1–2 mg/kg orally to a maximum of 40 mg, or hydrocortisone 4 mg/kg i.v. if the child is unable to tolerate orally.

5   Commence i.v. fluid administration if dehydration is present, but limit to 75% of maintenance requirements.

6   Refer all severe cases to the paediatric team.

    (i) Indications for ICU admission and possible ventilatory support include:

        (a) clinical deterioration

        (b) increasing exhaustion

        (c) persistent hypoxaemia

        (d) circulatory collapse.

    (ii) Discuss with ICU staff the administration of i.v. salbutamol, aminophylline and/or magnesium.

7   Discharge patients who have no breathing difficulty and do not require salbutamol more frequently than 6-hrly:

    (i) Provide a course of prednisone 1 mg/kg orally daily for 3–5 days.

    (ii) Ensure adequate inhaler technique with spacer.

    (iii) Arrange GP follow up within 24–48 hr, and start a written Asthma Action Plan if none exists.

BRONCHIOLITIS

DIAGNOSIS

1   This is a viral lower respiratory tract infection, which occurs in seasonal epidemics and usually affects children <1 year of age.

2   The most common infecting organism is the respiratory syncytial virus (RSV). Although other viruses are implicated, a routine nasopharyngeal aspirate (NPA) is **not** necessary in infants with a typical picture.

    (i) However, NPA can be useful for cohorting admitted patients.

3   Risk factors for severe bronchiolitis include prematurity, young <6 weeks, congenital heart disease and chronic lung disease.

4   It starts with fever and snuffles, but progresses rapidly to cough, fluid refusal, irritability, wheeze, chest hyperinflation and marked tachypnoea.

    (i) The illness usually peaks at day 2–3, with the wheeze and tachypnoea resolving by day 7. Cough may persist for weeks.

5 Listen for expiratory rhonchi and fine crepitations.
  (i) Look for irritability, lethargy and reluctance feeding, with a raised respiratory rate, tracheal tug, nasal flaring and intercostal recession in severe cases.
  (ii) Recurrent or prolonged apnoeic episodes also indicate severe disease.

6 Request a CXR in severe cases, or when there is diagnostic uncertainty such as possible heart failure.
  (i) Hyperinflation, parahilar peribronchial thickening and patchy areas of atelectasis and collapse are typical of bronchiolitis.

MANAGEMENT

1 Attach a pulse oximeter and give the child oxygen to maintain saturations above 94%.

2 Treat mild cases where the child is well perfused, feeding well and has oxygen saturations above 94% expectantly, and discharge for GP review the next day.

3 Admit moderate to severe cases with signs of lethargy, poor feeding, cyanosis, oxygen saturation less than 93%, or marked respiratory distress under the paediatric team.
  (i) Include any infant with recurrent apnoea, pre-existing lung disease, congenital heart disease or immunodeficiency, premature or aged <6 weeks. All are at highest risk of respiratory failure.
  (ii) Continue oxygen, and commence oral, nasogastric or i.v. fluid rehydration at 75% of maintenance requirement to reduce the risk from syndrome of inappropriate antidiuretic hormone secretion (SIADH).

PNEUMONIA

DIAGNOSIS

1 Up to 70% of pneumonias are caused by viruses such as influenza A or RSV.

2 Bacterial pneumonia is associated with high fever, localized findings on chest examination and lobar consolidation and pleural effusion on CXR.
  (i) Bronchopneumonia occurs more frequently in children with chronic illness, e.g. cerebral palsy, and may be bacterial or viral.
  (ii) However, bacterial and viral aetiologies cannot be reliably distinguished on either clinical or radiological criteria.

3 Lobar pneumonia commonly presents with sudden illness, fever, breathlessness and pleuritic chest pain. Wheeze and hyperinflation are more typically associated with asthma, bronchiolitis and croup.

4 The presentation of pneumonia in younger children is often atypical. Consider this diagnosis in infants and children with:
- (i) Cough, fever, dyspnoea and chest recession.
- (ii) Abdominal pain, vomiting and diarrhoea.
- (iii) Poor feeding, lethargy.
- (iv) Persistent fever.

5 Chest auscultation may be normal, especially in children under 12 months, or may reveal classic signs of bronchial breathing, crepitations and decreased breath sounds.
- (i) Tachypnoea with nasal flaring and intercostal recession are associated with respiratory compromise in infants.

6 Send blood for FBC, U&Es, blood sugar and blood cultures in severe cases. Attach a pulse oximeter.

7 Perform a CXR in every case to confirm lung pathology such as lobar consolidation, empyema or a pleural effusion, as clinical signs are unreliable.

MANAGEMENT

1 Give oxygen to maintain oxygen saturations above 94%.

2 Administer i.v. maintenance fluids to maintain hydration, particularly if the child is hypotensive or has difficulty feeding secondary to dyspnoea.

3 Administer antibiotic therapy according to local guidelines, and expert advice. Treatment regimens include:
- (i) *Birth to 1 week*
  - (a) benzylpenicillin 50 mg/kg i.v., 12-hourly for 7 days *plus* gentamicin (neonate less than 34 weeks postconceptional age: 4.5 mg/kg; 34 weeks or more postconceptional age: 4 mg/kg) i.v. daily for 7 days
  - (b) consider the possibility of HSV pneumonitis.
- (ii) *1 week to <3 months*
  - (a) afebrile but mildly unwell with signs of pneumonia, cover for *Bordetella pertussis* or chlamydial infection. Give azithromycin 10 mg/kg orally, daily for 5 days
  - (b) febrile, give benzylpenicillin 50 mg/kg i.v. 6-hourly for up to 7 days
  - (c) severe, give cefotaxime 50 mg/kg i.v. 8-hourly.
- (iii) *3 months to <5 years*
  - (a) non-severe, give amoxycillin 25 mg/kg orally, 8-hourly for 5 days, *or* benzylpenicillin 50 mg/kg i.v. 6-hourly for up to 5 days, if oral treatment not tolerated
  - (b) severe, give cefotaxime 50 mg/kg i.v. 8-hourly, or a combination of ceftriaxone 50 mg/kg i.v. daily *plus* flucloxacillin 50 mg/kg i.v. 6-hourly.

    (iv) *5–15 years*
        (a) non-severe, give amoxycillin 25 mg/kg up to 1 g orally, 8-hourly for 5 to 7 days, *or* if *Mycoplasma pneumoniae* is suspected, clarithromycin 7.5 mg/kg up to 500 mg orally, 12-hourly for 5 to 7 days
        (b) severe, give ceftriaxone 50 mg/kg up to 1 g i.v. daily, plus flucloxacillin 50 mg/kg up to 2 g i.v. 6-hourly *plus* azithromycin 10 mg/kg up to 500 mg i.v. daily.

4 Make certain to admit any child with respiratory compromise, altered level of consciousness, lethargy, difficulty feeding, cyanosis, or oxygen saturation <92% for i.v. antibiotics, and supportive care.

ANAPHYLAXIS

DIAGNOSIS

1 Anaphylaxis is an immediate-type hypersensitivity reaction to an ingested, inhaled, topical or injected substance. The most common agents include foods such as nuts, fish, milk, egg and food additives. Less frequent are medications, and wasp or bee stings.

2 Determine any history of asthma or atopy, the rapidity of symptom progression, previous reactions and prior response to medical management.

3 Look for an urticarial rash, conjunctival injection, erythema or pallor, stridor, hoarse voice, wheeze, cough and vomiting.

4 Symptoms and signs may rapidly progress to become potentially life-threatening, including stridor, severe wheeze and an altered conscious level. Shock is less common than in adult presentations.

MANAGEMENT

1 Stop or remove a precipitating agent such as an antibiotic or radiocontrast dye.

2 Assess and secure the airway and give high-flow oxygen by face mask.
    (i) Call the senior ED doctor for assistance if signs of upper airway obstruction secondary to laryngeal oedema occur, to prepare for possible endotracheal intubation.

3 Administer adrenaline (epinephrine).
    (i) Give 1 in 1000 adrenaline (epinephrine) 0.01 mg/kg (0.01 mL/kg) i.m.
    (ii) Give 1 in 1000 adrenaline (epinephrine) 5 mL nebulized if the airway is obstructing to reduce laryngeal oedema.

4 Insert an i.v. cannula and administer a fluid bolus of 20 mL/kg normal saline for shock with hypotension.

5 Give hydrocortisone 4 mg/kg i.v. for refractory bronchospasm and add regular nebulized salbutamol 2.5 mg if under 5 years of age, and 5 mg if over 5 years.

6 Refer all patients immediately to the paediatric team for admission, an Anaphylaxis Management Plan including EpiPen Junior or Anapen Junior containing 150 μg adrenaline if <20 kg (or EpiPen or Anapen containing 300 μg adrenaline if >20 kg), and immunology follow-up.

STRIDOR

This is an inspiratory noise originating from airway obstruction around or above the level of the larynx. Three important causes include:
- Croup (acute laryngotracheobronchitis)
- Inhaled foreign body
- Epiglottitis.

CROUP (ACUTE LARYNGOTRACHEOBRONCHITIS)

DIAGNOSIS

1 Croup is a viral infection primarily involving the larynx and subglottic area, most commonly due to parainfluenza viruses. It usually occurs in winter and affects children aged between 1 and 5 yr, with a peak at 2–3 yr.

2 It is characterized by a barking cough, harsh inspiratory stridor and hoarse voice. Symptoms often develop and are worse during the night and may follow a mild upper respiratory tract infection.

3 The child is febrile, irritable and tired, but lacks the drooling, dysphagia and toxic appearance of epiglottitis. Feeding and general activity is usually normal. In most cases of mild to moderate croup symptoms peak at 2–3 days and completely resolve within 1 week.

4 Severe disease is indicated by:
  (i) Hypoxia (late sign).
  (ii) Harsh inspiratory *and* expiratory stridor.
  (iii) Marked tachypnoea.
  (iv) Sternal recession.
  (v) Accessory muscle use.
  (vi) Increasing agitation and restlessness.
  (vii) Altered level of consciousness with lethargy.

5 Only attempt to examine the pharynx if the diagnosis remains unclear, providing epiglottitis or bacterial tracheitis are *not* suspected.

6 Croup is a clinical diagnosis and investigations are largely unhelpful and unnecessary.

MANAGEMENT

1 Nurse in an upright position with parents present and avoid distress with minimal handling.

2 Give dexamethasone 0.15 mg/kg orally or prednisolone 1 mg/kg orally, according to local policy.

3 Add nebulized 1 in 1000 adrenaline (epinephrine) 0.5 mL/kg to a maximum of 4 mL (4 mg) with oxygen in severe disease, and call the senior ED doctor.

4 Admit for observation patients with stridor at rest, persisting respiratory distress, patients who received adrenaline (epinephrine) and a patient presenting late at night.

5 Otherwise discharge milder cases with a letter for follow-up the next day by the general practitioner (GP).

INHALED FOREIGN BODY

DIAGNOSIS

1 This is most common in toddlers aged 1–3 years, frequently involving food products and usually affects the right main bronchus.

2 Children may present with upper airway obstruction, inspiratory stridor or with a new wheeze and persistent cough following a sudden choking episode.
   (i) However, the history of foreign body inhalation is not always present, or observed.

3 All symptoms may disappear if the object passes into the lower airways. Later, wheeze, recurrent or persistent pneumonia, or obstructive emphysema supervene, causing localized rhonchi, crepitations and breathlessness.

4 Request an anteroposterior and lateral CXR in the stable child with lower respiratory tract features.
   (i) Although an organic foreign body such as a peanut will not show, the secondary effects of compensatory hyperinflation on an expiratory film, collapse and consolidation will appear.

MANAGEMENT

1 *Complete airway obstruction*
   (i) Hold an infant or small child head down and deliver up to five blows to the back between the shoulder blades, followed by up to five chest thrusts.
   (ii) Perform abdominal thrusts after the back blows in an older child, but not in infants <1 year.
   (iii) Attempt removal of the impacted object under direct vision using a laryngoscope and a pair of long-handled forceps if the above measures fail, and the patient is unconscious, *or*
   (iv) Proceed directly to emergency cricothyroid puncture (see p. 469).

2   Stable airway obstruction
   (i)   Summon urgent anaesthetic and ENT help.

3   Disappearance of the symptoms of obstruction
   (i)   Consider the possibility that the foreign body has passed into the lower airways.
   (ii)   Refer the child to the paediatric team if the history is convincing, for consideration of rigid bronchoscopy even if the CXR appears normal.

EPIGLOTTITIS (SUPRAGLOTTITIS)

DIAGNOSIS

1   This now rare life-threatening infection of the supraglottic tissues usually affected children aged between 3 and 7 years in the winter months. The causative agent was classically *Haemophilus influenzae* type B (HiB), whose prevalence has markedly declined with immunization (see p. 309).
   (i)   Streptococci, staphylococci and viruses are now likely to be the cause of the infection, more so in adults.

2   Onset of symptoms occurs over 6–12 h and may rapidly progress to airway obstruction. These include:
   (i)   High fever: usually the first symptom.
   (ii)   Inspiratory stridor: softer than with croup.
   (iii) Severe sore throat: associated with dysphagia, inability to swallow saliva and drooling.
   (iv)   Muffled voice. Cough is usually absent.

3   The child looks anxious, pale and sick, and classically leans forwards drooling with an open mouth.

4   Do *not* perform any examination or procedure that might cause distress to the child. Allow the child to be nursed on the parent's lap, sitting upright with an oxygen mask held near its face.
   (i)   Never place an instrument in the child's mouth to examine the pharynx.

MANAGEMENT

1   Call the senior ED doctor, paediatric, anaesthetic and ENT teams urgently, and warn ICU.

2   Stay with the child until help arrives.

3   Be prepared to attempt intubation with a small endotracheal tube and an introducer if sudden respiratory arrest occurs, *or*
   (i)   Insert a large-bore i.v. cannula through the cricothyroid membrane if this fails, as an emergency airway (see p. 470).

4   Commence antibiotics i.v. with ceftriaxone 50–100 mg/kg/day (max 2 g).

ABDOMINAL PAIN, DIARRHOEA AND VOMITING

Abdominal pain may present acutely, or may become chronic and recurrent. Diarrhoea and vomiting are common problems that lead to dehydration.

ACUTE ABDOMINAL PAIN

DIAGNOSIS

1   Abdominal pain is a common paediatric presentation with an extensive differential diagnosis including surgical and non-surgical conditions.
2   An accurate history is essential. Ask about:
    (i)   Onset, nature, duration and radiation of the pain
          (a) a child >2 years should be able to indicate the site of the pain
          (b) in infants, pain may be inferred from spasms of crying, restlessness, drawing up of the knees and refusal to feed.
    (ii) Associated features such as vomiting, fever and rigors, dysuria or polyuria, and weight loss.
    (iii) Bowel habit: constipation, diarrhoea and the time of the last bowel motion or passage of flatus.
3   Significant features include pain >3 h, associated pyrexia and vomiting.
4   Check the vital signs and perform a full general examination looking for a raised temperature, rash and upper respiratory tract infection.
    (i)   Examine the abdomen for distension, palpable masses and signs of localized tenderness, guarding and rebound.
    (ii) Auscultate for bowel sounds and inspect the hernial orifices and genitalia.
5   Common causes of abdominal pain are best considered in two broad groups:
    (i)   *Surgical*
          (a) appendicitis
          (b) Meckel's diverticulitis
          (c) peritonitis
          (d) intestinal obstruction: adhesions, malrotation, intussusception and mid-gut volvulus
          (e) inguinal hernia with incarceration or strangulation
          (f) testicular torsion
          (g) pancreatitis
          (h) renal calculi
          (i) ectopic pregnancy
          (j) ovarian pathology
          (k) trauma, including child abuse.
    (ii) *Medical*
          (a) mesenteric adenitis
          (b) gastroenteritis
          (c) constipation

    (d) urinary tract infection (UTI)
    (e) hepatitis
    (f) Henoch–Schönlein purpura
    (g) diabetic ketoacidosis (DKA)
    (h) pneumonia
    (i) tonsillitis
    (j) inflammatory bowel disease.

6 Send bloods for U&Es if dehydrated, and FBC with blood cultures if sepsis or peritonitis is suspected.
    (i) Check a blood sugar for DKA.

7 Dipstick the urine and if UTI is suspected, send for microscopy and culture.
    (i) White cells are seen in the urine in peritonitis and appendicitis, as well as in UTI.
    (ii) Check a urinary β-hCG if sexually active.

8 Only request erect and supine abdominal X-rays when intestinal obstruction or perforation is suspected, or a CXR for pneumonia.

9 Request an ultrasound scan for pyloric stenosis, intussusception or renal pathology.

MANAGEMENT

1 *Suspected surgical abdomen*
    (i) Establish i.v. access and administer 20 mL/kg of normal saline i.v. for marked dehydration, hypoperfusion and shock.
    (ii) Give morphine 0.1 mg/kg or fentanyl 1.5 µg/kg for significant pain.
    (iii) Keep the patient fasted and refer for immediate surgical review.
    (iv) Place a nasogastric tube (NGT) if bowel obstruction is present.

2 Treat medical conditions according to the likely aetiology.

3 Arrange review within 24 h for a well child, if allowed home.

DIARRHOEA, VOMITING AND DEHYDRATION

DIAGNOSIS

1 Diarrhoea and vomiting are common problems that require investigation and treatment. Dehydration is a serious end result.

2 Causes of diarrhoea include:
    (i) *Gastroenteritis:*
        (a) viral: most common cause, including rotavirus, norovirus, astrovirus and adenovirus
        (b) bacterial: e.g. *Escherichia coli*, *Salmonella* or *Campylobacter*
        (c) protozoal: e.g. *Giardia lamblia*.
    (ii) *Infection:* septicaemia, UTI, pneumonia, tonsillitis, otitis media.
    (iii) *Surgical conditions:* appendicitis, intussusception and partial bowel obstruction.
    (iv) *Drugs:* particularly antibiotics such as ampicillin and erythromycin.

(v) *Chronic relapsing conditions* such as ulcerative colitis, Crohn's disease, and coeliac disease.

3 Vomiting is a common condition associated with a wide variety of causes:
   (i) *Causes in the newborn*
      (a) infection: meningitis and UTI
      (b) intestinal obstruction from duodenal atresia, Hirschsprung's disease, meconium ileus or necrotising enterocolitis
      (c) cerebral haemorrhage or oedema
      (d) metabolic: galactosaemia and congenital adrenal hyperplasia.
   (ii) *Causes in infants (up to 1 year)*
      (a) pyloric stenosis, typically in males aged 3–8 weeks presenting with projectile vomiting
      (b) infection: gastroenteritis, tonsillitis, otitis media, meningitis and UTI
      (c) intestinal obstruction from intussusception, an obstructed hernia, etc.
      (d) gastro-oesophageal reflux and hiatus hernia
      (e) feeding problems secondary to overfeeding or excessive wind
      (f) poisoning.
   (iii) *Causes after infancy*
      (a) infection: gastroenteritis, tonsillitis, otitis media, meningitis and UTI
      (b) intestinal obstruction or appendicitis
      (c) metabolic, such as ketoacidosis or uraemia
      (d) raised intracranial pressure or migraine
      (e) poisoning.

4 Take a careful history, recognizing that not all vomiting and diarrhoea in children is simply due to gastroenteritis. Serious features that indicate an alternative diagnosis to 'viral gastroenteritis' include:
   (i) Bloody diarrhoea.
   (ii) Vomiting bile, blood or faecal material
      (a) bilious vomiting in the neonate is a surgical emergency requiring immediate surgical referral.
   (iii) Systemic toxicity out of proportion to the degree of dehydration.
   (iv) Severe abdominal pain with significant tenderness, distension or a palpable mass.

5 Examine for evidence of an underlying cause and to determine the extent of dehydration.

6 **Assessment of dehydration**
Regardless of the suspected cause, assess and treat dehydration in its own right. Determine the approximate degree of dehydration on clinical assessment by estimated percentage change in body weight:
   (i) *Mild dehydration* (up to 5% body weight lost): there are no particular clinical signs and the child is in good

general condition, but with increased thirst and mild oliguria.
   (ii) *Moderate dehydration* (6–10% body weight lost): the child looks ill, is apathetic with sunken eyes and fontanelle, has a dry mouth, decreased skin tissue turgor, tachycardia, tachypnoea, marked thirst and oliguria.
   (iii) *Severe dehydration* (10% or more body weight lost): the child is drowsy, cool, cyanosed, tachypnoeic with deep acidotic breathing, tachycardic, hypotensive and may become comatose. There is a risk of sudden death.

7 Most children who can be orally rehydrated do not require blood tests.
   (i) Send blood for FBC, U&Es, blood sugar and venous blood gases in patients with moderate to severe dehydration.

8 Send urine for microscopy, culture and sensitivity if significantly dehydrated, febrile or in pre-school children with unexplained vomiting.

9 Collect a faecal sample only if the child has significant abdominal pain, persistent bloody diarrhoea or a history of recent overseas travel.

10 Order CXR and abdominal X-ray (AXR) if there is clinical evidence of respiratory tract infection or intestinal obstruction.

Warning: beware not to miss the diagnosis of dehydration in an overweight baby presenting with tachycardia alone.

MANAGEMENT

1 The aims of management are to:
   (i) Restore and maintain fluid and electrolyte balance.
   (ii) Restore nutrition.
   (iii) Replace ongoing losses (diarrhoea and vomiting).

2 Calculate the total amount of fluid needed over the next 24 h by adding together maintenance fluid requirements, estimated volume deficit and ongoing losses (see Table 8.5).

3 *Maintenance fluid requirements*
   These are:
   (i) 100 mL/kg per 24 h for the first 10 kg of body weight (4 mL/kg per h).
   (ii) 50 mL/kg per 24 h for the next 10 kg of body weight (2 mL/kg per h).
   (iii) 20 mL/kg per 24 h for each remaining kg of body weight (1 mL/kg per h).
   (iv) For example, a 24 kg child has a daily fluid maintenance requirement of:
   $(100 \text{ mL} \times 10) + (50 \text{ mL} \times 10) + (20 \text{ mL} \times 4) = 1580 \text{ mL per 24 h.}$

Table 8.5 Paediatric fluid and electrolyte requirements

Body weight	Fluid maintenance	
	mL/kg per hour	mL/kg per day
First 10 kg	4	100
Second 10 kg	2	50
Each subsequent kg	1	20
Potassium: maintenance	3 mmol/kg per 24 hours	
Fluid resuscitation: bolus	20 mL/kg crystalloid	
Deficit volume: estimation in dehydration (mL)	% body weight dehydration × weight (kg) × 10	
Burns: additional fluid requirement (mL per day)	% BSA burn × weight (kg) × 4	
Urine output: intended	Infants (<2 years): 2 mL/kg per hour Children (>2 years): 1 mL/kg per hour	

BSA, body surface area.

4 *Estimation of volume deficit*

Base this on the estimated percentage dehydration multiplied by the body weight, all multiplied by 10, that is:

Percentage dehydration × body weight (kg) × 10 in mL.

- (i) For example, a 24 kg child considered to be 5% dehydrated has a volume deficit of:

  $5 \times 24 \times 10 = 1200$ mL.
- (ii) Replace this fluid deficit over 24 h, if <5% dehydrated.
- (iii) Give half the fluids over the first 8 hours and the remaining half over the subsequent 16 hours, if >5% dehydrated and the sodium is normal.
- (iv) If the circulating volume has to be corrected in a shocked child (see below), dehydration is then assumed to be 10%, giving a maximum rehydration volume of 100 mL/kg.

5 *Treatment of severe dehydration*

Seek senior ED doctor help and refer the patient immediately to the paediatric team.

- (i) Give the shocked child 20 mL/kg normal saline i.v. (or i.o.) boluses as fluid resuscitation, until the circulation and hypoperfusion are restored.
- (ii) Aim to then replace the fluid deficit and maintenance requirements over 24 h with normal 0.9% saline in 5% dextrose, if the sodium level is between 130 and 150 mmol/L and the circulation is restored.
- (iii) Replace fluid and electrolytes more slowly over 2–3 days, if the sodium is <130 mmol/L or >150 mmol/L.

6 *Treatment of moderate dehydration*

Give rapid enteral (oral or nasogastric) rehydration with oral rehydrating solutions such as Gastrolyte™ or Pedialyte™ over 4-6 h, in frequent small amounts to replace the fluid deficit, and daily maintenance fluids over the following 18 h.

(i) Use oral rehydration, following an antiemetic such as ondansetron wafer 2 mg (8-15 kg), 4 mg (16-30 kg) and 8 mg (>30 kg) orally.

(ii) Otherwise, rapid nasogastric rehydration is safe and effective in most children even if the child is vomiting, as most children stop this once NGT fluids are started:

(a) consider particularly when i.v. access will be challenging, e.g. young chubby child

(b) commence NGT fluids at 25 mL/kg/h for the first 4 h.

(ii) A slower rehydration rate still is preferred in an infant <6 months of age, when co-morbidities are present or if a child has significant abdominal pain (seek senior doctor advice).

7 *Treatment of mild dehydration*

Oral rehydration:

(i) Continue milk and solid food during the diarrhoeal illness unless there is documented lactose intolerance. Continue breastfeeding, and supplement with extra water or glucose-electrolyte solution between feeds.

(ii) Oral glucose-electrolyte solutions:

(a) give 1–1.5 times the volume of their usual feed in infants

(b) give up to 200 mL of solution after each loose motion in older children, or enough to quench the thirst, given in frequent small amounts

(c) aim to replace the normal maintenance fluid requirement plus deficit volume over 24 h.

(iii) Discharge the child if they are tolerating oral fluids, have no clinical signs of dehydration, only occasional vomiting and a satisfactory social situation

(a) give the parents a letter for the GP, and instruct them to return if the child's condition deteriorates.

FEBRILE CHILD

Fever is the most common 'emergency' presentation in childhood. The normal oral temperature is 37°C, and the normal rectal temperature is 37.5°C. A fever is defined as a rectal temperature above 38°C.

Note that hypothermia or temperature instability may be a sign of serious bacterial infection, particularly in infants <3 mth.

DIAGNOSIS

1   A careful history and examination will identify the source of infection in the majority of cases. Look for the following common causes of fever in children:

   (i)   Respiratory: upper and lower respiratory tract infection.
   (ii)   Abdominal: gastroenteritis, appendicitis, UTI.
   (iii) ENT: otitis media, tonsillitis.
   (iv)   Exanthematous skin rash (see Table 2.13 on p. 118).

2   No obvious focus of infection is found following preliminary history and examination in a small number of children presenting with fever; e.g. a '*fever without focus*'. Most will have a viral infection, but the potential for significant bacterial infection must be evaluated.

   (i)   Ask about immunisations and whether they are up to date (see Figure 8.2 for an immunisation schedule).

3   The risk of a significant bacterial infection in fever without a focus is proportional to temperature and inversely proportional to age. Those most at risk are aged <3 years. Common bacterial infections *without* localizing signs can include:

   (i)   Meningitis and septicaemia.
   (ii)   Bone and joint infections.
   (iii) UTI.
   (iv)   Pneumonia.
   (v)   Occult bacteraemia (usually the patient is non-toxic and appears well).

4   Examine the child for signs of serious systemic compromise; i.e. that are potentially 'toxic':

   (i)   Lethargy, poor arousal and reduced activity.
   (ii)   Respiratory distress: nasal flaring, tachypnoea and grunting respirations.
   (iii) Circulatory impairment: poor peripheral perfusion, hypotension and tachycardia.
   (iv)   Signs of dehydration, reduced oral intake and reduced urine output.
   (v)   Sinister 'red flag' signs such as apnoea, cyanosis and convulsions.

5   Send blood for FBC, blood sugar, U&Es, blood cultures and urine culture if clearly unwell (lethargic, poorly interactive, difficult to rouse, inconsolable, tachypnoea, tachycardia, poor peripheral perfusion and any 'red flag' signs.)

   (i)   Obtain the urine sample by either clean catch (midstream urine [MSU]), suprapubic aspirate (SPA) ideally under ultrasound guidance, or a catheter specimen (CSU) and send for urgent microscopy, culture and sensitivity

   (a) UTI cannot be diagnosed on symptoms alone, nor by culture of urine from a bag specimen due to contaminants

   (b) urinary dipstick testing is a screening test only for UTI with poor sensitivity and specificity in young children, so always send a specimen for microscopy and culture if suspicion is high.

CHILD PROGRAMS	
Age	**Vaccine**
Birth	• Hepatitis B (**hepB**)[1].
2 mth	• Hepatitis B, diphtheria, tetanus, acellular pertussis (whooping cough), *Haemophilus influenzae* type b, inactivated poliomyelitis (polio) [**hepB-DTPa-Hib-IPV**] • Pneumococcal conjugate [**13vPCV**] • Rotavirus
4 mth	• Hepatitis B, diphtheria, tetanus, acellular pertussis (whooping cough), *Haemophilus influenzae* type b, inactivated poliomyelitis (polio) [**hepB-DTPa-Hib-IPV**] • Pneumococcal conjugate [**13vPCV**] • Rotavirus
6 mth	• Hepatitis B, diphtheria, tetanus, acellular pertussis (whooping cough), *Haemophilus influenzae* type b, inactivated poliomyelitis (polio) [**hepB-DTPa-Hib-IPV**] • Pneumococcal conjugate [**13vPCV**] • Rotavirus[2].
12 mth	• *Haemophilus influenzae* type b and meningococcal C [**Hib-MenC**] • Measles, mumps and rubella [**MMR**]
18 mth	• Measles, mumps, rubella and varicella (chickenpox) [**MMRV**]
4 yr	• Diphtheria, tetanus, acellular pertussis (whooping cough) and inactivated poliomyelitis (polio) [**DTPa-IPV**] • Measles, mumps and rubella [**MMR**] (to be given only if MMRV vaccine was not given at 18 months)
SCHOOL PROGRAMS	
10–15 yr	• Hepatitis B [**hepB**][3]. • Varicella [**chickenpox**][3]. • Human papillomavirus [**HPV**][4]. • Diphtheria, tetanus and acellular pertussis (whooping cough) [**dTpa**]

Legend:

[1] *Hepatitis B vaccine*: should be given to all infants as soon as practicable after birth. The greatest benefit is if given within 24 hr, and must be given within 7 days

[2] *Rotavirus vaccine*: third dose of vaccine is dependent on vaccine brand used. Contact your State or Territory Health Department for details

[3] *Hepatitis B and Varicella vaccine*: contact your State or Territory Health Department for details on the school grade eligible for vaccination.

[4] *HPV vaccine*: is for all adolescents aged between 12 and 13 yr. Contact your State or Territory Health Department for details on the school grade eligible for vaccination

Adapted with permission from Department of Health, Australian Government (2013) *The Australian Immunisation Handbook* 10th edition.

Figure 8.2 National Immunisation Program Schedule (Australia)

6 Request CXR in patients with respiratory distress, bradypnoea, abnormal breath sounds or oxygen saturations less than 95%.

7 Indications to perform a lumbar puncture are based on clinical grounds, and as part of a full sepsis work-up of an unwell infant <3 mth, or any temp over 38°C if aged <1 mth.

   (i) Only perform a lumbar puncture after consulting with the senior ED doctor.

   (ii) Lumbar puncture should not be done in a child with an impaired conscious state or focal neurological signs.

MANAGEMENT

1 Treat the unwell child symptomatically with oxygen via a face mask, an i.v. fluid bolus 10–20 mL/kg for hypotension and paracetamol 15 mg/kg orally or p.r., or ibuprofen 10 mg/kg orally for pain and distress. Involve the senior doctor early.

2 *Febrile child with no focus of infection*

   (i) Admit the following who may need empirical antibiotics:

   (a) febrile neonate <28 days old

   (b) systemically unwell child <36 months old with no discernable focus of infection

   (c) infants and young children with a non-blanching rash, signs of meningism or irritability.

   (ii) Infants and young children who display no overt toxic symptoms or signs:

   (a) most infants and small children <36 months of age who appear well, have no systemic toxic findings and have normal lab results including WCC $<15 \times 10^9$/L have a viral illness

   (b) discharge these patients with appropriate advice, and review after 12–24 h at the GP or in ED

   (c) <2% of these patients will turn out to have an *occult* bacteraemia, that is a positive blood culture, but negative urine and cerebrospinal fluid (CSF) culture:

   – admit patients with *Neisseria meningitidis* on blood culture for i.v. antibiotics

   – most patients with *Streptococcus pneumoniae* remain non-toxic and afebrile, will clear the organism themselves and require no further treatment. Advise parents to return if fever recurs within the first 7 days.

3 *Febrile child with a focus of infection*

   (i) Manage children with an identified focus of infection according to the individual condition and its severity based on the presence of systemic toxic signs.

   (ii) Admit under the paediatric team for management of the specific condition, if the child looks unwell.

    (iii) Discharge home if the child looks well with no toxic signs. Give symptomatic treatment and antibiotic therapy as indicated clinically
- (a) advise regular fluid intake 'little but often'
- (b) give paracetamol 15 mg/kg orally 4–6-hourly and/or ibuprofen 10 mg/kg orally 6–8-hourly
- (c) arrange review within 24–48 h in the ED or by the GP.

SEIZURES AND FEBRILE CONVULSIONS

SEIZURES

Seizures must be distinguished from other causes of brief loss of consciousness, such as syncope, pallid breath-holding, and cyanotic breath-holding.

DIAGNOSIS

The likely cause of a seizure can be related to the age of the child.

1   Newborn

Seizures tend to be mere twitching of a limb, fluttering of an eyelid or conjugate eye deviation. Causes include:
- (i)   Hypoglycaemia.
- (ii)   Hypocalcaemia.
- (iii) Hypoxia, especially from birth injury.
- (iv) Cerebral haemorrhage and subdural haematoma.
- (v)   Infection.
- (vi) Drug withdrawal.

2   Pre-school child

The commonest cause is a febrile convulsion.

Other possibilities include:
- (i)   Idiopathic epilepsy.
- (ii)   Meningitis or encephalitis.
- (iii) Head injury, including injury from child abuse.
- (iv) Dehydration from gastroenteritis etc.
- (v)   Hypoglycaemia.
- (vi) Poisoning.
- (vii) Sudden reduction in epilepsy medication.

3   Older child

Causes include:
- (i)   Idiopathic epilepsy.
- (ii)   Sudden reduction in epilepsy medication.
- (iii) Head injury.
- (iv) Meningitis or encephalitis.
- (v)   Hypoglycaemia.
- (vi) Poisoning, including theophylline, iron and tricyclic antidepressants.

MANAGEMENT

1 Clear the airway, place the child on their side, and give oxygen via a face mask. Attach electrocardiographic (ECG) monitoring and a pulse oximeter.

2 Check for hypoglycaemia using a blood-glucose test strip. Give 10% dextrose 5 mL/kg i.v. if the reading is low, and send blood for formal laboratory evaluation.

3 If the child has a further seizure or the seizure continues for up to 5 min:
  (i) Gain access and give midazolam 0.15 mg/kg i.v. or i.o., diazepam 0.25 mg/kg i.v. or i.o. at 1 mg/min up to a maximum of 0.5 mg/kg, or lorazepam 0.1 mg/kg i.v. or i.o.
    (a) monitor carefully for respiratory depression and record oxygen saturations every 2–5 min.
  (ii) Alternatively give midazolam 0.15 mg/kg i.m., or 0.5 mg/kg by the buccal or intranasal route; or rectal diazepam 0.5 mg/kg when i.v. or i.o. access fail.
  (iii) Give additional agents if seizures recur. Respiratory support may be needed and cardiac monitoring is essential:
    (a) phenytoin 20 mg/kg i.v. over 20 min, provided the child is not on oral phenytoin. Or:
    (b) phenobarbitone (phenobarbital) 20 mg/kg i.v. over 20 min if already on oral phenytoin.

4 Refer all children with an afebrile seizure to the paediatric team for further investigation. Admit children who have not fully recovered from the seizure or have focal neurological signs.

5 Advise parents that a child allowed home should be supervised when bathing, swimming, riding a bike and climbing trees until fully assessed and stabilized as an outpatient.

FEBRILE CONVULSION

DIAGNOSIS

1 These are common and occur in 2–5% of healthy pre-school children. They are benign with minimal morbidity and are usually associated with a viral infection.

2 Features that are consistent with the diagnosis of a febrile convulsion include:
  (i) Age between 6 months and 6 years.
  (ii) Brief generalized convulsion, <10 min in duration.
  (iii) Febrile child (temperature >38°C) with a prodromal illness.
  (iv) No focal neurological deficit or residual weakness such as a Todd's palsy.
  (v) No signs of meningitis or encephalitis.

3 Do **not** label the episode a 'febrile convulsion', when the features *differ* from those above i.e. a prolonged seizure with focal neurology.

4 The child will appear well following a simple febrile convulsion. Focus the examination on looking for the source of the fever, including in the throat, ears, chest, abdomen, urine, skin, etc.

5 Request a CXR, FBC and urinalysis, if no obvious source is identified.

(i) Consider the need for a lumbar puncture with a senior doctor, when no focus of infection is identified, or in a child <12 months of age, or an older child with prolonged febrile seizures.

MANAGEMENT

1 Manage the convulsion:

(i) Most convulsions are brief and do not require any specific treatment.

(ii) Position the child on their side, ensure a patent airway and use oropharyngeal suction if required.

(iii) Apply oxygen via face mask if the child is cyanosed.

(iv) Manage as for generalized seizures if the seizure lasts >5 min or is associated with focal neurology (see p. 312).

2 Treat the fever:

(i) Undress the child and reduce clothing to a minimum.

(ii) Administer an antipyretic analgesic such as paracetamol 15 mg/kg orally or as a suppository, or ibuprofen 10 mg/kg:

(a) however, the use of paracetamol has not been shown to prevent further febrile convulsions.

(iii) Treat appropriately if a focus is identified.

(iv) Investigate and treat as for 'fever without a focus' if no focus can be identified (see p. 310).

3 Consider other diagnoses if the child remains unwell or has an incomplete recovery, residual focal neurology or prolonged or multiple seizures.

4 Discharge if there is a full neurological recovery and no serious bacterial source is identified. Advise parents that:

(i) A repeat febrile convulsion will occur in 10–15% of children during the same illness.

(ii) The risk of developing further febrile convulsions during childhood is greater with younger children:

(a) the risk is 50% in a 1 year old

(b) the risk is 30% in a 2 year old.

(iii) Anticonvulsant treatment is not required.

(iv) The potential for developing epilepsy is the same as in the general population (1%), unless risk factors are present such as a family history of epilepsy, atypical or prolonged febrile convulsion, or neurodevelopmental problems

(a) there is a 2% risk of epilepsy, if the child has one of these risk factors, and 10% with two or more risk factors.

Most cases of acute poisoning in children are accidental, although rarely deliberate poisoning may occur as a form of child abuse, and adolescents may attempt suicide.

Obtain advice as necessary regarding toxic ingestions 24 h a day from the Poisons Information Centre on **13 11 26** (Australia), and in New Zealand on 03 479 7248 (or **0800 764 766** (24 h) within New Zealand).

Advice in the UK is available from the National Poisons Information Service (NPIS), which coordinates an Internet and telephone service to assist in the diagnosis, treatment and management of all types of poisonings.

- TOXBASE® is an online resource for the routine diagnosis, treatment and management of patients exposed to toxic substances. Use this as the first point of contact for poisons advice. It is available on http://www.toxbase.org/
- Specialist consultants are available for telephone advice in more complex clinical cases. A 24-h number **0844 892 0111** will direct callers to the relevant local centre in the UK.

DIAGNOSIS

1   Main categories of substances that may be taken include:
    (i)   Proprietary tablets and syrups, often prescribed for the parents.
    (ii)   Household and garden chemicals.
    (iii) Leaves, berries, seeds and fungi.
    (iv)   Alcohol, solvents and other illicit substances.

2   Ascertain what was taken, how much and when. If possible, the container the poison was in, or an example of the flora ingested, should be brought with the child.

3   Record baseline observations of temperature, pulse, blood pressure, respiratory rate, level of consciousness, and a blood glucose test stick for hypoglycaemia, particularly in alcohol and salicylate poisoning.

4   Send blood for U&Es, blood sugar and a serum drug level, which may include paracetamol, iron, salicylate, theophylline or alcohol as indicated clinically.

5   Perform an electrocardiogram for rate and conduction abnormalities, and commence ECG monitoring if abnormal.

MANAGEMENT

1   Clear the airway and give oxygen. Use a bag and mask if the gag reflex is absent, with an oropharyngeal airway, and call an airway-skilled doctor urgently to intubate the child.

2   Give 10% dextrose 5 mL/kg i.v. if the blood sugar level is low.

3   Give naloxone 10–40 μg/kg i.v., or i.m. if venous access is impossible, when there are pinpoint pupils and respiratory depression.

4 Start an i.v. infusion of normal saline and give 10–20 mL/kg for hypotension.

5 Activated charcoal 1–2 g/kg to reduce absorption of toxin has a limited role.

 (i) Reserve it for severe or life-threatening poisoning, where risk assessment suggests that supportive care or antidote treatment alone does not ensure a safe outcome.

 (ii) Charcoal is of most benefit within 1–2 h of ingestion, but is ineffective against certain substances (see p. 396).

 (iii) It is unpalatable and difficult to administer in children, but may be given mixed with ice cream or via an NGT

  (a) administration of activated charcoal via a misplaced NGT in the bronchial tree has resulted in death.

6 Ipecacuanha is not used in hospital in acute poisonings. Gastric lavage is now rare, unless the child presents within 1 h of ingesting a highly lethal drug, and/or is unconscious with the airway protected by an endotracheal tube.

7 Tablets that are particularly toxic even if just two tablets are ingested in a toddler (10 kg) are listed in Table 8.6.

8 Refer patients to the paediatric team for admission and observation if:

 (i) Symptomatic following significant ingestion.

 (ii) Potentially toxic ingestion.

 (iii) Presenting late at night and require overnight observation.

 (iv) Deliberate self-harm is suspected, for psychiatric assessment.

9 Specific poisonings and their treatments are described on pp. 397–417 in Section XIV, Toxicology.

Table 8.6 Highly toxic tablets, even if just *two* tablets are ingested by a 10 kg toddler

Agent	Features of severe toxicity
Amphetamines	Agitation, confusion, hypertension, hyperthermia
Calcium-channel blockers	Delayed onset of bradycardia, hypotension, cardiac conduction defects, refractory shock
Chloroquine/hydroxychloroquine	Rapid onset of coma, seizures and cardiovascular collapse
Dextropropoxyphene	Ventricular tachycardia
Opioids	Coma, respiratory arrest
Propranolol	Coma, seizures, ventricular tachycardia, hypoglycaemia
Sulfonylureas	Hypoglycaemia
Theophylline	Seizures, supraventricular tachycardia, vomiting
Tricyclic antidepressants	Coma, seizures, hypotension, ventricular tachycardia

LIMPING CHILD

DIAGNOSIS

1   This diagnostic dilemma presents frequently to the ED. The causes of limp range from serious conditions such as a bone tumour and septic arthritis to minor complaints including painful shoes or a plantar wart.

2   Remember to consider the abdomen and inguinoscrotal region, spine, pelvis, hip and lower limb as potential sources of pain or disability.

3   Ask about the onset of symptoms, any history of trauma, localized pain and associated systemic symptoms such as fever or rigors.

4   Check the vital signs, examine the abdomen and pelvis, evaluate gait and perform a lower limb musculoskeletal examination. Examine and treat the patient on a trolley with the parents present to alleviate anxiety. Test the full range of movement of all lower limb joints bilaterally.

   (i)   The hip is the most common source of pathology, but as pain is often referred to the knee, always examine both.

5   Age is the key factor in forming a list of differential diagnoses. Typical causes by age include:

   (i)   *Age 1–3 years*
      (a) infection: septic arthritis and osteomyelitis
      (b) developmental dysplasia of the hip
      (c) trauma: toddler's fracture, stress fracture, child abuse
      (d) cerebral palsy, neuromuscular disease, tumours and congenital hypotonia.

   (ii) *Age 4–10 years*
      (a) transient synovitis 'irritable hip'
      (b) Perthes' disease (up to 20% bilateral)
      (c) infection: septic arthritis and osteomyelitis
      (d) trauma: fractures, dislocations and ligamentous injuries
      (e) rheumatoid disease and Still's disease
      (f) leukaemia.

   (iii) *Age 11–15 years*
      (a) slipped upper femoral epiphysis (SUFE) – bilateral in up to 50%
      (b) trauma: overuse syndromes
      (c) arthritis, including Still's disease, juvenile rheumatoid arthritis and ankylosing spondylitis
      (d) infection: sexually transmitted disease (arthralgia and arthritis), septic arthritis and osteomyelitis / discitis.
      (e) neoplasia.

6   Transient synovitis and septic arthritis are difficult to differentiate and warrant urgent investigation.

7 Send blood for FBC, erythrocyte sedimentation rate (ESR), C-reactive protein (CRP) and blood culture, if infection is possible.

8 Request plain X-rays of the affected limb including 'frog lateral' X-rays of the hips if SUFE is suspected.

9 Arrange an ultrasound scan to demonstrate a hip effusion, if the X-rays are normal and pain is localized to the hip region.

    (i) Discuss the need for further tests such as CT, MRI or bone scan with the orthopaedic team.

MANAGEMENT

1 Administer oral pain relief, and immobilize a fracture and acute traumatic limb injury with a splint.

2 Disposition and further management is dependent on the underlying problem.

3 Patients with constitutional symptoms, fever, leucocytosis and elevated ESR and CRP require joint aspiration under anaesthesia to exclude a septic arthritis.

    (i) Refer these and traumatic fractures, slipped capital epiphysis, Perthes' disease and developmental dysplasia of the hip to the orthopaedic team.

4 Discharge for rest and analgesia if well with no serious cause found, and arrange follow up with the GP within 1–2 days.

    (i) Advise to return immediately if febrile, unwell or deteriorating.

SUDDEN UNEXPECTED DEATH IN INFANCY

DIAGNOSIS

1 Sudden unexpected death in infancy (SUDI) is used to describe any infant under the age of 1 year who dies suddenly or unexpectedly, and whose manner and cause of death are not immediately obvious prior to investigation.

    (i) It includes sudden infant death syndrome (SIDS) in >50%, deaths from medical problems including metabolic, occult infection or cardiac, and injuries such as neglect, suffocation and homicide.

2 SIDS is defined as the sudden death of any infant under the age of 1 year that is unexplained by history and in which a thorough post-mortem evaluation fails to demonstrate an adequate cause of death. It is becoming less frequent.

3 The cause of SIDS is unknown.

    (i) It is more common during winter, with a peak age of 3 months.

    (ii) Risk factors include tobacco exposure (before or after birth), sofa sharing, bed sharing with an intoxicated or smoker parent.

(iii) SIDS babies are more likely to be male, of lower gestational age at birth, low birth weight, lower APGAR scores, admitted to a special care baby unit and have congenital abnormalities.

(iv) Parents are more likely to be young, solo, have lower incomes, have a previous child with SIDS, previous stillbirths and higher parity.

(v) Protective factors include: sleeping supine (on the back), face uncovered, room sharing with parents, and in a safe cot that meets the relevant standards.

MANAGEMENT

1 Continue resuscitating in the resuscitation room, if the child is brought in by ambulance with CPR in progress. Call the senior ED doctor and paediatric team urgently (see CPR, p. 286).

2 Examine the child carefully for any signs of trauma or infection, including evidence of asphyxia or petechiae. Check the temperature and blood glucose.

3 Discuss the necessity for post-mortem blood tests for infection or a drug screen with the senior doctor. In addition, keep all clothes in a labelled hospital bag.

4 Check that the parents have full access to the resuscitation area, and encourage them to attend the resuscitation room if they want to. Provide a senior ED staff member to be with them at all times.

5 The senior doctor should then speak in private to the parents, to talk about the circumstances of the death and any recent illness in the child.

6 Encourage the parents to see and hold their child in privacy afterwards. They may derive benefit from the presence of the hospital chaplain and social worker, and may like a photograph or a lock of the child's hair.

7 Tell the parents that, because the death is sudden, the coroner (or procurator fiscal in Scotland) will be informed, and a post mortem may be required.

8 The coroner's officer or the police will then visit the parents later that day, and will take further details, possibly even removing the bedding for examination.

9 Write down and give the parents the details and phone number of the local SIDS help group (in Australia the SIDS and Kids website [http://www.sidsandkids.org/] and in the UK the Lullaby Trust (formerly Foundation for the Study of Infant Deaths) [http://www.lullabytrust.org.uk/]).

10 Make certain you also inform the following by telephone:

(i)   GP, to arrange for a home visit and to make sure all future clinic attendances for the deceased child are cancelled.

(ii) Health visitor.

(iii) Social work department.

(iv) Paediatric team, if the team was not present at the resuscitation.

(v)   Community Child Health Service, to cancel immunization appointments, etc.

DIAGNOSIS

1 Child abuse occurs when the adult responsible for the care of a child either harms the child, or fails to protect them from harm. It can manifest in different ways:
    (i)   Physical abuse including striking, shaking and burning.
    (ii) Emotional abuse often associated with delayed emotional development.
    (iii) Sexual abuse.
    (iv) Neglect including failure to provide shelter, clothing and nourishment.

2 Maintain a high index of suspicion in the following cases, especially if the child is <4 years old:
    (i) *History*
        (a) delay between the alleged injury and the presentation to the ED
        (b) inconsistency between the story and the actual injuries, or a changing story
        (c) abnormal parental behaviour, poor interaction with the child and apparent lack of parental concern
        (d) frequent attendance in the ED by the child or a sibling, often for little apparent reason
        (e) previous injuries on different dates
        (f) failure to thrive, or clinical signs of neglect.
    (ii) *Examination*
        (a) examine the child with the consent of at least one parent or the child's legal guardian. Undress the child fully in stages, and carefully document all the findings ideally using a body diagram
        (b) measure bruises, scratches, burns and other skin marks with a ruler. Arrange clinical photographs detailed in the medical notes to provide contemporaneous evidence. Look specifically for:
            – torn upper lip frenulum, or palatal haemorrhage from a feeding bottle or even a fist thrust into the mouth to prevent the baby crying, or from a direct blow
            – human bite marks, and bruising from a fist or slapping, which may rupture the tympanic membrane
            – bruising in unexpected locations such as buttocks or cheeks
            – cigarette burns, or scalds limited to the buttocks and genitalia or both feet, suggesting immersion in hot water

- fractured skull or long bone, particularly in a child not yet able to walk. A spiral fracture of a long bone is most suspicious, as are other healing fractures of differing ages on skeletal survey
- subconjunctival, vitreous or retinal haemorrhage, suggesting violent shaking, or from a direct blow
- signs of trauma to the genitalia or anus, perianal warts or other sexually transmitted diseases.

MANAGEMENT

1 Inform the senior ED doctor and paediatric team immediately if you have any suspicion of child abuse, and arrange for admission of the child.

2 Check whether the child is on the Child Protection Register already and involve the ED social worker early.

3 Do not confront the parents at this stage. Explain that you want a further opinion from a senior paediatric doctor, which necessitates admitting the child.

4 Make sure to accurately document in the medical notes the history, physical examination findings, timing and nature of consultations, and suspicion of child abuse.

5 Contact the social work department and follow local procedural policy with respect to the timing and involvement of additional agencies such as the police and social services, if the parent refuses admission.

6 Enlist the help of additional support groups such as the National Association for Prevention of Child Abuse and Neglect (NAPCAN. www.napcan.org.au) in Australia, or the National Society for Prevention of Cruelty to Children (NSPCC. www.nspcc.org.uk/) in the UK, if further advice or help is required.

 Tip: a similar presentation may be seen in osteogenesis imperfecta with multiple fractures, and idiopathic thrombocytopaenic purpura and leukaemia with widespread bruising and bleeding. However, these are rare compared with genuine cases of child abuse.

FURTHER READING

American Heart Association. https://eccguidelines.heart.org/index.php/circulation/cpr-ecc-guidelines-2/ (2015 CPR and ECC guidelines).

American Heart Association (2015) Part 12: Pediatric advanced life support: 2015 American Heart Association guidelines update for cardiopulmonary resuscitation and emergency cardiovascular care. *Circulation* **132**: S526–S542.

Australian Resuscitation Council. http://www.resus.org.au/ (resuscitation guidelines 2015).

European Resuscitation Council. http://cprguidelines.eu/ (ERC Guidelines 2015).

European Resuscitation Council (2015) European Resuscitation Council Guidelines for Resuscitation 2015 Section 6. Paediatric life support. *Resuscitation* **95**: 223–48.

Lullaby Trust. http://www.lullabytrust.org.uk/ (SIDS and SUDI).

Murray L, Little M, Pascu O, Hoggett K (2015) *Toxicology Handbook*, 3rd edn. Elsevier, Sydney.

Therapeutic Guidelines. eTG complete 2015. http://www.tg.org.au/

The Royal Children's Hospital Melbourne. Clinical Practice Guidelines. http://www.rch.org.au/clinicalguide/

Section IX

OBSTETRIC AND GYNAECOLOGICAL EMERGENCIES

GYNAECOLOGICAL ASSESSMENT AND MANAGEMENT

GENERAL PRINCIPLES

1   All gynaecological emergencies that present with abdominal pain or vaginal bleeding require a thorough history and examination. Be delicate and empathic when taking the history of the presenting complaint and discussing the patient's gynaecological and sexual history.

   (i)   Pay particular attention to the menstrual history, site of pain, presence of vaginal discharge, and urinary symptoms.

   (ii) Ascertain the patient's contraceptive history, her potential for being pregnant, and her gravida and parity. Also consider possible non-gynaecological conditions.

2   Perform a thorough examination including an abdominal examination, and vaginal examination with speculum and bimanual palpation. Allow the patient privacy to undress and **always** have a chaperone in attendance.

3   Send urgent blood samples to the laboratory, perform a urine or serum β-human chorionic gonadotrophin (hCG) pregnancy test, and institute resuscitative procedures as necessary.

PRESCRIBING IN PREGNANCY

1   Consult the prescribing information first before giving any drug to a pregnant patient, or breastfeeding mother. Look in the local drug formularies such as:

   (i)   *MIMS, Australian Medicines Handbook* (AMH), and the *British National Formulary* (BNF).

   (ii) Ideally, avoid all drugs in the first trimester of pregnancy unless absolutely necessary.

   (iii) Therefore, always enquire about the possibility of pregnancy in every female of reproductive age. This is also important when requesting X-rays

      (a) most hospital radiology departments have their own guidelines to minimize the risk of irradiation in early pregnancy.

GYNAECOLOGICAL CAUSES OF ACUTE ABDOMINAL PAIN

The following conditions present with acute abdominal pain in females:
- Ruptured ectopic pregnancy (see next section on Bleeding in Early Pregnancy)
- Pelvic inflammatory disease (acute salpingitis)
- Ruptured ovarian cyst
- Ovarian torsion
- Endometriosis.

PELVIC INFLAMMATORY DISEASE (ACUTE SALPINGITIS)

DIAGNOSIS

1 Pelvic inflammatory disease (PID) includes any combination of endometritis, salpingitis, tubo-ovarian abscess or pelvic peritonitis. It is usually a sexually transmitted disease caused principally by chlamydial or gonococcal infection.

  (i) Non-sexually acquired infection may follow instrumentation of the cervix, delivery, or recent insertion of an IUCD (10% of cases).

  (ii) Recurrent infections are increasingly likely to cause infertility, and an increased risk of ectopic pregnancy.

2 It presents acutely with fever (30%), malaise, bilateral lower abdominal pain, dyspareunia, menstrual irregularities and mucopurulent vaginal discharge.

3 On examination there is an elevated temperature with bilateral lower abdominal tenderness and guarding.

  (i) Vaginal examination reveals a cervical discharge, adnexal tenderness and cervical motion tenderness (excitation pain on moving the cervix).

4 Send an endocervical and urethral swab for gonococcal culture, and an endocervical swab for *Chlamydia* antigen, nucleic acid amplification by polymerase chain reaction (PCR) or culture.

5 Send blood for FBC and blood culture if there is a high fever. Perform a pregnancy test that should be negative.

6 Send an MSU for microscopy, culture plus gonococcal and chlamydial PCR.

7 Request an ultrasound to help identify a tubo-ovarian abscess, and to exclude other causes of lower pelvic pain.

Warning: PID is a notoriously difficult diagnosis to make, being easily missed or conversely diagnosed when not present. Laparoscopy is the gold standard but is reserved for complicated cases and when the diagnosis is unclear.

MANAGEMENT

1 Remove an IUCD if inserted within the last 3 weeks or if the infection is severe. Send it for culture and provide an alternate method for contraception.

2 Admit all patients who are systemically unwell, pregnant (unusual), intolerant to oral medication, have a confirmed tubo-ovarian abscess, or in whom the diagnosis is uncertain.

  (i) Start parenteral antibiotics according to local guidelines, such as ceftriaxone 2 g i.v. daily, plus azithromycin 500 mg i.v. daily, plus metronidazole 500 mg i.v. 12-hourly if infection was sexually acquired.

3   Otherwise, if the patient is clinically well and the infection was sexually acquired, give ceftriaxone 500 mg i.m., plus metronidazole 400 mg orally b.d. for 14 days, plus azithromycin 1 g orally once, then either azithromycin 1 g orally 1 week later or doxycycline 100 mg b.d. orally for 14 days.

4   Discharge the patient and arrange follow-up in gynaecology outpatients, or a genitourinary medicine clinic or GP to facilitate contact screening and treatment.
      (i)   Contact tracing of chlamydial- or gonococcal-positive patients is vital to prevent new and recurrent cases.
      (ii) Advise patients to abstain from sexual intercourse until the partner has been tested and treated.

RUPTURED OVARIAN CYST

DIAGNOSIS AND MANAGEMENT

1   There is sudden, moderate, lower abdominal and pelvic pain without gastrointestinal symptoms.

2   The patient is afebrile with localized tenderness, but no mass is felt.

3   A pregnancy test is negative, and pelvic ultrasound confirms the diagnosis.

4   Give analgesia as indicated and refer the patient to the gynaecology team.
      (i)   Laparoscopy may be indicated, particularly for signs of intraperitoneal haemorrhage with corpus luteal cyst rupture.

OVARIAN TORSION

DIAGNOSIS AND MANAGEMENT

1   A pathologically enlarged ovary or adnexal mass that twists or suddenly distends from a bleed causes abrupt lower abdominal pain, often with preceding episodes of milder pain.

2   The patient may have nausea and vomiting, a low-grade fever and localized abdominal tenderness with a palpable mass.

3   Send blood for FBC, collect an MSU, and exclude pregnancy with a pregnancy test.

4   Arrange a pelvic ultrasound, and refer the patient to the gynaecology team for possible laparoscopy.

ENDOMETRIOSIS

DIAGNOSIS AND MANAGEMENT

1   There is a preceding history of recurrent abdominal and flank pain, worse at the time of menstruation and immediately pre-menstrually. Other common symptoms include acquired dysmenorrhoea, dyspareunia, painful defecation (tenesmus) and infertility.

2   Examination is often normal, or may show adnexal or rectovaginal tenderness on internal examination.

3 Send blood for FBC, collect an MSU, and exclude pregnancy with a pregnancy test.

4 Arrange a pelvic ultrasound, and refer the patient to the gynaecology team.

    (i) This is a difficult diagnosis that requires review by the gynaecology team. A laparoscopy may be indicated, but there is poor correlation between symptoms and laparoscopic findings.

BLEEDING IN EARLY PREGNANCY

The two most important causes are ectopic pregnancy and spontaneous miscarriage.

The old term 'spontaneous abortion' has been replaced by 'spontaneous miscarriage' to diminish negative self-perceptions of women experiencing early pregnancy fetal demise.

RUPTURED ECTOPIC PREGNANCY

DIAGNOSIS

1 Ectopic pregnancy is more common in patients with a previous ectopic pregnancy, pelvic inflammatory disease, previous tubal surgery, assisted reproductive techniques, increased age, and in patients using an intrauterine contraceptive device (IUCD).

    (i) However 50% occur with no predisposing risk factors.

2 Ectopic pregnancy usually presents from the 5th to the 9th weeks of pregnancy. Patients may not realize they are pregnant, although have a history of breast tenderness, nausea or recent unprotected intercourse.

    (i) Consider an ectopic in every female patient with menstrual irregularities, vaginal bleeding, lower abdominal pain, shock or collapse.

3 The predominant feature on history is lower abdominal pain, which is present in over 90% of presentations. Vaginal bleeding is usually mild.

4 *Haemodynamically unstable patient:*

    (i) Unstable patients present with sudden abdominal pain, often referred to the shoulder tip, followed by scanty vaginal bleeding, proceeding to circulatory collapse and haemorrhagic shock.

    (ii) On examination the patient is pale, collapsed and hypotensive with a tender, rigid silent abdomen.

5 *Haemodynamically stable patient:*

    (i) Stable patients present with a recent history of a missed period or sometimes erratic periods, lower abdominal pain and slight vaginal bleeding that is typically dark brown ('prune juice'), although the bleeding can be fresh red.

(ii) There is localized lower abdominal tenderness and guarding to one side, and a smaller uterus than expected on bimanual palpation for the duration of apparent amenorrhoea.

6 Perform a pelvic examination.
   (i) Be gentle to avoid the potential for traumatic tubal rupture.
   (ii) Examine for discomfort and swelling in the lateral fornix.

7 Insert one or two large-bore i.v. cannulae and send blood for full blood count (FBC), urea and electrolytes (U&Es), blood sugar, β-hCG and group and save (G&S). Note the rhesus status.

8 Perform a pregnancy test.
   (i) A serum radioimmunoassay pregnancy test for β-hCG in blood is highly sensitive, with a negative test ruling out a recent ectopic or miscarriage, although it takes time to do and may not be available after hours.
   (ii) Alternatively, test for urinary β-hCG. This urine dipstick test can be done rapidly in the emergency department (ED), and may be positive even before the first missed period. Again, a negative test virtually rules out an ectopic.

9 Request an ultrasound scan:
   (i) Transabdominal (TA) ultrasound scan can demonstrate a gestational sac within the uterus, which should be reliably identified by 6 weeks. It may also show free intraperitoneal fluid in free rupture
      (a) absence of a gestational sac is suggestive of an ectopic pregnancy
      (b) the exception to this rule is the rare heterotopic pregnancy, with an intrauterine *plus* an ectopic pregnancy
      (c) this occurs particularly in women undergoing assisted reproductive technology treatment such as *in vitro* fertilization (IVF).
   (ii) Transvaginal (TV) ultrasound scan is more sensitive, and should be able to show a gestational sac if the β-hCG is >1000 IU, or if the pregnancy is around 5 weeks, when the pregnancy is intrauterine
      (a) again, absence of a gestational sac is suggestive of an ectopic pregnancy
      (b) in addition, it should be able to identify most signs of the extrauterine pregnancy itself.
   (iii) Thus, ultrasound features suggesting an ectopic pregnancy include an empty uterus, intrauterine pseudosac, a tubal ring, adnexal mass and fluid in the pouch of Douglas.

Tip: a patient presenting with a positive pregnancy test, abdominal pain, scanty vaginal bleeding and absence of intrauterine pregnancy on ultrasound scan has an ectopic pregnancy until proven otherwise.

MANAGEMENT

1 Unstable ectopic pregnancy:
- (i) Give high-flow oxygen by face mask and organize urgent cross-match of 4 units of blood.
- (ii) Commence an infusion of crystalloid such as normal saline or Hartmann's then blood, and refer the patient immediately to the gynaecology team
  - (a) inform theatre and the duty anaesthetist.

2 Stable ectopic pregnancy:
- (i) Stratify these patients on the basis of the ultrasound and β-hCG findings
  - (a) admit patients with a positive pregnancy test, empty uterus on TV ultrasound examination and clinical signs of an ectopic for a laparoscopy (or medical management in selected patients)
  - (b) follow up those patients with a positive pregnancy test, an empty uterus but no ultrasound signs of an ectopic with serial β-hCG examinations every 48 h, and a repeat ultrasound.
- (ii) Ultimately, a laparoscopy or laparotomy confirms the condition and allows definitive management, although the occasional case can be managed medically with i.m. methotrexate.
- (iii) Therefore refer all cases to the gynaecology team.

3 Give all rhesus-negative mothers RhD immunoglobulin 250 units i.m. to prevent maternal formation of antibodies from isoimmunization.

SPONTANEOUS MISCARRIAGE

Spontaneous miscarriage (failed pregnancy) is the expulsion of the products of conception before the 20th week of pregnancy. It is most common in the first trimester and occurs in 10–20% of all diagnosed early pregnancies. There are five recognized stages of spontaneous miscarriage.

DIAGNOSIS

1 *Threatened miscarriage*
- (i) This is most common up to 14 weeks gestation, causing mild cramps and transient vaginal bleeding. These symptoms indicate a possible miscarriage.
- (ii) The uterine size is compatible with the duration of pregnancy. As a rough guide, the expected size of the uterus is:
  - (a) abdominal palpation: the fundus reaches the symphysis pubis at 12 weeks and the umbilicus at 20 weeks
  - (b) bimanual examination: the uterus is the size of a hen's egg at 7 weeks, an orange at 10 weeks, and a grapefruit at 12 weeks.
- (iii) The external cervical os is closed on speculum examination.

2 *Inevitable miscarriage*
- (i) This represents a spontaneous miscarriage that cannot be arrested.

      (ii) The bleeding is heavier, followed by lower abdominal cramps that are more persistent.

      (iii) The external cervical os is open 0.5 cm or more

          (a) products of conception may be found in the vagina, or protruding from the cervical canal in which case there will be ongoing pain, bleeding and bradycardia ('cervical shock').

      (iv) Symptoms and signs of pregnancy such as amenorrhoea, nausea, vomiting, breast enlargement, tenderness, tingling, areolar pigmentation and frequency of micturition will disappear.

3   Incomplete miscarriage

      (i)   Parts of the fetus or placental material are retained in the uterus.

      (ii) The bleeding remains heavy and the cramps persist, even following the passage of clots and the products of conception.

4   Complete miscarriage

      (i)   All the fetal and placental material has been expelled from the uterus.

      (ii) The bleeding and cramps stop after the conceptus has been passed and the signs of pregnancy disappear.

      (iii) The cervical os is closed.

5   Missed miscarriage

      (i)   An early pregnancy fetal demise in which all the products of conception are retained.

      (ii) Cramps and bleeding are replaced by an asymptomatic brownish vaginal discharge.

      (iii) The uterus is small and irregular, and ultrasound fails to detect fetal heart motion.

      (iv) Infection and disseminated intravascular coagulation (DIC) may occur.

6   Gain i.v. access and send blood for FBC and G&S if the bleeding is heavy. Note the rhesus antibody status.

7   Perform a quantitative serum β-hCG to confirm the pregnancy, and as a baseline for subsequent serial testing to monitor for a continued pregnancy or fetal demise.

8   Arrange a pelvic ultrasound to assess fetal size and viability, and to rule out an ectopic pregnancy.

MANAGEMENT

1   Commence an infusion of normal saline.

2   Remove the products of conception with sponge forceps if they are blocking the cervical canal, to relieve the pain, bradycardia and hypotension.

      (i)   Send them for histology to exclude a hydatidiform mole.

3 Give rhesus-negative mothers RhD immunoglobulin 250 units i.m. within 72 hours, and 625 units i.m. after the first trimester (500 IU i.m. in the UK at or after 20 weeks gestation).

    (i) The role and need for RhD immunoglobulin in a threatened miscarriage before 12 weeks gestation is unclear.

    (ii) RhD immunoglobulin is no longer recommended in the UK for any miscarriage before 12 weeks, provided there is no instrumentation.

4 Refer patients with a threatened miscarriage to the EPEU (Early Pregnancy Evaluation Unit) or similar for ongoing management.

    (i) 85–90% will progress to term if ultrasound confirms a live intrauterine gestation.

5 Admit all other patients under the gynaecology team for surgical (evacuation of retained products of conception – ERPC), medical (misoprostol) or expectant management of uterine evacuation for an inevitable, incomplete or silent miscarriage.

 Tip: miscarriage can be associated with significant psychological sequelae. An empathic approach to medical care, and provision of counselling and psychological support are important.

SEPTIC ABORTION

DIAGNOSIS AND MANAGEMENT

1 This is the result of 'backstreet' abortion or occasionally therapeutic uterine evacuation.

    (i) Incomplete uterine emptying with haemorrhage, infection and/or instrumentation injury occur.

2 There is rapidly spreading pelvic infection, with salpingitis, peritonitis, pelvic and pulmonary thrombophlebitis, which can lead to septicaemia, DIC, shock and death.

3 The patient presents unwell with fever, abdominal pain, foul-smelling vaginal discharge and bleeding. The patient will progress to hypotension, oliguria, confusion and coma if untreated.

4 Give the patient high-flow oxygen by face mask.

5 Gain i.v. access, send blood for FBC, coagulation profile, U&Es, liver function tests (LFTs), blood sugar, two sets of blood cultures and G&S for rhesus D antigens. Start rapid normal saline i.v.

6 Commence gentamicin 5 mg/kg i.v., ampicillin 2 g i.v. and metronidazole 500 mg i.v., and refer the patient urgently to the gynaecology team for evacuation of the uterine contents or emergency hysterectomy.

CONDITIONS IN LATE PREGNANCY

Ideally, all patients >18–20 weeks pregnant should be sent straight to the labour ward. Occasionally, they are too unstable or there is not time to get them there. Thus the following conditions may be seen, all requiring prompt obstetric help.

TERMINOLOGY

Two terms are easy to confuse in obstetric practice:
- *Gravida* is the number of times a woman has been pregnant, with twins counting as one. A first pregnancy is a 'primigravida'.
- *Parity* is defined as the number of times a woman has given birth to a fetus with a gestational age of 24 weeks or more.

ANTEPARTUM HAEMORRHAGE

DIAGNOSIS AND MANAGEMENT

1   Vaginal bleeding after 24 weeks gestation can be a life-threatening emergency, particularly if associated with placenta praevia, placental abruption or uterine rupture.

2   **Placenta praevia**
    (i)   This is classically associated with painless vaginal bleeding and uterine hypotonia, although mild abdominal cramping pain may occur if a small abruption coexists.
    (ii) Abdominal examination confirms a 'soft' uterus with a high presenting part.
    (iii) The fetal condition is usually good and obstetric management is often conservative.

3   **Placental abruption**
    (i)   This is associated with minor trauma, pre-eclampsia, essential hypertension, a history of previous abruption, and use of cocaine.
    (ii) Patients present with severe lower abdominal pain and vaginal bleeding if the abruption is 'revealed'. Examination shows a hard 'woody' uterus, which is painful to palpate.
    (iii) There is a high incidence of fetal demise prior to delivery.

4   **Never** perform a vaginal or speculum examination in the ED on a patient with an antepartum haemorrhage, as this may precipitate torrential vaginal haemorrhage from a low-lying placenta.
    (i)   Such examination should only be performed by an experienced obstetrician in an operating theatre prepared for an immediate caesarean section, preferably after an urgent ultrasound scan.

5   Give oxygen, place the patient in the left lateral position, insert two large-bore i.v. cannulae and send blood for FBC and coagulation profile, and cross-match 4 units. Start an i.v. infusion if the patient is hypotensive or shocked.

6 Give non-sensitized rhesus-negative mothers RhD immunoglobulin 625 IU i.m. (500 units i.m. in the UK).

7 Request an ultrasound to differentiate the potential causes of antepartum haemorrhage. It can localize the placental position and determine the presence and size of a concealed abruption bleed.

8 Refer the patient immediately to the obstetric team.

PRE-ECLAMPSIA AND ECLAMPSIA

DIAGNOSIS AND MANAGEMENT

1 Pre-eclampsia is defined clinically by hypertension and proteinuria, with or without pathological oedema, which develop after 20 weeks gestation including in labour and post-partum.

2 Hypertension includes:
  (i) A systolic blood pressure >140 mmHg and diastolic blood pressure >90 mmHg on two successive measurements 4–6 h apart in the third trimester of pregnancy.
  (ii) A rise in blood pressure of >25–30 mmHg systolic or 15 mmHg diastolic compared with early pregnancy (booking) blood pressure.

3 Fulminant or severe pre eclampsia is associatcd with:
  (i) Systolic blood pressure (BP) >160 mmHg, diastolic BP >110 mmHg.
  (ii) Headache, visual symptoms.
  (iii) Nausea, vomiting and abdominal pain.
  (iv) Oliguria (<500 mL/24 h).
  (v) Irritability and hyper-reflexia.

4 Complications of severe pre-eclampsia include:
  (i) Acute pulmonary oedema.
  (ii) HELLP syndrome – haemolysis, elevated liver enzymes and low platelets.
  (iii) Disseminated intravascular coagulation.
  (iv) Ccrebral haemorrhage.
  (v) Seizures (eclampsia).

5 Call the senior ED doctor and obstetric team urgently. Give oxygen, gain i.v. access and send blood for FBC, U&Es, LFTs, blood sugar, coagulation profile and uric acid. Commence a normal saline infusion.

6 Catheterize the patient. Place a wedge under the right hip, or nurse in the left lateral position.

7 Magnesium sulphate is the drug of choice for seizure prophylaxis in pre-eclampsia, and for eclampsia:
  (i) Give an initial dose of magnesium 4 g (16 mmol) i.v. over 5–10 min, then commence an infusion of magnesium 1 g/h (4 mmol/h) for at least 24 h.

    (ii)   Treat any seizure with a further bolus of magnesium 2 g (8 mmol) i.v.

8 Give diazepam 0.1–0.2 mg/kg i.v. if seizures persist, or magnesium is not readily available.

9 Treat severe hypertension with hydralazine 5 mg i.v. bolus every 20 min (to a maximum cumulative dose of 20 mg) or labetalol 20 mg i.v. bolus escalating to 40 mg bolus every 10 min (to a maximum cumulative dose of 300 mg).

    (i)   Aim for a diastolic blood pressure of 90–100 mmHg to reduce the risk of cerebrovascular accident and further seizures.

10 The only definitive treatment of eclampsia is delivery, once seizures are controlled, hypoxia is corrected and treatment of the severe hypertension is under way.

EMERGENCY DELIVERY

MANAGEMENT

1 Call the obstetric team and paediatric or neonatal team immediately.

2 Allow the mother to lie or sit semi-upright, and give her 50% nitrous oxide with oxygen (Entonox™) during the first half of the contractions.

3 A mediolateral episiotomy may be needed in primiparous women, but is not routine.

4 Ask the mother to pant and thus to stop pushing as the head crowns, usually with the occiput upwards/face down, which is followed by rotation (restitution) of the head laterally.

5 Clamp and cut the cord immediately if it is wound tightly around the baby's neck.

    (i)   Otherwise the cord can be clamped off or tied with two 2/0 silk ties at leisure at least 1 min after delivery, and divided.

6 The next contraction delivers the anterior shoulder by gentle downward traction on the head, which is followed by the posterior shoulder and trunk.

7 Deliver the baby by lifting the head and trunk up and over the symphysis pubis, to lie on the mother's abdomen.

8 Wipe or suction mucus from the baby's nose and mouth, then dry and wrap in a blanket. Be prepared to mask ventilate initially with air if there is apnoea.

    (i)   Make certain to maintain newborn temperature between 36.5–37.5°C.

9 Avoid the temptation to pull on the cord in the routine management of the third stage of labour, for fear of causing uterine inversion.

    (i)   Palpate the abdomen to exclude the possibility of a second fetus, and gently massage the uterus to stimulate uterine contraction.

    (ii)   Give oxytocin 10 units i.m. This helps prevent post-partum haemorrhage and aids delivery of the placenta.

  (iii) An alternative is oxytocin 5 units with ergometrine (Syntometrine™) 500 µg (1 mL) i.m., but this is associated with nausea, vomiting and hypertension, and has little advantage over oxytocin alone.

10 Encourage the mother to commence suckling her baby immediately, as this will naturally stimulate uterine contraction, help to expel the placenta and reduce the risk of haemorrhage.

TRAUMA IN LATE PREGNANCY

Treatment priorities for trauma in a pregnant patient are the same as for the non-pregnant patient. The best treatment for the fetus is to rapidly stabilize the mother.

MANAGEMENT

1 Follow the immediate management guidelines as for multiple injuries (see p. 168), but note the following additional considerations:

  (i) Tilt the supine, third trimester patient laterally using a wedge or pillow under the right hip, and manually displace the gravid uterus upwards and to the left to minimize impaired venous return from inferior vena caval compression.

  (ii) Protect the airway from the increased risk of gastric regurgitation and pulmonary aspiration

   (a) remember as minute ventilation increases in late pregnancy, hypocapnoea with $PaCO_2$ 32 mmHg (4.2 kPa) is normal.

  (iii) Larger amounts of blood may be lost before obvious signs of hypovolaemia such as tachycardia, hypotension and tachypnoea occur, as both maternal blood volume and cardiac output increase in pregnancy

   (a) common mistakes are to fail to recognize shock despite normal vital signs, and to then fail to treat aggressively with crystalloid and blood.

  (iv) Observe and monitor *every* pregnant woman with a potentially viable fetus of >24 weeks gestation with cardiotocography (CTG) for at least 6 h, looking particularly for evidence of placental abruption with fetal distress and frequent uterine contractions

   (a) fetal distress occurs readily even without signs of maternal shock, as blood is shunted preferentially away from the uterus to maintain the maternal circulation following blood loss.

  (v) Also arrange an abdominal ultrasound to evaluate both the mother and the fetus. It is highly sensitive for detecting free intraperitoneal fluid (blood) following blunt trauma.

  (vi) Retroperitoneal bleeding with pelvic fracture after blunt trauma may be massive from the engorged pelvic veins.

2 Assess the fetus during the secondary survey after initial resuscitation of the mother.

    (i) Examine fundal height, uterine tenderness, fetal movement, fetal heart rate and strength of contractions.

    (ii) Use a fetal stethoscope, Doppler ultrasound or cardiotocograph to assess the fetal heart rate. Fetal distress is indicated by:

        (a) bradycardia <110 beats/min (normal 120–160 beats/min)

        (b) loss of fetal heart acceleration to fetal movement, or late deceleration after uterine contractions.

3 Important causes of fetal distress or fetal death in trauma include maternal hypovolaemia, placental abruption and uterine rupture.

    (i) Signs of placental abruption vary from vaginal bleeding, abdominal pain, tenderness, increasing fundal height and premature contractions, to maternal shock.

    (ii) Signs of traumatic uterine rupture, which occurs more commonly in the second half of pregnancy, range from abdominal pain, to maternal shock or a separately palpable uterus and fetus.

4 Continue fetal monitoring with CTG for a minimum of 6 h, even after apparently minor maternal trauma.

5 Give all rhesus-negative mothers RhD immunoglobulin 625 IU i.m. (500 units i.m. in the UK).

6 Call the obstetric team to review and admit every pregnant trauma case. Call the paediatric team in addition if the fetus is >24–26 weeks gestation and immediate delivery is indicated.

CARDIOPULMONARY RESUSCITATION IN LATE PREGNANCY

DIAGNOSIS

1 Causes of cardiac arrest in late pregnancy include cardiac disease and aortic dissection, pulmonary embolism, psychiatric disorders including drug overdose, hypertensive disorders of pregnancy, sepsis, uteroplacental bleeding (ante- and post-partum), amniotic fluid embolus and cerebrovascular haemorrhage.

MANAGEMENT

1 Key interventions in cardiac arrest in pregnancy:

    (i) Tilt the patient laterally using a wedge or pillow under the right side, and displace the uterus by lifting it manually upwards and to the left off the great vessels.

    (ii) Give 100% oxygen and administer a fluid bolus.

2 Modifications to basic life support (BLS) in pregnancy:

    (i) Apply cricoid pressure whenever administering positive-pressure ventilation as there is increased risk of regurgitation and pulmonary aspiration.

    (ii)   Place hands higher on the chest wall, slightly above the centre of the sternum when performing external cardiac compressions.

    (iii) Effective external chest compression is more difficult due to flared ribs, raised diaphragm, breast enlargement and inferior vena caval compression.

    (iv) Remember, defibrillation shocks are not a risk to the fetus.

3   Modifications to advanced life support (ALS):

    (i)   Hypoxaemia is common due to reduced functional residual capacity and increased oxygen demand.

    (ii)   Intubation is more difficult during pregnancy secondary to some of the physical factors outlined in (2) (iii) above

        (a) be prepared to use an endotracheal tube that is 0.5–1.0 mm smaller in diameter than expected, as the airway may be narrower secondary to laryngeal oedema.

    (iii) Do not use the femoral veins for venous access. Drugs administered via this route may not reach the maternal heart until after the fetus has been delivered.

    (iv) Continue to use all the usual recommended resuscitation procedures and drugs for circulatory support.

4   Consider immediate caesarean section if the resuscitation is not rapidly successful with ROSC within 4 min, having called the obstetric and paediatric teams on the arrival of the patient.

    (i)   Ideally, perimortem caesarean section should be within 5 min of cardiac arrest for optimum maternal and neonatal survival.

    (ii)   Continue cardiopulmonary resuscitation throughout the procedure and afterwards until a stable rhythm with a sustained cardiac output is obtained.

WOMEN'S MEDICINE CRISES

EMERGENCY CONTRACEPTION

Occasionally, patients present for emergency contraceptive measures after unprotected intercourse. There are two possibilities:

1   *Intrauterine contraceptive device (IUCD)*

    (i)   A copper device may be used up to 5 days after unprotected intercourse and is more effective than hormonal methods of emergency contraception.

    (ii)   Test for sexually transmitted diseases on IUCD insertion and consider a single dose of azithromycin 1 g orally prophylactically in the casual sexual encounter, if the patient is concerned.

2   *Post-coital 'morning after' pill*
This may be used up to 72 h after unprotected intercourse. Taking the dose as soon as possible increases the efficacy.
- (i) Give levonorgestrel 1.5 mg as a single dose
  - (a) do not prescribe in women with undiagnosed vaginal bleeding, breast cancer or severe liver disease
  - (b) give 2.25 mg levonorgestrel (1.5 mg taken immediately and 750 μg taken 12 hours later) in patients taking enzyme-inducing drugs such as carbamazepine, rifampicin, phenytoin and phenobarbitone (phenobarbital).
- (ii) Give a repeat levonorgestrel dose if vomiting occurs within 2 hours, with an antiemetic such as metoclopramide 10–20 mg i.v. or domperidone 20 mg orally.
- (iii) Explain to the patient that:
  - (a) her next period may be early or late
  - (b) a barrier method of contraception must be used until this next period.
- (iv) Refer all patients for follow-up to their general practitioner (GP) or a family planning clinic to check that:
  - (a) the pregnancy test is negative 3–4 weeks later
  - (b) the patient receives proper contraceptive advice for the future.

MISSED ORAL CONTRACEPTIVE PILL

The critical time for loss of contraceptive protection is at the beginning or end of the menstrual cycle, due to extension of the 'pill-free' interval.

1   *Combined oral contraceptive pill*
- (i) *Up to 12 hours late*: Take the missed pill and carry on as usual.
- (ii) *Over 12 hours late*:
  - (a) continue normal pill taking, but for the next 7 days either abstain from sex or use an alternative barrier method of contraception such as the condom
  - (b) start the next packet immediately the present one is over, if these 7 days run beyond the end of the packet; i.e. no gap between packets
    - this will mean that no period may occur until the end of two packets
  - (c) miss out the seven inactive pills if the everyday pills are the ones being taken
  - (d) emergency contraception is recommended if more than two pills are missed from the first seven tablets in a packet.

2   *Progestogen-only pill*
Over 3 h late, continue normal pill taking, but abstain from sex or use an alternative barrier method of contraception for the next 7 days.

DOMESTIC VIOLENCE TO FEMALES

DIAGNOSIS

1 Domestic violence affects women of every class, race and religion. It may commence at times of acute stress such as unemployment, first pregnancy or separation.

2 The victim may present with injury, abdominal or other pain, substance abuse, attempted suicide, sexual assault or with multiple somatic complaints.

3 Victims may delay attending, and may be evasive and embarrassed. Their partner may answer for them or act unconcerned.

MANAGEMENT

1 Ensure privacy by interviewing alone without the partner. Ask gently but directly about the possibility of violence, which may initially be denied.

2 Record all injuries, measuring bruises or lacerations with a ruler, and institute any urgent treatment to save life.

3 Enquire about any additional risk of physical or sexual abuse to other members of the household, particularly children (see p. 319).

4 Call the duty social worker. Offer admission if it is unsafe for the patient to return home or if acute psychiatric illness is present, e.g. depression.

5 However, if the patient wishes to return home, give written contact numbers, including:
- (i)   GP.
- (ii) Women's refuge.
- (iii) Domestic violence 24-h specialist helpline.
- (iv) Local police.

 Tip: a similar management approach to domestic violence is applicable to both sexes, as well as in the elderly.

SEXUAL ASSAULT

Follow a standard procedure in all cases of alleged sexual assault in which the patient requests or accepts police involvement.

MANAGEMENT

1 Be accompanied by a senior female nurse escort at all times.

2 Record a careful history of exactly what occurred and when, and a description of the assailant.

3 Institute any urgent treatment to save life, e.g. cross-match and starting a transfusion for haemorrhage.

4 Contact the police and inform the sexual assault service, duty government medical officer or police surgeon. He or she will perform the forensic examination aimed at meticulously collecting evidence.

   (i) Make certain informed written consent is obtained in advance.

5 Meanwhile, examine the patient for associated injuries, measuring bruises or lacerations with a ruler. Again obtain informed, written consent to keep all clothing for later forensic analysis.

   (i) Ask the patient to undress on a sheet to collect any debris.

   (ii) Wear gloves and wrap each garment in a brown paper bag fastened with tape and labelled with the patient's name, the date, the nature of the sample, and the name of the person taking the sample.

6 Request a senior gynaecology doctor to perform the examination of the external genitalia and vagina, when the sexual assault service, duty government medical officer or police surgeon is unavailable.

7 Check whether the police have been able to arrange for a designated sexual offences unit to attend (usually non-uniformed female police officers with special training).

8 Call the duty social worker or give the patient written contact telephone numbers/addresses if a social worker is not available immediately.

9 Offer admission to the patient if indicated and discuss the following issues:

   (i) Emergency contraception.

   (ii) Exclusion of a sexually transmitted disease or to provide prophylactic treatment and follow-up.

   (iii) Specialist counselling from various external organizations based in most regional centres, e.g. rape crisis lines.

10 Provide written aftercare instructions with details of all the tests performed, treatments provided, and other arrangements made, as the patient's memory at this time of intense stress will not be reliable.

FURTHER READING

American Heart Association (2015) Part 10: Special circumstances of resuscitation: 2015 American Heart Association guidelines update for cardiopulmonary resuscitation and emergency cardiovascular care. *Circulation* **132**: S501–S518.

American Heart Association (2015) Part 13: Neonatal resuscitation: 2015 American Heart Association guidelines update for cardiopulmonary resuscitation and emergency cardiovascular care. *Circulation* **132**: S543–S560.

European Resuscitation Council (2015) European Resuscitation Council Guidelines for Resuscitation 2015 Section 7. Resuscitation and support of transition of babies at birth. *Resuscitation* **95**: 249–63.

European Resuscitation Council (2015) European Resuscitation Council Guidelines for Resuscitation 2015 Section 4. Cardiac arrest in special circumstances. *Resuscitation* **95**: 148–201.

National Blood Authority. http://www.blood.gov.au/system/files/documents/glines-anti-d.pdf (RhD prophylaxis).

National Institute for Health and Care Excellence. http://www.nice.org.uk/ (antenatal care and emergencies).

Royal College of Obstetricians and Gynaecologists. https://www.rcog.org.uk/en/guidelines-research-services/ (RhD prophylaxis, pre-eclampsia).

Society of Obstetric Medicine of Australia and New Zealand (SOMANZ). https://somanz.org/ (pre-eclampsia).

Therapeutic Guidelines. eTG complete 2015. http://www.tg.org.au/

OPHTHALMIC EMERGENCIES

Ophthalmic emergencies may be grouped into traumatic or non-traumatic, and subdivided according to whether the eyelids are affected, or if the eye is red, painful or has diminished visual acuity.

VISUAL ACUITY

Always record visual acuity, with distance glasses if they are worn, at the start of every eye examination before any drops or dyes have been introduced.

- Acuity is measured by reading a Snellen chart at a distance of 6 m.
- Each eye is tested separately, and the lowest line that can be read accurately is recorded. Normal vision is 6/6.

Ask patients with refractive errors who have left their glasses at home to look through a pinhole to optimize their visual acuity.

TOPICAL OPHTHALMIC PREPARATIONS

The following preparations are referred to in the text:
- Antibiotic drops: 0.5% chloramphenicol solution, two drops every 2–3 h.
- Antibiotic ointment: 1% chloramphenicol ointment, one application to the lower lid conjunctival sac every 4 h, or at night (if drops are used during the day).
- Local anaesthetic: 1% amethocaine (tetracaine) solution or 0.4% oxybuprocaine solution, one or more drops as required.
  - The patient must then wear a protective eye pad for 1–2 h until corneal sensitivity returns
  - **Never** allow the patient to take the drops home.
- Fluorescein corneal stain: fluorescein sodium strips, or 2% fluorescein solution (do not use with soft contact lenses).
- Short-acting mydriatic and cycloplegic dilating drops to examine the fundus: 1% tropicamide, two drops repeated after 15 minutes if necessary (do not use in patients with narrow anterior chambers, to avoid precipitating glaucoma).
- Cycloplegic to paralyse the ciliary body: 1% cyclopentolate two drops lasts 6–24 h, or 2% homatropine two drops can last from 8–12 h to 1–2 days.
- Miotic to constrict the pupil or reverse a mydriatic: 2% pilocarpine one or two drops.

> **Warning:** steroid preparations should not be used except by an experienced ophthalmologist. Any condition diagnosed that requires steroids also needs an ophthalmic opinion first.

PERIORBITAL HAEMATOMA ('BLACK EYE')

DIAGNOSIS AND MANAGEMENT

1 This is caused by a direct blow. If bilateral, suspect local trauma to the nose or a basal skull fracture (see p. 31).

2 Perform a thorough stepwise assessment:
  - (i) Check that the patient can still see, if necessary by opening the eyelids manually, and record the visual acuity.
  - (ii) Systematically assess the eye for damage:
    - (a) examine the cornea for abrasions, the anterior chamber for hyphaema, the sclera for perforation, the pupil size and reactions, and the globe for loss of eye movements
    - (b) check for the presence of a normal red reflex through the pupil, or an afferent pupillary defect abnormality (Marcus Gunn pupil - see page 356).
  - (iii) Refer any abnormal findings suggestive of one of the above complications immediately to the ophthalmology team.
  - (iv) Palpate to see whether the bony margin of the orbit is intact
    - (a) test that the eye movements are full and the eyeball is not tethered, suggesting a 'blow-out' fracture of the orbital floor (see p. 380).

3 Request appropriate facial X-rays if a 'blow-out' or a malar fracture is suspected, and refer the patient to the maxillofacial surgery team.

4 Otherwise, give the patient an analgesic such as paracetamol 500 mg and codeine phosphate 8 mg two tablets q.d.s. and chloramphenicol eye ointment if the eye is shut.

5 Review the patient within 48 h when the swelling has decreased to re-confirm the absence of significant ocular damage.

SUBCONJUNCTIVAL HAEMATOMA

DIAGNOSIS AND MANAGEMENT

Two types are recognized – spontaneous and traumatic.

1 *Spontaneous*
  - (i) This may arise from coughing or from atherosclerotic vessels, particularly in the elderly, and is occasionally associated with hypertension or a bleeding diathesis.
  - (ii) Measure the blood pressure and reassure the patient that the subconjunctival blood will disperse within 2 weeks. No treatment is needed.

2   *Traumatic*

    (i)   This may be due to a surface conjunctival foreign body, or a more serious penetrating foreign body and/or bulging scleral perforation

        (a) gentle digital assessment may reveal reduced eyeball tone in penetration of the globe.

    (ii) Refer all patients immediately to the ophthalmology team if a serious cause is suspected.

    (iii) Consider a basal skull fracture when the posterior margin of the haematoma cannot be seen

        (a) arrange a computed tomography (CT) head scan and refer the patient to the neurosurgical team (see p. 31).

    (iv) Otherwise, minor cases require reassurance only.

EYELID LACERATION

DIAGNOSIS AND MANAGEMENT

1   Refer the patient directly to the ophthalmology or plastic surgery team if the laceration involves the tarsal plate, upper eyelid, lid margin or the medial canthus and the lacrimal apparatus.

2   Otherwise, suture the eyelid under local anaesthesia using fine 6/0 non-absorbable monofilament nylon or polypropylene sutures. Remove after 4 days.

EYELID BURN

DIAGNOSIS AND MANAGEMENT

1   Examine the eye carefully for evidence of corneal or scleral damage before oedema makes the examination impossible, although the blink reflex usually protects the globe.

2   Give the patient antibiotic drops, analgesia and tetanus prophylaxis, and refer immediately to the ophthalmology team.

CHEMICAL BURNS TO THE EYE

DIAGNOSIS AND MANAGEMENT

1   Alkalis are more deeply penetrating and dangerous than acids, and include common agents such as cement, plaster powder, and oven or drain cleaners.

2   The mainstay of treatment is immediate, copious, prolonged irrigation (up to 30 min) with normal saline from an i.v. giving set. Instil local anaesthetic drops to open the eye initially.

3   Give additional analgesia if necessary with morphine 5 mg i.v. plus an antiemetic such as metoclopramide 10 mg i.v.

4   Take care to irrigate all corners of the eye and to evert the upper eyelids to remove any particulate matter, and to irrigate the superior fornix of the conjunctiva.

5   Refer the patient immediately to the ophthalmology team, unless fluorescein staining reveals no corneal damage and the surrounding conjunctiva appears normal and is pain-free, i.e. no injury is apparent.

CONJUNCTIVAL FOREIGN BODY

DIAGNOSIS AND MANAGEMENT

1   Usually a piece of grit blows into the eye causing pain, redness and watering, and is easily seen on direct vision.

2   Remove with a moistened cotton-wool bud after instilling local anaesthetic. Provide an eye pad to be worn for 1–2 h until the return of normal sensation.

3   The object may have impacted on the upper subtarsal conjunctiva if nothing is seen immediately. The eye will be red and painful to blink, and fluorescein staining will reveal multiple linear corneal abrasions.

4   Evert the upper eyelid.
    (i)   Stand behind the patient to evert the upper lid, supporting the head against your body.
    (ii) Instruct the patient to look downwards, pull the upper lid eyelashes down and then up and over the tarsal plate, which is held depressed by a glass rod or orange stick (see Fig. 10.1).
    (iii) Remove the foreign body with a moistened cotton-wool bud.

5   Give the patient antibiotic drops for 2 days if fluorescein shows signs of corneal abrasion.

6   Always consider intraocular penetration, with any high velocity injury, e.g. by a metal fragment from drilling or hammering, or a stone from mowing (see p. 350).

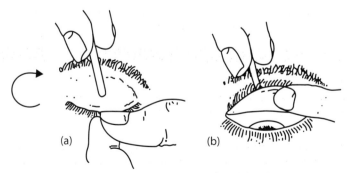

Figure 10.1 Eversion of the upper eyelid.
(a) Lifting the tarsal plate up and over, and (b) demonstrating the underside of the upper eyelid (subtarsal conjunctiva).

CORNEAL FOREIGN BODY

DIAGNOSIS AND MANAGEMENT

1   The foreign body may be obvious, or revealed by fluorescein staining.

2   Instil local anaesthetic drops and attempt removal of the foreign body with a moistened cotton-wool bud or the bevel of a hypodermic needle, introduced from the side.

3   However, leave deep or recalcitrant foreign bodies, and those with an extensive rust ring alone.
    (i)   Refer the patient to the ophthalmology team to avoid causing further damage during attempted removal.

4   As local anaesthetic was used, pad the eye for 1–2 h until the return of normal sensation. Treat any corneal epithelial defect demonstrated on fluorescein staining as for a corneal abrasion (see below).

5   Review the patient within 2 days to exclude infection, but ask them to return earlier if pain increases or vision deteriorates.
    (i)   Refer the patient immediately to the ophthalmology team if there is then evidence of an infected corneal ulcer.

CORNEAL ABRASION

DIAGNOSIS AND MANAGEMENT

1   Corneal abrasion is due to a foreign body or to direct injury from a finger, stick or a piece of paper.

2   There is intense pain, watering and blepharospasm. Local anaesthetic drops may be needed before the eye can be opened properly.

3   Use fluorescein staining to reveal the damage.

4   Give the patient 0.5% chloramphenicol eye drops and cycloplegic drops, and review within 2 days.

5   An eye pad is not needed, other than for 1–2 h following local anaesthetic use.

6   The cornea should be fully recovered by 2 days, so refer the patient to the ophthalmology team if there is delayed healing or a recurrence.

FLASH BURN (ARC EYE)

DIAGNOSIS AND MANAGEMENT

1   Exposure to ultraviolet light from welding without using protective goggles, or from a sun lamp, causes a superficial keratitis.

2   There is intense pain, watering and blepharospasm occurring after a few hours. Fluorescein staining reveals a pitted corneal surface due to a superficial punctate keratitis.

3 Instil local anaesthetic drops and mydriatic/cycloplegic drops. Double-pad the eyes shut until the return of normal sensation and the blepharospasm settles.

4 Give an analgesic such as paracetamol 500 mg and codeine phosphate 8 mg two tablets q.d.s. Recovery occurs within 12–24 h.

BLUNT TRAUMA TO THE EYE

DIAGNOSIS AND MANAGEMENT

1 Always consider injury to the eye in any trauma to the face. Eye examination must not be omitted just because other injuries appear more dramatic or periorbital oedema obscures the eye.

2 Blunt trauma may cause a sequence of injuries from the front to the back of the eye. Systematically exclude each one:

(i) Periorbital haematoma or subconjunctival haemorrhage.

(ii) Corneal abrasion or laceration.

(iii) Bleeding into the anterior chamber, called hyphaema. This may be microscopic or macroscopic with formation of a fluid level.

(iv) A fixed pupil or torn iris, known as traumatic mydriasis and iridodialysis, respectively.

(v) A dislocated lens or subsequent traumatic cataract.

(vi) Vitreous haemorrhage, causing a dull or absent red reflex and obscuring the fundus.

(vii) A retinal tear, with retinal detachment seen as a dark, wrinkled, ballooned area diametrically opposite any resultant visual field defect.

(viii) Retinal oedema (*commotio retinae*) seen as whitish areas of oedema, usually associated with haemorrhage.

(ix) Optic nerve damage, causing blindness with no direct pupillary response to light.

(x) Ruptured globe, with marked visual loss, a soft eye, and shallow anterior chamber.

(xi) Retrobulbar haematoma, with pain, proptosis and a fixed, dilated pupil.

(xii) Orbital fracture, usually a 'blow-out' fracture of the orbital floor (see p. 380).

3 Refer a patient with any of the complications above from (ii) through to (xi) directly to the ophthalmology team. Do not allow the patient home in the meantime, but arrange for them to lie quietly and semi-upright, pending expert assessment.

(i) Ideally, pad both eyes and give appropriate analgesia.

(ii) Protect a suspected ruptured globe with an eye shield, not an eye pad.

PENETRATING TRAUMA TO THE EYE

DIAGNOSIS AND MANAGEMENT

1   Penetrating trauma is usually obvious, although on occasions it may be diffi-cult to recognize initially and must be thought of after a high-velocity injury mechanism such as drilling or mowing.

2   Look for the following injuries:
   (i)   Corneal laceration, often with prolapse of the iris into the defect.
   (ii) Scleral perforation with chemosis or bulging local haemorrhage. This must be differentiated from a trivial subconjunctival bleed.
   (iii) Collapse of the anterior chamber, hyphaema or vitreous haemorrhage, pupil irregularity and lens dislocation.

3   Intraocular foreign body:
   (i)   This is usually a metal fragment from using a hammer and chisel, metal drill or grinding wheel.
   (ii) Sudden sharp pain is followed by localized redness, or the outside of the eye may appear deceptively normal and the incident forgotten.
   (iii) Examine carefully for a puncture wound, and use an ophthalmoscope to inspect the inner eye, although a traumatic cataract may preclude this.
   (iv) X-ray the orbit if there is the remotest possibility of penetration. Request two soft-tissue films, with the eye looking up and down, to identify a radiodense intraocular foreign body
         (a) request a CT of the orbit if the X-ray is negative, but suspicion remains high.

4   Instil antibiotic eye drops (not ointment), protect the eye from further damage with an eye shield, and give tetanus prophylaxis.
   (i)   Provide analgesia if required, e.g. morphine 5 mg i.v. with an antiemetic such as metoclopramide 10 mg i.v.
   (ii) Give gentamicin 5 mg/kg i.v. plus ceftriaxone or cefotaxime 1 g i.v.

5   Refer all cases of documented penetrating injury to the eye, and actual or suspected intraocular foreign body immediately to the ophthalmology team.

CONDITIONS AFFECTING THE EYELIDS

BLEPHARITIS

DIAGNOSIS AND MANAGEMENT

1   Blepharitis is an infection of the eyelid margin, causing red, itchy, crusted lids, which may become chronic with seborrhoeic dermatitis, rosacea or allergy. Styes and chalazions are commonly associated.

2 Prescribe antibiotic ointment, but refer the patient to the ophthalmology clinic for follow-up if this condition becomes persistent or recurrent.

STYE (EXTERNAL HORDEOLUM)

DIAGNOSIS AND MANAGEMENT

1 This is due to an infection of a lash follicle pointing on the lid margin.
2 Give the patient antibiotic ointment and remove any protruding eyelash. Warm bathing may help.

MEIBOMIAN ABSCESS (INTERNAL HORDEOLUM)

DIAGNOSIS AND MANAGEMENT

1 This is an infected Meibomian gland within the tarsal plate. It does not discharge as easily as an external stye, and it may leave a residual Meibomian cyst.
2 Alternatively, it may point and discharge inwards through the tarsal plate, causing conjunctivitis and discharge.
3 Commence flucloxacillin 500 mg orally q.d.s. and refer the patient to the ophthalmology clinic. Warm bathing is unhelpful.

MEIBOMIAN CYST (CHALAZION)

DIAGNOSIS AND MANAGEMENT

1 This feels like a hard pip within the tarsal plate, usually from chronic inflammation causing granuloma formation.
2 Refer the patient to the ophthalmology clinic for incision and curettage.

DACRYOCYSTITIS

DIAGNOSIS AND MANAGEMENT

1 Dacryocystitis is inflammation of the lacrimal sac in the inner canthus of the lower eyelid. Dacryoadenitis is inflammation of the lacrimal gland in the outer upper eyelid.
2 There is a localized, tender, red swelling and watering of the eye due to the blocked lacrimal duct.
3 Start a systemic antibiotic such as flucloxacillin 500 mg orally q.d.s. after sending a swab of any exuding pus.
4 Refer the patient to the next ophthalmology clinic.

ORBITAL AND PERIORBITAL CELLULITIS

DIAGNOSIS AND MANAGEMENT

1 Infection may be:
    (i) Preseptal 'periorbital cellulitis', often related to locally infected or traumatized skin.
    (ii) Post-septal or true 'orbital cellulitis', which is less common and more serious. It arises from the paranasal sinuses or orbital trauma.

2   There is generalized malaise, and a red, warm, oedematous or discharging eye.

    (i)   Orbital cellulitis also causes limited or painful eye movements, reduced vision and proptosis.

    (ii) Adjacent sinuses are tender when associated with the infection.

3   Take blood for full blood count (FBC) and two sets of blood cultures and give flucloxacillin 2 g i.v. plus ceftriaxone 2 g i.v. or cefotaxime 2 g i.v.

4   Refer the patient immediately to the ophthalmology team and obtain a CT scan. Request an ENT opinion if the paranasal sinuses are involved.

5   Complications, particularly in children, can occur within hours, including central retinal vein occlusion, optic nerve compression, cavernous sinus thrombosis and meningitis.

BASAL CELL CARCINOMA (RODENT ULCER)

DIAGNOSIS AND MANAGEMENT

1   Basal cell carcinoma is the most common malignancy of the eyelid, more frequent on the lower lid and following prolonged exposure to sunlight.

2   An early, opalescent pink papule with surface telangiectasia progresses slowly to an ulcerated nodule with a pearly, rounded edge that is locally invasive.

3   Refer the patient to the next ophthalmology clinic for treatment by excision, curettage, cryotherapy or radiotherapy in the elderly.

OPHTHALMIC SHINGLES (HERPES ZOSTER OPHTHALMICUS)

DIAGNOSIS AND MANAGEMENT

1   This presents as a vesicular rash over the distribution of the ophthalmic division of the trigeminal (V) cranial nerve. Pain and tingling often precede the rash.

2   The patient is usually unwell and in pain. The eye may be involved, resulting in blepharitis, conjunctivitis, keratitis, uveitis, secondary glaucoma, ophthalmoplegia or optic neuritis.

3   Treatment of the varied ocular problems is awkward, as eyelid swelling makes topical therapy difficult and pain may be incapacitating. Ideally it should be begun within 72 h of onset.

4   Start famciclovir 250 mg orally t.d.s., valaciclovir 1 g orally t.d.s, or aciclovir 800 mg orally five times a day to decrease pain, corneal damage and uveitis.

5   Refer the patient to the ophthalmology team for inpatient care.

Important causes to consider include:
- Acute conjunctivitis
- Acute keratitis
- Acute iritis
- Acute episcleritis and scleritis
- Acute glaucoma.

ACUTE CONJUNCTIVITIS

DIAGNOSIS

1 The causes are:
  (i) Allergic or irritative, e.g. from dry eyes.
  (ii) Viral, particularly adenovirus or enterovirus.
  (iii) Common bacterial, e.g. staphylococci, streptococci or *Haemophilus*.
  (iv) Uncommon bacterial, e.g. gonococcal or chlamydial.

2 There is generalized conjunctival injection, with gritty discomfort, mild photophobia and variable discharge. Vision should be normal.

MANAGEMENT

1 Advise the patient to clean away the discharge with moist cotton-wool balls, and avoid irritating cosmetics and eye lotions.

2 Allergic conjunctivitis responds to sodium cromoglycate (cromoglicate), non-steroidal anti-inflammatory drugs (NSAIDs), or steroid eye drops, but the latter two should *only* be prescribed by an ophthalmologist.
  (i) Initially prevent secondary bacterial infection with antibiotic drops and refer the patient to the ophthalmology clinic.

3 Viral conjunctivitis, due to the adenovirus ('pink eye') or enterovirus, is highly contagious. Person-to-person spread is rapid unless scrupulous care is taken with hand hygiene and towel or face washer use.
  (i) Give antibiotic drops and ointment to prevent secondary bacterial infection.
  (ii) Refer the patient to the next ophthalmology clinic for a definitive diagnosis and to monitor for the development of keratitis.

4 Bacterial conjunctivitis requires frequent antibiotic drops, as often as hourly in severe cases, and ointment at night. Refer the patient to the ophthalmology clinic if the infection does not settle.

5   Gonococcal or chlamydial conjunctivitis usually occurs in young adults, causing chronic bilateral conjunctivitis with mucopurulent discharge. The cornea may be involved (keratitis).

(i)   The diagnosis is difficult but should be suspected when conventional antibiotic therapy fails.

(ii)   Associated urethritis or salpingitis may suggest the aetiology.

(iii)   Take special swabs for antigen detection, polymerase chain reaction (PCR) or culture, and treat with ceftriaxone 1 g i.v. for gonococcus and/or azithromycin 1 g orally for chlamydia.

(iv)   Refer the patient to the ophthalmology clinic and remember the need for further contact screening and treatment

(a) this can be coordinated with a genitourinary medicine clinic (Special Clinic) or the GP.

ACUTE KERATITIS

DIAGNOSIS

1   There are many possible causes of inflammation of the cornea, including viruses such as herpes simplex virus (HSV) and the adenovirus, bacterial infection of a corneal ulcer, wearing contact lenses (*Pseudomonas aeruginosa* or rarely fungal), secondary to blepharitis (marginal keratitis), abrasion and exposure.

2   The main distinguishing feature from conjunctivitis is the prominent pain, with diminution of vision if there is a central ulcer or a hypopyon (pus in the anterior chamber).

3   Use fluorescein staining to demonstrate a marginal or central ulcer, or the typical branching, dendritic ulcer of herpes simplex keratitis.

MANAGEMENT

1   Commence antibiotic drops or 3% aciclovir ointment five times daily for herpes simplex ulceration.

2   Refer the patient immediately to the ophthalmology team, particularly if a bacterial ulcer or herpes simplex are suspected.

3   Steroid eye drops are absolutely forbidden.

ACUTE IRITIS

DIAGNOSIS

1   Although most cases are idiopathic, iritis is occasionally due to exogenous infection from a perforating wound or corneal ulcer.

2   Otherwise, ill-understood endogenous mechanisms, some linked with HLA-B27 and seronegative arthropathy, may be causally related such as ankylosing spondylitis, Reiter's syndrome, ulcerative colitis, Crohn's disease, and Still's disease.

(i)   Rarer causes include sarcoidosis, toxoplasmosis, Behçet's, tuberculosis (TB) and herpes zoster ophthalmicus.

3   There is circumcorneal ciliary injection, constant pain, photophobia and impaired vision.

4   The pupil contracts, and tiny aggregates of cells, known as keratic precipitates (KPs) may be seen on the inner (posterior) surface of the cornea.

5   Pus forms in the anterior chamber causing a hypopyon in severe cases, and the iris may adhere to the anterior lens surface causing posterior synechiae.

MANAGEMENT

1   Refer the patient immediately to the ophthalmology team for treatment with steroid drops and a cycloplegic such as homatropine.

2   Attacks may become recurrent and progress to secondary glaucoma.

ACUTE EPISCLERITIS AND SCLERITIS

DIAGNOSIS

1   Episcleritis is localized inflammation beneath the conjunctiva adjacent to the sclera that usually resolves spontaneously in 1–2 weeks.

2   Scleritis is a more painful inflammation of the sclera itself. Rheumatoid arthritis, systemic lupus erythematosus (SLE), Wegener's, polyarteritis and other systemic illnesses such as sarcoid and TB may be associated.

3   The eye is locally red in episcleritis; and diffusely red and tender with reflex tearing but minimal discharge in scleritis.
   (i)   Progression to scleral thickening and discolouration then eyeball perforation may occur in scleritis.

4   Send blood for full blood count (FBC), erythrocyte sedimentation rate (ESR), rheumatoid factor and anti-CCP, antinuclear antibody (ANA) and DNA antibodies.

MANAGEMENT

1   Commence an NSAID such as ibuprofen 200–400 mg orally t.d.s. or naproxcn 250 mg orally t.d.s.

2   Refer the patient to the ophthalmology team for definitive treatment, including steroid eye drops.

ACUTE GLAUCOMA

DIAGNOSIS

1   Acute angle-closure glaucoma causes a unilateral red painful eye, associated with a narrowed anterior chamber with obstruction to the outflow of aqueous humour.

2   It is more common in middle-aged or elderly hypermetropes (long-sighted people), and may be precipitated by pupillary dilation including drug related.

3 There is severe throbbing, boring pain accompanied by headache, nausea, vomiting and prostration.

(i) Vision is reduced with haloes around lights, and the cornea becomes hazy with a fixed, semi-dilated oval pupil. On gentle palpation the eye feels hard.

MANAGEMENT

This is an ocular emergency requiring urgent referral to the ophthalmology team. On their advice commence:

1 Topical drops such as pilocarpine one every 5 min for 15 min, then half-hourly; and/or 0.5% timolol one.

2 Acetazolamide 500 mg slowly i.v. then 250 mg i.v. or orally t.d.s. – but contraindicated in sulphonamide allergy.

3 An antiemetic such as metoclopramide 10 mg i.v. and analgesia such as morphine up to 2.5 mg i.v. for severe pain.

SUDDEN LOSS OF VISION IN THE UNINFLAMED EYE

Conditions to be considered include:
- Central retinal artery occlusion.
- Central retinal vein occlusion.
- Vitreous haemorrhage.
- Retinal detachment.
- Optic neuritis.

CENTRAL RETINAL ARTERY OCCLUSION

DIAGNOSIS

1 This condition is most common in the elderly arteriosclerotic patient, but it may occur due to emboli or in association with temporal arteritis.

2 There is sudden blindness associated with a relative afferent pupillary defect (RAPD), known as a Marcus Gunn pupil.

3 Testing for a relative afferent pupillary defect (RAPD), Marcus Gunn pupil:

(i) Direct a swinging light into one eye then briskly into the other. This produces apparent dilation of the pupil in the affected eye, as the relaxing consensual reflex in the good eye is dominant.

(ii) It is an excellent sign of a unilateral or asymmetrical optic nerve or retinal lesion.

4 The fundus is milky white, the optic disc is pale and oedematous, and a cherry-red spot develops at the macula in 1–2 days.

5   A preceding history of transient episodes of monocular visual loss 'amaurosis fugax' suggests embolic branch retinal artery occlusion.

   (i)   Perform a work-up for a transient ischaemic attack including a duplex carotid ultrasound, and commence aspirin – see page 94.

6   Alternatively, a prodromal history of headache, scalp tenderness and malaise suggest temporal arteritis causing anterior ischaemic optic neuropathy (AION).

   (i)   Measure an urgent ESR and, if raised, immediately give the patient prednisolone 60 mg orally to prevent the other eye becoming involved (see p. 103).

MANAGEMENT

1   Commence acetazolamide 500 mg slowly i.v. or orally to reduce intraocular pressure.

2   Give gentle pulsed ocular massage with sustained pressure on the globe for 5–10 s, followed by sudden release repeated for 10–15 min.

3   Refer the patient urgently to the ophthalmology team, as treatment within 1–2 h including anterior chamber paracentesis may restore the retinal circulation.

CENTRAL RETINAL VEIN OCCLUSION

DIAGNOSIS

1   This condition is most common in elderly patients with atherosclerosis, hypertension and simple glaucoma. Diabetes and hyperviscosity also predispose to this.

2   Visual loss is less abrupt but may be noticed suddenly. An RAPD (Marcus Gunn pupil) occurs in more extensive cases.

3   The fundus is dramatic and shows congested veins with scattered flame haemorrhages and optic disc swelling.

MANAGEMENT

1   There is no specific treatment, although predisposing conditions must be looked for particularly diabetes and hypertension.

2   Refer the patient to the ophthalmology clinic to monitor for the development of secondary acute glaucoma (some weeks later) from neovascularization.

VITREOUS HAEMORRHAGE

DIAGNOSIS

1   This may be traumatic; or spontaneous associated with proliferative diabetic retinopathy, posterior vitreous detachment ± a retinal tear particularly in high myopia (short-sighted person), various blood disorders, and branch or central retinal vein occlusion.

2   There is a reduced or absent red reflex and diminution in vision, preceded by a history of 'cobwebs' or 'floaters'.

MANAGEMENT

1 Refer the patient to the ophthalmology team to look for the predisposing conditions, and to exclude a retinal tear or detachment.

2 Vitrectomy may be necessary if the haemorrhage fails to clear.

RETINAL DETACHMENT

DIAGNOSIS

1 This may be traumatic; or spontaneous in myopes (short-sighted people), or may follow a vitreous haemorrhage such as associated with proliferative diabetic retinopathy.

2 There is peripheral visual loss, like a curtain, which may be profound if the macula is affected. A preceding history of sudden flashes of light or floaters is common.

3 The retina is dark, wrinkled and ballooned, and the choroid may appear as a red tear, although peripheral detachments may not be seen.
  - (i) An RAPD (Marcus Gunn pupil) occurs only if the detachment is large.

4 Request an ultrasound scan, but this must not delay ophthalmology referral.

MANAGEMENT

1 Refer the patient immediately to the ophthalmology team for a time-critical repair technique.

OPTIC NEURITIS

DIAGNOSIS

1 This may be autoimmune, post-viral or associated with demyelination from multiple sclerosis. It is more commonly unilateral but may occasionally be bilateral.

2 There is progressive loss of central, particularly colour vision over hours to days, with pain on moving the eye.

3 Visual acuity is reduced, and a RAPD (Marcus Gunn pupil) is seen.

4 Look at the fundus for papillitis if the optic disc is involved. This must be distinguished from papilloedema:
  - (i) Papilloedema tends to be bilateral and pain-free with normal pupil responses.
  - (ii) There is little or no visual loss, but an enlarged blind spot is found on field testing in papilloedema.

5 Examine the patient for other signs of demyelination.
  - (i) Never inform him or her of your suspicions at this early stage.
  - (ii) One in three will show clinically definite signs of MS within 5 yr of a first episode of idiopathic optic neuritis.

MANAGEMENT

1 Refer the patient to the ophthalmology clinic.

2 A lumbar puncture or MRI followed by parenteral steroid treatment such as methylprednisolone 250 mg i.v. q.d.s. for 3 days may be indicated for severe visual loss associated with demyelination.

FURTHER READING

Cochrane Collaboration. http://www.cochrane.org/search/site/Eyes%20and%20 vision/ (Cochrane review topics: Eyes and vision).

NSW Agency for Clinical Innovation (ACI). *Eye Emergency Manual. An Illustrated Guide*, 2nd edn 2009. http://www.aci.health.nsw.gov.au/resources/ ophthalmology/eye-emergency-manual/eem

Therapeutic Guidelines. eTG complete 2015. http://www.tg.org.au/

ENT EMERGENCIES

TRAUMATIC CONDITIONS OF THE EAR

SUBPERICHONDRIAL HAEMATOMA

DIAGNOSIS

1. Blunt trauma to the ear causes bleeding between the perichondrium and auricular cartilage, known as a subperichondrial haematoma.
2. This can lead to a 'cauliflower ear' deformity from proliferative fibrosis if left untreated.

MANAGEMENT

1. Refer the patient with a large and extensive bleed directly to the ENT team for immediate surgical drainage.
2. Otherwise, aspirate small clots under local anaesthesia, and apply firm pressure by packing around the interstices of the ear with cotton-wool under a turban dressing.
   (i) Refer the patient to the next ENT clinic, because the bleeding may recur.
3. Give the patient flucloxacillin 500 mg orally q.d.s. for 5 days to protect against perichondritis.

WOUNDS OF THE AURICLE

MANAGEMENT

1. Perform minimal debridement of devitalized tissue under local anaesthesia.
2. Refer the patient to the ENT team or plastic surgeons if there are extensive lacerations, skin loss or exposed cartilage.
3. Otherwise, suture the skin with 6/0 non-absorbable monofilament nylon or polypropylene and apply a firm dressing. Remove the sutures after 5 days.
4. Give the patient flucloxacillin 500 mg orally q.d.s. for 5 days to protect against perichondritis, and administer tetanus prophylaxis.

FOREIGN BODY IN THE EXTERNAL EAR

DIAGNOSIS AND MANAGEMENT

1. A foreign body in the external ear causes pain, deafness and discharge if left.
2. Attempt gentle removal if the foreign body is superficial, with a suction catheter, angled probe or alligator forceps.
3. Do not attempt any further manoeuvres if the object is not freed instantly, or if the patient is uncooperative, as the object may be pushed further in, and cause extreme pain and eardrum damage.
   (i) Refer the patient to the next ENT clinic.

PERFORATED EARDRUM

DIAGNOSIS

1 The eardrum may be perforated by direct injury from a sharp object, such as a hairpin, or indirectly by pressure from a slap, blast injury, scuba diving, or from a temporal bone fracture (see below).

2 There is pain, conductive deafness and sometimes bleeding.

3 Suspect inner ear involvement if there is tinnitus, vertigo or severe hearing loss.

MANAGEMENT

1 Refer the patient immediately to the ENT team if inner ear damage is suspected.

2 Otherwise, do not put anything into the ear or attempt to clean it out. Advise the patient to keep water out of the ear canal.

3 Give an antibiotic such as amoxycillin 500 mg orally t.d.s., and refer the patient to the next ENT clinic.

TEMPORAL BONE FRACTURE

Most basal skull fractures (see also p. 31) involve the temporal bone. Fractures may be divided into tympanic bone fractures, longitudinal fractures and transverse fractures.

DIAGNOSIS

1 The temporal bone forms the glenoid fossa of the temporomandibular joint, and is damaged if the mandibular condyle is driven upwards into the middle ear or external auditory canal, causing bleeding or laceration of the canal.

2 Alternatively, a longitudinal fracture of the temporal bone will tear the eardrum and cause dislocation of the ossicular chain, with conductive deafness, haemotympanum and cerebrospinal fluid (CSF) leakage.

    (i) Occasionally, delayed facial nerve damage is seen.

3 A transverse fracture of the temporal bone results in complete sensorineural deafness associated with tinnitus, vertigo and nystagmus.

    (i) Facial nerve palsy is more common than with longitudinal fractures.

4 Do not insert an auriscope to examine obvious bleeding from the external auditory meatus, as infection may then be introduced.

5 Remember that a temporal bone fracture may be a clinical diagnosis, if X-rays have to wait until the patient is stable and other injuries to the head, neck and chest have been assessed fully.

    (i) Request an immediate CT head scan once the patient has been stabilized.

MANAGEMENT

1   Admit the patient under the surgical team for head injury care and advice from the neurosurgical unit or ENT specialist.

NON-TRAUMATIC CONDITIONS OF THE EAR

All these conditions present with pain and/or hearing loss.

OTITIS EXTERNA

DIAGNOSIS

1   A bacterial or fungal infection is usually responsible, often following repeated use of cotton-wool buds, or exposure to water ('swimmer's ear').

2   There is extreme pain, desquamation of skin, and on otoscopy an oedematous, narrowed ear canal, often containing debris and discharge.

MANAGEMENT

1   Attempt aural toilet using a cotton wick or fine aspiration tube on suction to gently remove the debris, although pain may preclude this.

2   Insert a Merocel™ wick to maintain external ear canal patency.
    (i)   Add a proprietary anti-infective and steroid preparation such as Kenacomb Otic™, Sofradex™ or Locorten-Vioform™ three drops two to four times daily into the external auditory canal, and onto the wick.

3   Refer the patient to the ENT clinic for formal aural toilet.

4   Refer the patient directly to the ENT team if the otitis externa is severe with painful occlusion of the external ear canal.

FURUNCULOSIS OF THE EXTERNAL EAR

DIAGNOSIS

1   A furuncle may develop in the outer part of the external auditory canal causing extreme pain.

2   Movement of the pinna and introduction of a speculum exacerbate the pain. Deafness is minimal.

3   Remember to test the urine for sugar.

MANAGEMENT

1   Insert a wick soaked in 10% ichthammol in glycerin to encourage discharge of the pus, start flucloxacillin 500 mg orally q.d.s. and give an analgesic such as paracetamol 500 mg and codeine phosphate 8 mg two tablets orally q.d.s.

2   Refer the patient to the ENT clinic for follow-up.

ACUTE OTITIS MEDIA

DIAGNOSIS

1 This is common in children, due to viral or bacterial infection such as pneumococcus, *Moraxella catarrhalis* or *Haemophilus influenzae*, which is now rapidly decreasing in children under 6 years with HiB immunization.

2 There is acute onset of intense earache, variable fever, conductive deafness, and on examination of the eardrum in the early stages there is loss of the light reflex and injected vessels are seen around the malleus.

3 As the infection progresses, a bulging, immobile drum is seen, which may perforate, discharging pus.

MANAGEMENT

1 Most cases settle spontaneously with regular analgesia such as paracetamol 15 mg/kg orally q.d.s. or ibuprofen 10 mg/kg orally t.d.s.

2 The role of antibiotics is contentious. If systemically unwell with fever and vomiting, or no better by 48 h give amoxycillin 250–500 mg orally t.d.s. for 5 days with the analgesia.

    (i) Give cefuroxime 125–250 mg orally b.d. for 5 days if the patient is allergic to penicillin.

MASTOIDITIS

DIAGNOSIS AND MANAGEMENT

1 There is extension of infection from acute otitis media into the mastoid air-cell system.

2 The patient is ill and feverish, with local redness and tenderness over the mastoid, and the pinna is pushed down and forwards.

3 Complications include cranial nerve palsy, meningitis and subperiosteal abscess.

4 Refer the patient immediately to the ENT team for X-ray, CT scan and parenteral antibiotics.

VERTIGO

DIAGNOSIS

1 Two main groups occur:

    (i) *Peripheral vertigo* (85%)

       This is due to lesions in the vestibular nerve and inner ear, such as acute labyrinthitis, vestibular neuronitis, Ménière's disease with accompanying sensorineural deafness and tinnitus, benign paroxysmal positional vertigo (BPPV), otosclerosis, cholesteatoma, ototoxic drugs such as gentamicin and rapid, high-dose frusemide (furosemide), or trauma.

(ii) *Central vertigo* (15%)
This is due to lesions in the CNS, such as a vertebrobasilar transient ischaemic attack (TIA), a cerebellar or brainstem stroke, cerebello-pontine angle tumour, demyelination, vertebrobasilar migraine, or alcohol and drug toxicity.

2 *Peripheral vertigo* is usually acute, intermittent, positional and associated with nystagmus, deafness, tinnitus, nausea, vomiting and sweating.

3 *Central vertigo* is more gradual in onset, constant and dominated by the associated neurological signs such as headache, weakness, ataxia and/or dysarthria.

MANAGEMENT

1 Give patients with incapacitating vertigo midazolam 0.05–0.1 mg/kg i.v. or diazepam 0.1 mg/kg i.v. as symptomatic treatment, with bed rest until the vertigo has gone.

(i) Alternatively, give prochlorperazine 12.5 mg i.m. or i.v., but beware that it may cause extrapyramidal side effects including akathisia – an unpleasant 'intolerable sense of restlessness' in up to one-third of patients.

2 Refer patients with peripheral causes of vertigo that do not settle to the ENT team, and with central causes of vertigo to the medical team.

(i) A computed tomography (CT) scan or magnetic resonance imaging (MRI) is indicated for focal neurological signs.

FACIAL NERVE PALSY

DIAGNOSIS

1 *Lower motor neurone paralysis*

(i) There is weakness of the whole side of the face, including the forehead muscles.

(ii) Causes include:

(a) Bell's palsy with an abrupt onset sometimes associated with postauricular pain, hyperacusis and abnormal taste in the anterior two-thirds of the tongue

(b) trauma to the temporal bone or a facial laceration in the parotid area

(c) tumours, such as an acoustic neuroma or parotid malignancy

(d) infection, such as acute otitis media, chronic otitis media with cholesteatoma or geniculate herpes zoster, the Ramsay–Hunt syndrome

(e) miscellaneous, including Guillain–Barré syndrome, sarcoidosis, diabetes and hypertension.

2 Upper motor neurone paralysis

    (i)   There is weakness of the lower facial muscles sparing the forehead, often associated with other neurological signs such as hemiplegia.

    (ii) The cause is usually a stroke.

3 Examine the external auditory canal, eardrum, parotid region and make a full neurological assessment.

MANAGEMENT

1 Refer all acute cases with associated signs immediately to the medical, surgical or ENT team according to the likely aetiology.

2 Give prednisolone 50 mg orally once daily for 5 days, in a patient with Bell's palsy if seen within 3 days of onset.

    (i)   Add hypromellose artificial tears, tape or pad the eye closed at night, and refer to the next ENT clinic.

    (ii) The role of additional antiviral therapy is inconclusive.

TRAUMATIC CONDITIONS OF THE NOSE

FRACTURED NOSE

DIAGNOSIS

1 This injury is usually obvious following a direct blow, causing swelling, deformity and epistaxis.

2 Exclude a more serious facial bone fracture, e.g. with cerebrospinal fluid rhinorrhoea from cribriform plate damage (see p. 31).

3 Look carefully for a septal haematoma which, if left, leads to necrosis of the nasal cartilage and septal collapse.

    (i)   The nasal passage is blocked by a dull-red swelling replacing the septum, associated with marked nasal obstruction.

4 Do **not** take a nasal X-ray as this does not alter the clinical management.

MANAGEMENT

1 Refer any patient with a grossly deformed or compound fracture, or a septal haematoma to the ENT team.

    (i)   Refer more serious facial bone fractures to the maxillofacial surgery team.

2 Otherwise, refer the patient to the ENT clinic within the next 5–10 days, if the patient requests operative treatment to straighten the nose for cosmetic reasons.

FOREIGN BODY IN THE NOSE

DIAGNOSIS AND MANAGEMENT

1   This may be quite asymptomatic, or it may lead to a serosanguineous, offensive, unilateral nasal discharge.

2   Attempt removal with a bent probe or pair of forceps if the object is easily accessible in the anterior part of the nose, after the patient has vigorously blown the nose (which may dislodge the object anyway).

3   However, refer immediately to the ENT team if removal is difficult, or a child is uncooperative.

   (i)   Sudden posterior dislodgement with inhalation of the foreign body into the airway is a real danger.

NON-TRAUMATIC CONDITIONS OF THE NOSE

EPISTAXIS

DIAGNOSIS

1   This is usually spontaneous in children, occurring from vessels in Little's area on the anterior part of the septum, possibly precipitated by rhinitis or minor trauma such as picking.

2   The bleeding occurs posterior to Little's area in adults and may be associated with a bleeding diathesis, including anticoagulant or antiplatelet drugs.

3   Bleeding originates higher in the posterior part of the nose in the elderly from arteriosclerotic vessels, and rapidly leads to haemorrhagic shock if profuse.

4   Send blood for full blood count (FBC), clotting study and group and save (G&S) in any patient with profuse bleeding. Establish an i.v. infusion with normal saline 10 mL/kg, before the patient becomes hypotensive, and restore the circulation.

   (i)   Call the senior ED doctor immediately in these cases.

MANAGEMENT

1   *Bleeding from Little's area*

   (i)   Pinch the anterior part of the nose for 10 min with the patient sitting forward until the bleeding stops. Forbid the patient to pick, blow or sniff through the nose to prevent recurrence of the epistaxis.

   (ii)   Identify with suction or by swabbing if a bleeding point persists, and anaesthetize the area with a cotton-wool pledget soaked in 4% lignocaine (lidocaine) with adrenaline (epinephrine).

(iii) Cauterize the bleeding point with a silver nitrate stick touched onto the area for <10 s. Avoid overzealous application or cauterization to both sides of the septum, as these will lead to septal necrosis.

2   Persistent anterior bleeding and failed cautery

(i) *Anterior nasal tamponade*
Insert an epistaxis balloon catheter or Merocel™ nasal tampon, both of which are far easier and less distressing to insert than formal packing.

(ii) *Anterior nasal pack*
   (a) cover the patient and yourself with protective drapes when no nasal tamponade device is available, and wear a face mask and goggles
   (b) apply further local anaesthetic with cotton-wool pledgets soaked in 4% lignocaine (lidocaine) with adrenaline (epinephrine). The maximum dose is 7 mg/kg or 12 mL, i.e. approximately 500 mg lignocaine (lidocaine) with adrenaline (epinephrine) in a 65 kg patient
   (c) use 2 cm petroleum-jelly gauze or a calcium alginate (Kaltostat™) 2 g pack
   (d) insert successive layers horizontally along the floor of the nose using Tilley's nasal dressing forceps (see Fig. 11.1)
   (e) remember in adults the nose extends 6.5–7.5 cm backwards to the posterior choanae.

(iii) Give the patient amoxycillin 500 mg orally t.d.s. and refer to the ENT team for admission with removal of the pack within 48 h.

3   Severe posterior bleeding

(i) *Anterior and posterior nasal tamponade*
Stem posterior nasal bleeding by inserting a double epistaxis-balloon device, with separate balloons for anterior plus posterior tamponade. Tape securely to the cheek.

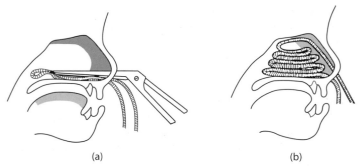

(a)   (b)

Figure 11.1 Anterior nasal packing.
(**a**) Introducing the first loop horizontally along the floor of the nose, and (**b**) building the layers horizontally upwards until pack is in place.

(ii) Use a Foley urethral catheter if tamponade is unavailable, and insert far back along the floor of the nose, inflate the retaining balloon with air, and pull the catheter forwards to occlude the back of the nose. Tape the catheter securely to the cheek to prevent it slipping backwards
   (a) then insert an anterior nasal pack as described previously
   (b) occasionally both sides of the nose require packing to stop the bleeding.
(iii) Refer the patient immediately to the ENT team for admission.

TRAUMATIC CONDITIONS OF THE THROAT

See Section V, Surgical Emergencies: Neck Injuries, p. 174.

NON-TRAUMATIC CONDITIONS OF THE THROAT

TONSILLITIS

DIAGNOSIS AND MANAGEMENT

1   This is more frequently viral than bacterial, but differentiating the two clinically is difficult.
   (i) Fever above 38°C (100°F), tender cervical adenopathy, tonsillar exudate and absence of cough favour β-haemolytic *Streptococcus*, particularly in children aged 3–14 years.
   (ii) Glandular fever (EBV) presents with a grey, exudative tonsillitis typically in late adolescence.
   (iii) Other less common causes include CMV, herpes simplex, *Mycoplasma pneumoniae,* gonococcus and *Chlamydia*.

2   There is fever, fetor, sore throat and dysphagia.
   (i) A febrile convulsion may be precipitated in a child <5 years old.

3   Send blood for FBC, electrolyte and liver function tests (ELFTs) and Epstein–Barr virus (EBV) serology including IgM and IgG.
   (i) IgM positive result indicates acute infection; IgG only positive indicates past infection.
   (ii) LFTs may be mildly deranged in EBV infection.

4   Give an antipyretic analgesic, and consider penicillin V 500 mg orally b.d. for 10 days, particularly when the patient is systemically unwell or has peritonsillar cellulitis, or is immunosuppressed or underprivileged.

      (i)   Add prednisone 50 mg orally daily for 2–3 days if pain or swelling are marked.

5   Return the patient to the care of his or her GP.

QUINSY (PERITONSILLAR ABSCESS)

DIAGNOSIS AND MANAGEMENT

1   This may follow tonsillitis and is more common in adults.

2   There is a worsening of the illness, with high temperature, muffled voice, dysphagia, referred earache and trismus.

3   Examination shows unilateral swelling of the soft palate, with displacement of the tonsil downwards and medially, and deviation of the uvula to the unaffected side.

4   Give benzylpenicillin 1.2 g i.v. q.d.s. and metronidazole 500 mg i.v. t.d.s.
      (i)   Add prednisone 50 mg orally daily for 2–3 days particularly for any peritonsillar cellulitis.

5   Refer the patient immediately to the ENT team for operative drainage.

FOREIGN BODY IN THE PHARYNX

DIAGNOSIS

1   Fish or meat bones are the most common objects to cause symptoms.

2   Usually, a fish bone will impact in the tonsil, base of the tongue or posterior pharyngeal wall.
      (i)   Depress the tongue to look at the tonsil, or use a laryngeal mirror to visualize the back of the tongue and posterior pharynx.

3   Request a lateral soft-tissue X-ray of the neck if no bone is seen despite symptoms.
      (i)   Calcification of superimposed hyoid, thyroid, cricoid and laryngeal cartilages often cause confusion in the diagnosis.

MANAGEMENT

1   Refer the patient immediately to the ENT team for oesophagoscopy if oesophageal impaction is suspected with dysphagia, excessive salivation, local tenderness or pain.

2   Otherwise, attempt to remove a fish bone from the tonsil or the back of the tongue using Tilley's curved forceps.
      (i)   Refer the patient immediately to the ENT team if this fails in a patient with pain or who is salivating excessively.

3   Alternatively, the pharyngeal mucosa may only have been scratched. If symptoms are minimal, prescribe an antibiotic such as amoxycillin 500 mg orally t.d.s. and ask the patient to return in 24 h for review.

SWALLOWED FOREIGN BODY

DIAGNOSIS

1 Coins are the most common objects swallowed by pre-school children, although small children swallow almost anything, and the elderly may swallow their dentures.

2 Oesophageal impaction, usually around the cricopharyngeus at the level of C6, causes dysphagia, excessive salivation, local tenderness or retrosternal pain, but may be asymptomatic.

3 Occasionally, airway obstruction occurs from upper oesophageal impaction, or the object may in fact have been inhaled, not swallowed (see p. 300).

4 ***Button batteries***

These pose a particular risk, as they cause local corrosive effects or mucosal perforation with later stenosis, particularly in the oesophagus, and sometimes in the stomach if they disintegrate.

5 Request X-rays of the neck and chest to look for oesophageal impaction.
   (i) Include anteroposterior (AP) and lateral views to avoid missing a radio-opaque object superimposed over the skeletal or cardiac shadows on the AP view, and to differentiate tracheal lodgement.
   (ii) Also request an abdominal X-ray in button-battery ingestion and/or for symptoms such as abdominal pain, distension, diarrhoea or gastrointestinal bleeding.

MANAGEMENT

1 Refer the following patients *immediately* to the ENT team:
   (i) Airway obstruction or foreign body inhalation (rather than ingestion).
   (ii) Oesophageal impaction suspected clinically.
   (iii) Oesophageal lodgement seen on X-ray or inferred from pre-vertebral soft-tissue swelling, soft-tissue gas, or air in the upper oesophagus.
   (iv) Button battery lodged in the oesophagus, or stomach
      (a) all oesophageal batteries need immediate removal, while those in the stomach may be managed expectantly if asymptomatic.

2 Allow the patient home, if the patient is asymptomatic, and neck and chest X-rays are normal.
   (i) Reassure the parents that most objects will pass spontaneously.
   (ii) Request immediate review if symptoms develop.
   (iii) Otherwise, repeat X-rays are only required if the patient develops symptoms.

STRIDOR

See Section VIII, Paediatric Emergencies, p. 299.

FURTHER READING

Cochrane Collaboration. http://www.cochrane.org/search/site/ear%20nose%20 throat (Cochrane review topics: Ear, nose and throat disorders).

Drotts D, Vinson D (1999) Prochlorperazine induces akathisia in emergency patients. *Annals of Emergency Medicine* **34**: 469–75.

Therapeutic Guidelines. eTG complete 2015. http://www.tg.org.au/

MAXILLOFACIAL AND DENTAL EMERGENCIES

LACERATIONS

MANAGEMENT

1 Face

    (i)   Meticulously debride facial cuts under local anaesthesia, and suture using fine 5/0 non-absorbable monofilament nylon or polypropylene sutures, removed by 4 days.

2 Lips

    (i)   Use 3/0 or 4/0 absorbable sutures such as polydioxanone or polyglactin for intraoral lesions, and 5/0 non-absorbable monofilament nylon or polypropylene sutures for external lacerations.

    (ii) Refer the patient to the oral surgery team if the full thickness of the lip is lacerated vertically, breaching the vermilion border, to avoid cosmetic deformity from inexperienced repair.

3 Tongue

    (i)   Leave most lacerations unless they are >1 cm or through the edge, or bleeding profusely. In those cases repair with an absorbable suture such as 3/0 polydioxanone or polyglactin.

    (ii) Advise regular mouthwash of warm saline.

TOOTH INJURIES

MANAGEMENT

1 Chipped tooth

    (i)   *Enamel or dentine damage:* the tooth will be sensitive but viable. Advise the patient to avoid hot and cold drinks and refer to the patient's own dentist within 24 hours.

    (ii) *Pulp space exposed:* the tooth may be bleeding from the pulp, and sensitive to temperature and/or touch. Refer the patient immediately to the oral surgery team, as there is a risk of pulp infection or necrosis.

2 Displaced tooth

    (i)   Do not manipulate unless the tooth is about to fall out, in which case it should be firmly replaced in its socket.

    (ii) Refer the patient to a dental surgeon as soon as possible for immobilization of the tooth.

3 Avulsed permanent incisor tooth

The best chance of successful re-implantation is by reposition of an avulsed tooth within 30 min outside its socket, or up to 2 h if stored in milk or saline, which help preserve the delicate periodontal ligament cells.

(i) Transport the tooth in milk or saline if immediate re-implantation is not possible
  (a) the patient's own buccal sulcus is not ideal due to the presence of bacteria and incompatible osmolarity and pH.

(ii) Handle the tooth only by the crown on arrival in the emergency department (ED), rinse it in saline, and replace back into the socket with firm pressure. No analgesia is necessary.

(iii) Splint the tooth with aluminium foil, give the patient an antibiotic such as amoxycillin 500 mg orally t.d.s., and tetanus prophylaxis
  (a) an avulsed tooth is considered a 'tetanus-prone' wound (see p. 269).

(iv) Refer the patient to a dental surgeon as soon as possible.

4   Avulsed primary (deciduous) incisor tooth
Do **not** replace these, but refer the patient to a dental surgeon for follow-up.

> **Warning:** when a tooth or denture is found to be missing following trauma, perform an anteroposterior (AP) and lateral chest radiograph (CXR) to exclude inhalation into the lung, or AP and lateral neck X-rays to exclude lodgement in the upper oesophagus.

5   Bleeding tooth socket
(i) This can be post-traumatic or post-extraction.

(ii) Clear out clots and arrest haemorrhage using a calcium alginate (Kaltostat^{TM}) dressing or gauze roll. Ask the patient to bite on it for 15–30 min.

(iii) Infiltrate with 1% lignocaine (lidocaine) with 1 in 200 000 adrenaline (epinephrine) if the bleeding persists, and close the mucosa over the socket using 3/0 absorbable polydioxanone or polyglactin sutures.

(iv) Refer the patient to the oral surgery team if this fails.

6   Broken denture
(i) Always save a broken denture as it will be invaluable to the maxillofacial surgeon to aid in the fixation of any jaw fracture, or if a splint is needed.

FRACTURED MANDIBLE

DIAGNOSIS

1   This is due to a blow on the jaw causing a unilateral or frequently bilateral fracture. Occasionally, the temporomandibular joint may be dislocated or the condylar process driven up into the temporal bone, causing bleeding and deformity of the external auditory canal.

2   Look for localized pain, particularly on attempted jaw movement, and malocclusion.

3   Examine inside the mouth for bruising or bleeding of the gum and discontinuity of the teeth, if there is a displaced fracture.

   (i)   Assess for numbness of the lower lip if the inferior dental nerve has been damaged in its course through the mandible.

4   Request X-rays including an anteroposterior view, with a panoramic orthopantomogram (OPG) or lateral views of the mandible.

MANAGEMENT

1   Clear the airway of any clots or debris, and ensure that the tongue or a portion of the mandible does not slip back and occlude the pharynx.

2   Refer any unstable or grossly displaced injuries immediately to the maxillofacial surgery team.

3   Otherwise, give the patient tetanus prophylaxis and antibiotics for an un-displaced fracture, as many fractures are compound into the mouth.

   (i)   Give amoxycillin 875 mg and clavulanic acid 125 mg one tablet orally b.d. for 5 days.

4   Refer the patient to the next maxillofacial surgery clinic.

DISLOCATED MANDIBLE

DIAGNOSIS

1   Dislocation may occur spontaneously after yawning or it may follow a blow to the jaw. It may be unilateral or more commonly bilateral and may become recurrent.

2   The mouth is stuck open and is painful.

3   Exclude drug-induced dystonia to metoclopramide or phenothiazines on direct questioning, as this may mimic or even predispose to dislocation.

   (i)   Give benztropine (benzatropine) 1–2 mg i.v. followed by 2 mg orally once daily for up to 3 days if this is a dystonic reaction (see p. 276).

4   Request an AP and lateral X-ray of the temporomandibular joints to exclude an associated fracture, unless the dislocation was spontaneous or recurrent.

MANAGEMENT

1   Try to gently reduce without sedation if recurrent in the absence of a fracture.

   (i)   Give midazolam 0.05–0.1 mg/kg i.v. or diazepam 0.1–0.2 mg/kg i.v. with a second doctor and full resuscitation facilities available if unsuccessful.

2   Reduction of the dislocation:

   (i)   Stand in front of the patient and place your gauze-wrapped thumbs inside the mouth over the posterior molar area, with your fingers under the chin.

(ii) Press firmly downwards to distract the condyle applying pressure to the angle of the jaw, then push backwards and up to relocate the condyle in the fossa.

(iii) Reduce one side at a time in bilateral dislocations.

(iv) Repeat the X-ray to confirm reduction, and refer to the next maxillofacial surgery clinic. Advise the patient to avoid excessive mouth opening.

(v) Apply a barrel bandage to discourage wide opening if the dislocation is recurrent or required midazolam or diazepam i.v.

FRACTURE OF THE ZYGOMA OR ZYGOMATICOMAXILLARY (MALAR) COMPLEX

DIAGNOSIS

1 This injury is due to a direct blow to the cheek, which may fracture the zygomatic arch in isolation, or cause a 'tripod' fracture to the zygomaticomaxillary (malar) complex that extends through three structures:

(i) Superiorly through the zygomaticofrontal suture.

(ii) Laterally through the zygomatic arch or zygomaticotemporal suture.

(iii) Medially through the zygomaticomaxillary suture or the infraorbital foramen region.

2 There is flattening of the cheekbone (malar process) best seen from above which may become masked by oedema, epistaxis, subconjunctival haemorrhage extending posteriorly, and infraorbital nerve paraesthesia.

(i) Jaw movement may be limited if the coronoid process is obstructed under the zygomatic arch.

3 Although these fractures are best diagnosed clinically by finding focal bony tenderness, request facial X-rays including occipitomental views (OM 10° and OM 30°).

(i) Look carefully for the fractures, comparing with the normal side, or

(ii) Look for secondary evidence of injury, e.g. opacity of the maxillary antrum from bleeding into the maxillary sinus or overlying soft-tissue swelling.

(iii) Request a computed tomography (CT) scan for more complex injuries to the zygomaticomaxillary (malar) complex, or for an associated 'blow-out' fracture of the orbital floor.

MANAGEMENT

1 Advise the patient **not** to blow his or her nose, as subcutaneous emphysema may develop if the paranasal sinuses are involved.

2 Commence amoxycillin 500 mg orally t.d.s. (or cefuroxime 500 mg orally b.d. if the patient is allergic to penicillin) for 5 days, as most fractures are compound into the maxillary sinus, with an analgesic such as paracetamol 500 mg and codeine phosphate 8 mg two tablets orally q.d.s.

3 Refer the patient to the maxillofacial surgery team within 24 hours for elevation of the depressed cheekbone within 7 days.

ORBITAL FLOOR 'BLOW-OUT' FRACTURE

DIAGNOSIS

1 This uncommon fracture is due to blunt trauma to the eye from a small object about the size of a squash ball, that drives the eyeball backwards and ruptures the weak bony floor of the orbit.

    (i) Orbital fat and occasionally the inferior rectus muscle herniate through the defect into the maxillary sinus.

2 Exclude blunt trauma to the eye initially (see p. 349). The fracture itself causes enophthalmos, which may be masked by periorbital oedema, infra-orbital nerve loss to the side of the nostril and upper lip, and diplopia from restricted upwards gaze due to trapping of the inferior rectus muscle or orbital fat.

3 Request facial X-rays, although these may not show the fracture itself.

    (i) This can be inferred from an opaque maxillary sinus or a fluid level from bleeding, and a 'tear drop' soft-tissue opacity hanging from the roof of the sinus.

4 Request a CT scan if there is doubt, as this demonstrates the fractures clearly.

MANAGEMENT

1 Refer a patient with blunt eye damage immediately to the ophthalmology team.

2 Commence amoxycillin 500 mg orally t.d.s. and 1% chloramphenicol eye ointment 4-hourly.

3 Refer the patient to the maxillofacial surgery team within 24 h.

LE FORT MIDDLE-THIRD OF FACE FRACTURES

DIAGNOSIS

These complicated fractures are usually bilateral and are divided into three broad groups:

1 *Le Fort I*

    (i) This is due to a blow to the maxilla causing a horizontal fracture separating the alveolar bone and teeth from the maxilla.

    (ii) There is epistaxis and malocclusion, and crepitus may be elicited.

2 *Le Fort II*

    (i) This is a pyramidal fracture extending up from a Le Fort I fracture to involve the nasal skeleton and the middle of the face. The middle of the face is thus 'stove in', elongating the face and causing malocclusion.

    (ii) The airway may be compromised and cerebrospinal fluid (CSF) may leak from the nose.

3 *Le Fort III*

    (i)   This fracture displaces the entire mid-facial skeleton from the base of the skull (craniofacial dysjunction).

    (ii)   There is massive facial swelling and bruising, and often brisk pharyngeal bleeding that may cause haemorrhagic shock. The airway is again in danger.

4 Remember that the blow to the face may have caused an additional head, base of skull or cervical spine injury.

    (i)   Stabilize the airway and treat shock as a priority.

    (ii)   Request a head, cervical spine and facial bones CT scan as indicated, once the patient has been stabilized.

MANAGEMENT

1 Attend urgently to the airway and bleeding.

    (i)   Sometimes, if the face is stove in, manually lifting the whole segment forwards relieves the airway.

    (ii)   Call immediately for senior ED doctor help if there is difficulty maintaining an adequate airway, and prepare for orotracheal intubation or even a cricothyrotomy.

    (iii)   Pack inside the oral and/or nasal cavity if bleeding is torrential.

2 Refer all mid-face fractures immediately to the maxillofacial surgery or ENT team.

NON-TRAUMATIC CONDITIONS OF THE MOUTH

TOOTHACHE

DIAGNOSIS AND MANAGEMENT

1 Toothache is usually due to inflammation of the pulp space in a carious tooth.

2 Exclude a dental abscess (see below) and give the patient an analgesic such as paracetamol 500 mg and codeine phosphate 8 mg two tablets orally q.d.s.

3 Return the patient to his or her own dentist.

DENTAL ABSCESS

DIAGNOSIS AND MANAGEMENT

1 An apical or periapical abscess is an extension of a pulp space infection.

    (i)   The tooth is tender on tapping, with associated soft-tissue swelling and continuous pain.

2 A periodontal abscess follows periodontitis from poor dental hygiene particularly in smokers and diabetics. Halitosis, increasing pain and swelling occur.

  (i) There may be systemic malaise and fever, with a risk of spread to deeper fascial spaces.

3 Refer the patient to the oral surgery team if the abscess is pointing extraorally.

4 Otherwise, commence an antibiotic such as amoxicillin 875 mg and clavulanic acid 125 mg one tablet orally b.d. for 5 days with an analgesic (e.g. codeine phosphate 30–60 mg orally q.d.s.), and return the patient to his or her own dentist.

LUDWIG'S ANGINA

DIAGNOSIS AND MANAGEMENT

1 This condition is a bilateral, fulminant, brawny cellulitis of the sublingual and submandibular areas, associated with poor dental hygiene or dental instrumentation. It is uncommon, and may spread into the retropharyngeal and superior mediastinal spaces.

2 There is trismus with reduced mouth opening, dysphagia, with elevation and firmness of the tongue associated with submandibular pain and swelling.

  (i) The risk is sudden respiratory obstruction from displacement of the tongue and submandibular tissues.

  (ii) Do **not** send for an x-ray without expert airway supervision.

3 Call immediately for senior ED doctor help, and prepare for orotracheal intubation or even a cricothyrotomy.

4 Give benzylpenicillin 1.8 g i.v. and metronidazole 500 mg i.v. and admit the patient immediately under the ENT team for careful observation of the airway.

5 Request a CT scan **only** if the airway is protected, or not considered at risk.

SUBMANDIBULAR SWELLINGS

DIAGNOSIS AND MANAGEMENT

Look for the following possible causes:

1 *Submandibular stone*

  This intermittently blocks the submandibular duct, causing pain and swelling aggravated by food. The stone is palpable on bimanual examination in the floor of the mouth and is seen on X-ray. Refer the patient to the oral surgery team.

2 *Submandibular abscess*

  The pain is constant with associated malaise, swelling in the angle of the jaw, and trismus. Refer the patient to the oral surgery team.

3   *Dental abscess*

This may point downwards from a molar tooth to the submandibular area. Treat with antibiotics and analgesia and refer to the oral surgery team.

4   *Lymph node enlargement*

The most common causes of cervical adenopathy in this area are tonsillitis and pharyngitis.

5   *Mumps*

This affects the parotids and is usually bilateral, but can affect the submandibular glands. Remember the association with orchitis. Give the patient paracetamol elixir, and reassure them.

6   *Rare*

These include carcinoma, lymphoma, sarcoid, tuberculosis, osteomyelitis, and a bony cyst or fibrous dysplasia. Refer to the appropriate specialty team.

FURTHER READING

Cochrane Collaboration. http://www.cochrane.org/search/site/Oral%20health (Cochrane review topics: Oral Health).

Therapeutic Guidelines. eTG complete 2015. http://www.tg.org.au/

PSYCHIATRIC EMERGENCIES

DIAGNOSIS

1 The most common method of deliberate self-harm is by acute poisoning.
- (i) This may be admitted freely, or may be evident from finding an empty bottle beside the patient or a suicide note.
- (ii) The possibility should also be remembered in any unconscious or confused patient, or in patients with unexplained metabolic, respiratory or cardiac problems (see p. 24).

2 More violent methods of self-harm include cutting the wrists or throat, shooting, hanging, suffocation, gassing, jumping from a height or in front of a vehicle, and drowning.
- (i) These are more common in completed suicide.

3 Perform a formal psychiatric assessment when the patient has made a full recovery, is alert and orientated, and all necessary medical therapy is completed. This will help plan the further management of the patient with the psychiatric team.
- (i) Assessment of current suicidal intent. Enquire specifically about:
  - (a) present suicidal thoughts
  - (b) previous deliberate self-harm
  - (c) evidence of a pre-meditated act without the intention of being found
  - (d) feeling of hopelessness.
- (ii) Determine other high-risk factors for completed suicide:
  - (a) mental illness including depression and schizophrenia; severe anxiety
  - (b) violent self-harm attempt, such as jumping, hanging or shooting
  - (c) previous self-harm attempt
  - (d) chronic alcohol abuse, drug dependence, unemployment, homelessness
  - (e) older, single, urban, lonely male
  - (f) chronic, painful or terminal physical illness
  - (g) puerperium.
- (iii) Record a general mental state examination:
  - (a) general appearance, behaviour, attitudes
  - (b) speech including pressure of speech, neologisms
  - (c) mood and affect, appropriateness
  - (d) thought processes for content and form

    (e) perception including delusions and hallucinations (especially auditory)

    (f) cognition with a Mini-Mental State Examination (see Table 2.10 on p. 84)

    (g) insight and judgement

    (h) impulsivity.

MANAGEMENT

1 Perform the necessary investigations and resuscitative procedures to save life, and refer the patient directly to the medical, surgical or orthopaedic team if there is serious illness or injury, with a clear alert as to the underlying intention.

2 A medically unimportant acute poisoning, including a patient also intoxicated with alcohol, may still have been a serious self-harm attempt.

    (i) Admit the patient for 24 h, possibly to the emergency department's own observation ward.

3 Then refer any patient considered to have a continuing suicide risk or mental illness behaviour immediately to the psychiatric team.

4 Alternatively, make a psychiatric outpatient appointment for the patient if there is no current suicidal intent, no high-risk factor for completed suicide and a normal mental state examination.

5 Refer problems with a domestic or social basis to the social work team.

6 Inform the general practitioner (GP) by fax and letter in every case, if the patient is allowed home. The patient should ideally be accompanied by a relative or friend when they go.

VIOLENT PATIENT

DIAGNOSIS

1 Much violence encountered by staff in the emergency department will be the result of alcohol intoxication, either by the patient or sometimes by relatives or friends, who may be irritated and angry at having to wait when the department is busy.

2 Other causes for violent behaviour include:

    (i) Drugs, such as cocaine and freebase 'crack' cocaine, amphetamines including methylamphetamine 'Ice' and 'Ecstasy', or phencyclidine 'PCP'.

    (ii) Mental illness flares up particularly mania and paranoid schizophrenia, personality disorder.

(iii) Withdrawal syndromes from alcohol or barbiturates.
(iv) Hypoglycaemia, including as the patient recovers from a hypoglycaemic episode after i.v. dextrose administration.
(v) Post-ictal state.
(vi) Hypoxia.
(vii) Other organic confusional state (see p. 82).

MANAGEMENT

1 Explain what is happening at all times, keep reassuring the patient, and avoid confrontation.
   (i) Never turn your back on a patient or allow them between you and the cubicle door.
   (ii) Call the police immediately if a weapon is involved. Await their arrival before proceeding.

2 Attempt verbal de-escalation by defining acceptable and unacceptable behaviour and their likely consequences. Speak firmly with courtesy and respect.
   (i) Offer oral medication such as diazepam 5–10 mg and/or olanzapine 5–10 mg.

3 Move on to show of force then physical restraint if verbal de-escalation fails:
   (i) Call the hospital security guards, and await adequate numbers, ideally five or six people, as a 'show of force'.
   (ii) Never try to restrain a patient single-handedly.
   (iii) Conversely, never remove physical restraints until a full evaluation has been made and help is at hand.

4 Move on to rapid tranquilisation if physical restraint fails.
   (i) Give diazepam 5–10 mg i.v. or midazolam 5–10 mg i.v., supplemented with haloperidol or droperidol 5–10 mg i.m. or slowly i.v.
   (ii) Such treatment may be given without consent under common law in an emergency if the patient is a danger to others or themselves.

5 Monitor every patient once sedated in a resuscitation area until the risks of respiratory depression and hypotension have passed.
   (i) Complete a full physical examination, looking for evidence of organic disease including abnormal vital signs.
   (ii) Observe the patient until fully awake and alert.

6 Record exact details of events and the necessary action taken in the notes.

7 Admit the patient under the medical or psychiatric team if further treatment is indicated.

8 Debrief staff in the emergency department, and consider immediate support for staff injury or intimidation.
   (i) Plan future team strategies for violence prevention and management.

ALCOHOL AND DRUG WITHDRAWAL

DIAGNOSIS AND MANAGEMENT

1 Patients may be seen who are dependent on or abuse the following classes of drugs:

   (i) Alcohol.

   (ii) Opiates.

   (iii) Stimulants including amphetamines and cocaine.

   (iv) Sedatives including benzodiazepines and barbiturates.

   (v) Miscellaneous substances including cannabis, solvents and petrol.

2 Abrupt withdrawal of many of these drugs causes acute symptoms.

   (i) Alcohol withdrawal causes agitation, irritability, tremor and seizures, then delirium tremens (see p. 88)

      (a) give a benzodiazepine i.v. or orally if symptoms are distressing

      (b) seek help for the patient from an expert drug and alcohol dependency unit.

   (ii) Opiate withdrawal causes restlessness, excitability, muscle cramps, diarrhoea, tachycardia and sweating – known as 'cold turkey'

      (a) give a benzodiazepine i.v. or orally if symptoms are distressing

      (b) seek help for the patient from an expert drug and alcohol dependency unit.

   (iii) Benzodiazepine withdrawal causes a rebound increase in tension, anxiety and apprehension, with anorexia, insomnia, irritability, myoclonic jerks and seizures

      (a) seek help for the patient from an expert drug and alcohol dependency unit.

PROBLEM DRINKING

DIAGNOSIS

1 Alcohol misuse is related to many emergency department presentations, from falls, collapse, head injury and assault to non-specific gastrointestinal problems, psychiatric problems and the 'frequent attender'.

2 Ask the patient directly if they drink alcohol, how much on a regular daily basis and whether their attendance is related to alcohol.

3 Use a validated screening questionnaire such as the CAGE (see Table 13.1).

4 Sometimes, alcohol-dependent patients themselves request help or may be brought in by concerned others to stop drinking.

Table 13.1 CAGE screening questionnaire for alcohol abuse

C	Have you ever felt you should **C**ut down on your drinking?
A	Have people **A**nnoyed you by criticizing your drinking?
G	Have you ever felt bad or **G**uilty about your drinking?
E	Have you ever had a drink as an **E**ye-opener first thing in the morning to steady your nerves or help get rid of a hangover?

"Yes" to two or more indicates probable chronic alcohol abuse or dependence.

MANAGEMENT

1   Refer the patient immediately to the psychiatric team if there is suicidal ideation or overt depression.

2   Otherwise, refer the patient to the appropriate hospital or community clinic for outpatient assessment, or
    (i)   Refer to the social work department or a special alcohol health worker for a brief intervention programme, including advice and management on alcohol-related harm to health.

3   Meanwhile, give the patient the telephone number of local support organizations to contact, such as Alcoholics Anonymous and Al-Anon. These provide help and advice to both the problem drinker and their family and friends.

4   Always write to or fax the general practitioner (GP) to enlist their help and support.

OPIATE AND INTRAVENOUS DRUG ADDICTION

MANAGEMENT

1   Admit opiate and intravenous drug-use patients under the medical team, if they present with any of the following addiction-associated emergency medical complications, apart from simple acute intoxication (usually managed in the emergency department alone):
    (i)   Cellulitis or abscess.
    (ii)   Pulmonary or cerebral infection.
    (iii) Septicaemia.
    (iv)   Bacterial endocarditis.
    (v)   Hepatitis B, C or D, and, increasingly, human immunodeficiency virus (HIV) infection.

2   Otherwise, if a regular opiate user requires admission to the emergency department observation ward, perhaps following an orthopaedic or minor operative procedure:
    (i)   Give salicylate or paracetamol for mild to moderate pain, and methadone orally or i.m. for severe pain.
    (ii)   Give the patient diazepam 5–10 mg orally if signs of opiate withdrawal occur, repeated as required.

3 Refer patients wishing to stop their habit and seeking help to:
  (i)   Drug and Alcohol Dependency Unit.
  (ii) Social work department.
  (iii) Drug dependency 24-h emergency organization such as Narcotics Anonymous.
  (iv) GP.

> **Warning:** if a patient should demand a controlled drug, explain that it is an offence for a doctor to administer or authorize the supply of a drug of addiction, except in the treatment of an organic disease or injury, unless licensed to do so.

BENZODIAZEPINE AND SOLVENT ADDICTION

MANAGEMENT

1 Patients who are addicted to these groups of drugs all require referral to a specialist drug and alcohol dependency clinic to coordinate their withdrawal regimen. Help and advice is available from:
  (i)   Social work department.
  (ii) Drug dependency organization including self-help groups.
  (iii) GP.

INVOLUNTARY ADMISSION

1 It is sometimes necessary to detain a patient against his or her will in or through the emergency department under the prevailing local Mental Health Act (MHA).
  (i)   Always request the help and advice of the psychiatric team in such circumstances. It is unusual to have to act in their absence.

2 Generic criteria that must be fulfilled for instigating involuntary admission for assessment include:
  (i)   The person appears to have a mental illness that requires immediate assessment at an authorized mental health service.
  (ii) There is a risk the person may cause harm to self or another, or might suffer serious mental or physical deterioration.
  (iii) There is no less restrictive way of ensuring the patient is assessed.
  (iv) The person is lacking the capacity to consent to be assessed or has unreasonably refused to be assessed.

3 Various broad types of orders or Sections for regulated (compulsory) admission exist according to the MHA policy in use locally.
   (i) Make sure you know details of the local policy, which varies from country to country, and state to state.
   (ii) Most include an emergency examination order signed by a police or ambulance officer; and a short (24 h–3 day) assessment order signed by two different persons that will include a medical practitioner or authorized mental health practitioner.
   (iii) A longer 21-day, or 28-day or more admission period usually needs to be supported by two medical recommendations. Again details vary locally.

4 All regulated patients admitted involuntarily are then subject to mandatory psychiatric review according to the local MHA legislation.

5 Make certain you know who can sign which order, when the order lapses, and what it allows the medical practitioner to do.

6 Make sure you also understand the distinction between involuntary detention for assessment, and administering emergency treatment under common law without the patient's consent if they pose a serious threat to themselves or others.

FURTHER READING

ACEP Emergency Medicine Practice Committee (2014). Care of the psychiatric patient in the Emergency Department - A review of the literature. http://www.acep.org (evaluation, medical clearance and disposition).

Crawford MJ, Patton R, Touquet R *et al.* (2004) Screening and referral for brief intervention of alcohol-misusing patients in an emergency department: A pragmatic randomised controlled trial. *Lancet* **364**: 1334–9.

Phillips G, Mason S, Baston S (2015) Mental health and the law: The Australasian and UK perspectives. In: Cameron P, Jelinek G, Kelly A-M *et al. Textbook of Adult Emergency Medicine*, 4th edn. Churchill Livingstone, Edinburgh, pp. 808-817. (mental health legislation, involuntary admission).

Therapeutic Guidelines. eTG complete 2015. http://www.tg.org.au/

TOXICOLOGY

ACUTE POISONING: GENERAL PRINCIPLES

Most cases of acute poisoning are acts of deliberate self-harm in the adult, but are usually accidental in children. Cases should initially be managed as medical emergencies and require substance identification, risk assessment, resuscitation, general supportive and specific treatment, with a period of observation.

Thereafter, cases will require psychiatric assessment. Remember that an apparently trivial act of self-harm may still indicate serious suicidal intent (see p. 386).

DIAGNOSIS

1   Consider acute poisoning in the unconscious patient or one exhibiting bizarre behaviour, or in unexplained metabolic, respiratory or cardio-vascular problems.

2   Obtain specific information from the patient, witnesses, and ambulance personnel regarding:
   (i)   Pharmaceutical agent or toxin ingested:
      (a) remember that two or more drugs are taken in 30% of cases
      (b) alcohol is a common adjunct.
   (ii) Quantity of agent ingested (look for empty blister packets or bottles).
   (iii) Time since ingestion.
   (iv) History of any toxic effects experienced from the poisoning.
   (v)   Specific events prior to arrival in the emergency department (ED), such as:
      (a) deterioration in conscious level
      (b) seizures.
   (vi) Clinical features on presentation.

3   Corroborate the history in the cooperative patient, but do not be misled, as information supplied may be incomplete or deliberately false.

4   Focus the examination on immediate life threats, identification of clinical signs specific to certain drugs, and obtaining baseline vital signs.
   (i)   Rapidly assess airway patency, respiratory function and conscious level.
   (ii) Record the pulse, blood pressure, respiratory rate, temperature and blood sugar level, and attach a cardiac monitor and pulse oximeter to the patient
      (a) hypoglycaemia and hyperthermia are common findings in the collapsed patient with a drug overdose, and are often overlooked.
   (iii) Look for signs of seizure activity, assess upper and lower limbs for signs of hypertonicity and clonus, and examine the pupils.
   (iv) Look for clues to the substance taken ('toxidrome'):
      (a) *dilated pupils:* tricyclics, amphetamine, antihistamines, anticholinergic agents

       (b) *pinpoint pupils:* opiates, organophosphates

       (c) *nystagmus:* alcohol, benzodiazepines, phenytoin

       (d) *hyperventilation:* salicylates

       (e) *seizures:* antidepressants, tramadol, sulphonylureas, theophylline, isoniazid, sympathomimetics such as cocaine and amphetamines, withdrawal states

       (f) *nasal bleeding or perioral sores:* solvent abuse.

5 Gain i.v. access and send blood for FBC, U&Es, LFTs and a paracetamol level in **all** poisonings.

     (i) Only send a salicylate level if symptomatic of salicylism or when comatose (see p. 400).

6 Perform an arterial or venous blood gas to rapidly determine metabolic acidosis, respiratory function and electrolyte imbalance, if the patient is significantly unwell.

     (i) Metabolic acidosis is associated with many poisonings including salicylates, methanol, iron and ethylene glycol.

7 Request other measurable specific serum drug levels in suspected ingestion of phenytoin, sodium valproate, digoxin, carbamazepine, iron, lithium, ethanol, methanol or ethylene glycol and theophylline.

8 Perform an electrocardiogram (ECG) to look for tachycardia, bradycardia and potential cardiac conduction abnormalities such as QT prolongation and widening of the QRS complex.

9 Request a chest X-ray (CXR) if clinical signs of aspiration are present.

10 Request an abdominal X-ray (AXR) when potentially radiopaque tablets such as iron or potassium have been ingested.

MANAGEMENT

1 Start immediate resuscitation if risk assessment indicates ingestion of a potentially lethal drug, or if the patient is obtunded with signs of cardio-respiratory distress.

2 *Unconscious or collapsed patient*

     (i) Clear the airway by extending the head, remove dentures, vomit or blood by a quick sweep round the mouth with a Yankauer suction catheter, and give oxygen via a face mask.

     (ii) Insert an oropharyngeal Guedel airway if the patient is not breathing or the gag reflex is reduced, and use a bag–valve mask system to ventilate the patient, aiming for an oxygen saturation above 94%.

     (iii) Call an airway-skilled doctor urgently to pass a cuffed endotracheal tube to protect and maintain the airway and to optimize ventilation.

3 Administer the following without delay:

     (i) 50% dextrose 50 mL i.v. if the blood sugar level is low.

     (ii)   Naloxone 0.1–0.4 mg i.v. slowly if the pupils are pinpoint, the respiratory rate is below 10/min and opioid intoxication is suspected (see p. 404)

        (a) beware that larger doses of naloxone may precipitate opioid withdrawal and severe agitation in an opioid-dependent patient.

    (iii) Normal saline to treat hypotension and maintain the circulation. If hypotension is secondary to an arrhythmia or myocardial depression, specific drug therapy and inotropic support may be needed.

4   Treat toxic seizures with:

     (i)   Midazolam 0.05–0.1 mg/kg i.v., diazepam 0.1–0.2 mg/kg i.v. or lorazepam 0.07 mg/kg up to 4 mg i.v.

     (ii) Second-line treatment such as phenobarbitone (phenobarbital) 10–20 mg/kg i.v. at no faster than 100 mg/min. Phenytoin is contraindicated in the treatment of toxic seizures.

5   ***Gastrointestinal decontamination***

This is **not** routine, and is only instituted once basic resuscitative and supportive care have been performed and the airway is secure.

     (i)   *Activated charcoal*:

        (a) is used to reduce the absorption of many drugs. Consider in patients presenting within 1 h of taking a potentially toxic overdose of an agent known to be adsorbed to charcoal

        (b) give 50 g for adults (1 g/kg body weight in children) in 100–200 mL water administered orally or via a nasogastric tube. Warn the patient that charcoal is unpalatable and will turn the stools black

        (c) charcoal administration is contraindicated when:

           – an oral antidote such as methionine is to be given

           – the patient has an altered level of consciousness or an unprotected airway

           – the patient has ingested substances not adsorbed to charcoal, such as iron, lithium, alcohols, acid, alkali, petroleum, pesticides or cyanide.

     (ii) *Whole bowel irrigation* (WBI):

        (a) is not used routinely, but may be helpful in poisonings with:

           – toxic ingestion of agents such as iron, lithium and calcium-channel blockers

           – sustained-release or enteric-coated medications

           – 'body-packers' who have ingested wrapped illicit drugs

        (b) is contraindicated in patients with:

           – an unprotected airway

           – haemodynamic instability

           – bowel obstruction, perforation or ileus

           – vomiting, or inability to pass NG tube.

6   *Enhanced elimination*

Consider for specific poisonings in consultation with the ICU. Obtain additional advice from a Poisons Information Service.

(i)   Multiple-dose activated charcoal (MDAC): give repeated 25–50 g charcoal every 4 h. This may be useful in severe dapsone, carbamazepine, phenobarbitone (phenobarbital), quinine and theophylline poisoning and possibly salicylate poisoning.

(ii)   Haemodialysis, charcoal haemoperfusion and urinary pH modification are alternatives in certain severe poisonings.

7   *Antidotes*

These drugs counter the effects of a poison, but are available for only a few specific agents.

8   Admit the patient following ED resuscitation, supportive care, decontamination and antidote administration to the ED observation unit, medical team or ICU, depending on the clinical severity of poisoning.

9   All patients will require psychiatric evaluation and management following this medical care.

Warning: gastric lavage is rarely if ever used, and induced emesis is positively contraindicated.

SPECIFIC POISONS

Obtain advice as necessary regarding toxic ingestions 24 h a day from the Poisons Information Centre on **13 11 26** in Australia, and in New Zealand on 03 479 7248 (or **0800 764 766** (24 h) within New Zealand).

Advice in the UK is available from the National Poisons Information Service (NPIS), which coordinates an internet and telephone service to assist in the diagnosis, treatment and management of all types of poisonings.

- TOXBASE® is an online resource for the routine diagnosis, treatment and management of patients exposed to toxic substances. Use this as the first point of contact for poisons advice. It is available on http://www.toxbase.org/
- Specialist consultants are available for telephone advice in more complex clinical cases. A 24-h number **0844 892 0111** will direct callers to the relevant local centre in the UK.

PARACETAMOL

DIAGNOSIS

1   Paracetamol overdose is common and potentially lethal.

2   Hepatocellular necrosis is the major complication of paracetamol toxicity.

Factors that enhance the potential for hepatotoxicity, and therefore morbidity and mortality, include:

    (i)   Late presentation with delayed antidote administration, especially if over 24 h.

    (ii)   Staggered overdose: multiple supra-therapeutic ingestions over a number of days.

    (iii)   Glutathione deficiency in starvation and debilitating illness such as AIDS.

    (iv)   Enzyme-inducing drugs such as carbamazepine, phenobarbitone (phenobarbital), rifampicin or isoniazid.

    (v)   Regular alcohol use.

3 Determine the time since ingestion, total paracetamol consumed and the patient's weight:

    (i)   Patients who have taken >10 g (20 tablets) or >200 mg/kg over a period of <8 h are considered at risk from severe liver damage.

    (ii)   The greatest risk of hepatotoxicity is related to the extent of delay beyond 8 h until antidote treatment with *N*-acetylcysteine (NAC) is commenced.

    (iii)   Hepatotoxicity may also occur in patients who take repeated or staggered doses, or sustained-release preparations.

4 The patient is usually asymptomatic, but can present in fulminant hepatic failure with abdominal pain, vomiting, jaundice, tender hepatomegaly and encephalopathy.

    (i)   Coagulopathy, hypoglycaemia and metabolic acidosis occur in severe poisoning.

5 Gain i.v. access and send bloods for full blood count (FBC), urea and electrolytes (U&Es), liver function tests (LFTs), prothrombin index (PTI) (international normalized ratio [INR]) and a blood sugar level.

    (i)   These bloods become more important if the patient presents over 8 h after ingestion, and are essential if presentation is delayed beyond 24 h or more.

    (ii)   Send a paracetamol level once 4 h or more have elapsed since overdose.

MANAGEMENT

1 Resuscitation is rarely required unless the patient is in fulminant hepatic failure.

    (i)   Administer 50% dextrose 50 mL i.v. if the patient is hypoglycaemic.

2 Review the blood results:

    (i)   Plot the serum paracetamol level on the paracetamol nomogram for all patients presenting between 4 and 24 h after an acute, single ingestion of paracetamol (Fig. 14.1)

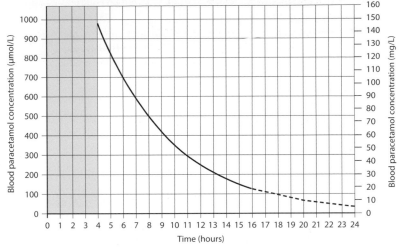

Figure 14.1 Treatment nomogram for paracetamol poisoning. Treat any patient with a serum paracetamol level above the nomogram treatment line. (Make certain the correct units are used).

Reproduced with permission from Daly FFS, Fountain JS, Murray L et al. (2008) Guidelines for the management of paracetamol poisoning in Australia and New Zealand – explanation and elaboration. *Medical Journal of Australia* **188**: 296–301.

        (a) the treatment nomogram has been simplified to a single treatment line now for all patients

        (b) this line has been lowered by 25% from previous standard lines.

    (ii) Treat all patients who have a serum paracetamol level above the nomogram treatment line.

    (iii) A raised PTI (INR) >2.0 or alanine aminotransferase (ALT) levels >1000 IU/L indicate significant hepatotoxicity.

3   NAC, the antidote for paracetamol, is highly effective when commenced within 8 h of poisoning. Administer NAC in the following circumstances:

    (i) Patients presenting within 8 h of ingestion, with a 4–8-h serum paracetamol level above the nomogram treatment line (see Fig. 14.1).

    (ii) Potentially toxic ingestion of paracetamol (more than 20 tablets or 200 mg/kg) in a patient presenting 8– 24 h after overdose, or if the serum paracetamol level will not be available within 8 h of the original ingestion:

        (a) commence treatment immediately without waiting for the blood results

        (b) cease treatment if the serum paracetamol level turns out to be below the relevant treatment line, and the ALT and PTI (INR) are normal.

     (iii) Patients presenting with deranged ALT and PTI (INR) more than
          24 h after acute overdose, or following staggered overdose
          (a) serum paracetamol levels are difficult to interpret in cases
               of staggered ingestion. Monitor the PTI (INR) and ALT
               regularly instead and seek specialist toxicologist advice
               (see below).

4   Consult a clinical toxicologist for patients presenting with a staggered overdose, with delayed presentation of more than 24 h, and patients with severe liver dysfunction and an elevated PTI (INR).

5   Use the adult infusion protocol for NAC below.
     (i)   Take care with the dose calculation:
         (a) 150 mg/kg (0.75 mL/kg) in 5% dextrose 200 mL i.v. over
             15–60 min
         (b) 50 mg/kg (0.25 mL/kg) in 5% dextrose 500 mL i.v. over 4 h
         (c) 100 mg/kg (0.5 mL/kg) in 5% dextrose 1000 mL i.v. over 16 h.
     (ii) Or read from the drug-insert infusion dosage guide the volume
          in millilitres of NAC 200 mg/mL to be added to the 5% dextrose,
          according to the patient's weight in kg.

6   Side effects are mostly from non-allergic anaphylactic reactions, occurring in the first 30 min of administering high-dose NAC. These include nausea, flushing, itching, urticaria, wheeze and hypotension.
     (i)   Stop the infusion.
     (ii) Give promethazine 12.5–25 mg i.v. or chlorphenamine 10 mg i.v.
     (iii) Once symptoms have settled, re-commence the initial infusion at
          a slower rate over 1–2 h.

SALICYLATES

DIAGNOSIS

1   The clinical features of salicylate toxicity following acute ingestion are dose related:
     (i)   Ingested dose <150 mg/kg: usually asymptomatic.
     (ii) 150–300 mg/kg: moderate symptoms such as tachypnoea, nausea,
          vomiting and tinnitus (salicylism).
     (iii) 300–500 mg/kg: severe toxicity with metabolic acidosis,
          dehydration, agitation, confusion and an altered level of
          consciousness leading to coma.
     (iv) More than 500 mg/kg ingested is associated with pulmonary and
          cerebral oedema and may be fatal.

2   Gain i.v. access and send bloods for U&Es, blood sugar and a salicylate level.
     (i)   Perform arterial blood gases (ABGs) to detect respiratory
          alkalosis or a metabolic acidosis in symptomatic patients.

MANAGEMENT

1   Call an airway-skilled doctor immediately to pass a cuffed endotracheal tube if the patient is obtunded, unconscious or unable to protect their airway.

2   Commence a normal saline infusion to replace insensible losses associated with hyperthermia, hyperventilation and vomiting.

3   Administer charcoal as soon as possible, even in patients with a delayed presentation, as salicylates cause delayed gastric emptying. Consider repeat-dose activated charcoal every 4 h to reduce salicylate absorption in the following situations:
   (i)   Overdose of sustained-release aspirin.
   (ii) Evidence of continued absorption with rising serum salicylate levels.

4   Urinary alkalinization may reduce salicylate elimination from 20 to 5 h. Consider in patients with signs and symptoms of salicylate toxicity, or a serum salicylate level of >300 mg/L (2.2 mmol/L).
   (i)   Give a bolus of 8.4% sodium bicarbonate 1 mmol/kg (1 mL/kg) i.v.
   (ii)   Follow with an infusion of 8.4% sodium bicarbonate 100 mmol (100 mL) in 5% dextrose solution 1 L, at a rate of 100–250 mL/h.
   (iii) Titrate this bicarbonate infusion to maintain urinary pH >7.5 and urine output >1 mL/kg per h.

5   Monitor serum electrolytes, salicylate level and urinary pH every 2–4 h.
   (i)   Salicylate level:
          (a) symptoms occur at 300 mg/L (2.2 mmol/L)
          (b) significant toxicity occurs at 500 mg/L (3.6 mmol/L)
          (c) repeat the level at least once. Rising levels indicate continued drug absorption.
   (ii)   Potassium: significant hypokalaemia hinders salicylate elimination so potassium must be replaced.

6   Patients with no clinical evidence of salicylate toxicity, normal venous or ABGs with falling serum salicylate levels 4 h apart in the therapeutic range may be medically cleared for psychiatric review.

7   Otherwise observe all patients with clinical salicylate toxicity for a minimum of 12 h until they demonstrate resolution of symptoms and a falling serum salicylate level, before considering them medically stable.

8   Consult a clinical toxicologist for patients with salicylate levels >500 mg/L (3.6 mmol/L), severe symptoms or obtunded.
   (i)   Consider haemodialysis for severe poisoning with a metabolic acidosis or a salicylate level >700 mg/L (5.1 mmol/L).

TRICYCLIC ANTIDEPRESSANTS

DIAGNOSIS

1   Tricyclic antidepressant (TCA) overdose is associated with significant mortality. Ingestion of ≥15–20 mg/kg is potentially fatal.

2   The onset of symptoms is usually rapid, and in large overdoses deterioration occurs within 1–2 h. Significant toxicity is heralded by cardiotoxicity, convulsions and coma.

3   Clinical features include:
   (i)   *Anticholinergic*: warm dry skin with absent sweating, dilated pupils, urinary retention, sinus tachycardia, and delirium.
   (ii) *Central nervous system (CNS)*: seizures usually associated with an altered level of consciousness and rapid development of coma, especially with a large overdose.
   (iii) *Cardiovascular*: cardiac arrhythmias are common and occur as a result of sodium-channel blockade, associated with hypotension.

4   Perform an ECG. Look for tachycardia, heart block, junctional rhythms and ventricular tachycardia (VT) with progressive QRS widening, and QTc prolongation.
   (i)   A QRS interval of >100 ms and a positive R wave >3 mm amplitude in aVR indicate cardiotoxicity and are predictive of ventricular arrhythmias.

5   Gain i.v. access and send blood for FBC, U&Es and a paracetamol level and attach a cardiac monitor and pulse oximeter to the patient.

6   Perform an ABG or VBG to monitor for hypoxia and acidosis, both of which exacerbate cardiotoxicity.

MANAGEMENT

1   Give high-dose oxygen and commence a normal saline infusion.

2   Call an airway-skilled doctor to pass an endotracheal tube in patients with a reduced conscious level, inadequate respiratory effort or convulsions, with or without cardiac arrhythmias.
   (i)   The patient should be hyperventilated to a pH of 7.5, as alkalaemia decreases the risk of cardiotoxicity.

3   Administer activated charcoal as soon as possible once the airway is secured, to all patients with significant TCA ingestion, even with a delayed presentation.

4   Give a loading dose of 8.4% sodium bicarbonate 1–2 mmol/kg (1–2 mL/kg), followed by an infusion of 20–100 mmol/h (20–100 mL/h) to maintain an arterial pH of between 7.50 and 7.55.
   (i)   Sodium bicarbonate is a specific antidote in TCA poisoning and provides high concentrations of sodium ions, which reduce cardiotoxicity.
   (ii) Indications for sodium bicarbonate administration include:
       (a) cardiac arrhythmia or cardiac arrest
       (b) widened QRS interval of >120 ms
       (c) persistent hypotension despite saline or colloid fluid administration.

5   Repeat the ABGs or VBG and electrolytes regularly to ensure maintenance of alkalaemia and avoid hypernatraemia.

6   Perform repeated ECGs to monitor for cardiac arrhythmias and to observe the resolution of any QRS prolongation.

7   Refer patients with significant cardiovascular or CNS toxicity to the intensive care unit (ICU) for ECG monitoring and supportive care.

8   Observe patients with drowsiness alone and non-progressive or absent ECG changes in the ED observation unit, until any clinical signs of sedation or anticholinergic delirium have resolved.

BENZODIAZEPINES

DIAGNOSIS

1   These are comparatively safe if taken alone. Reported deaths are associated with mixed overdoses with other CNS depressants such as opioids and alcohol.

2   Clinical manifestations include drowsiness, respiratory depression, ataxia and dysarthria.

3   Coma is unusual unless combined with other sedatives or alcohol, or in the elderly.

4   Gain i.v. access and send blood for U&Es and a paracetamol level. No specific investigations are required unless co-ingestion is suspected. Attach a cardiac monitor and pulse oximeter to the patient.

5   Perform a baseline ECG.

MANAGEMENT

1   Give high-dose oxygen and nurse in the left lateral position to prevent aspiration, unless the airway is protected.

2   Administer normal saline to maintain a normal blood pressure (BP).

3   Gastrointestinal decontamination is rarely necessary unless there is co-ingestion or the patient is deeply unconscious, in which case protect the airway *first* by endotracheal intubation.

4   Admit the patient to the ED observation unit overnight, followed by subsequent psychiatric evaluation.

5   Flumazenil, a specific benzodiazepine receptor antagonist, is **rarely** if ever indicated.
    (i)   Flumazenil may induce VT, elevate intracranial pressure, precipitate benzodiazepine withdrawal in chronic abusers, and may invoke seizures, particularly with co-ingestion of TCAs.
    (ii) Potential role for flumazenil is thus restricted to:
        (a) reversal of excessive benzodiazepine sedative effect following procedural sedation, particularly in the elderly.

OPIOIDS

DIAGNOSIS

1 Opioid drugs include opium alkaloids such as morphine and codeine; semi-synthetic opioids such as heroin (diamorphine) and oxycodone and fully synthetic opioids such as pethidine and methadone.

2 Opioids produce euphoria, pinpoint pupils, sedation, respiratory depression and apnoea with increasing doses.

3 Other complications of opioid intoxication include hypotension, convulsions, non-cardiogenic pulmonary oedema and compartment syndrome from prolonged immobility.

4 Perform a thorough examination to evaluate potential complications, and to exclude alternative causes of an altered mental state with bradypnoea such as sepsis, neurotrauma, stroke and metabolic disease (see p. 24).

5 Send bloods for U&Es, blood sugar and serum paracetamol level. Perform an ECG.

MANAGEMENT

1 Commence supportive care with oxygen and assisted ventilation.

2 Give naloxone 0.1–0.4 mg i.v. as a bolus or in 0.1 mg increments. Carefully titrate response to achieve improved airway control and adequate ventilation, without precipitating an acute agitated withdrawal state.

   (i) Naloxone is a short-acting opioid antagonist that may be administered by the i.m., i.v., s.c. or endotracheal routes.

   (ii) It is safe and rarely associated with complications, but may cause acute withdrawal and severe agitation in the opioid-dependent individual.

   (iii) Use it to reverse severe respiratory depression, apnoea and oversedation, or for cases of undifferentiated coma with respiratory depression and pinpoint pupils.

3 Continue to monitor for respiratory depression and hypoxia. Further doses of naloxone or an infusion may be required due to its short half-life.

4 Observe all patients for a period, because re-sedation with respiratory depression may occur as the naloxone wears off, particularly with sustained-release preparations or long-acting methadone.

IRON

DIAGNOSIS

1 Acute iron overdose is a potentially life-threatening condition, particularly in children who mistake iron tablets for sweets.

2 The clinical course following iron overdose includes:

   (i) *Gastrointestinal toxicity:* haemorrhagic gastroenteritis with vomiting, abdominal pain and bloody diarrhoea. Failure to develop significant gastrointestinal symptoms within 6 h of ingestion effectively rules out significant iron poisoning.

(ii) *Systemic toxicity*: hypotension, shock, lethargy, metabolic acidosis, seizures, coma, and acute liver and renal failure.

3 Toxicity is determined by the quantity of elemental iron ingested:
   (i) <20 mg/kg: usually asymptomatic.
   (ii) 20–60 mg/kg: gastrointestinal symptoms predominate.
   (iii) 60–120 mg/kg: systemic toxicity.
   (iv) >120 mg/kg: potentially fatal.

4 Send blood for FBC, U&Es, LFTs, blood glucose, lactate, a serum iron level and venous blood gas (VBG).
   (i) Serum iron levels peak at 4–6 h after ingestion.
   (ii) Levels >90 μmol/L are associated with systemic toxicity.

5 Request a plain AXR to look for residual whole tablets or a concretion, as most iron preparations are radio-opaque.
   (i) A negative AXR does not rule out ingestion.

MANAGEMENT

1 This depends on the initial assessment and clinical manifestations, and the potential amount of elemental iron ingested.

2 Start aggressive fluid resuscitation in patients with signs of gastrointestinal or systemic toxicity, and institute decontamination and chelation measures. Discuss these with the senior ED doctor or a clinical toxicologist:
   (i) Decontamination:
      (a) do not administer charcoal or attempt to induce vomiting
      (b) perform whole bowel irrigation if there are significant numbers of tablets beyond the pylorus.
   (ii) Chelation therapy:
      (a) Start a desferrioxamine infusion at 2 mg/kg per h and increase to 15 mg/kg per h in severe cases.

3 Most patients will remain asymptomatic, or develop mild gastrointestinal symptoms only.
   (i) Give i.v. fluids to replace vomiting and diarrhoea losses, provide supportive care and observe for a minimum of 6 h.

4 Refer all moderate-to-severe cases to the ICU team.

DIGOXIN

DIAGNOSIS

1 Toxicity occurs from acute overdose or secondary to long-term therapy. Foxglove and oleander ingestion will also cause acute cardiac glycoside poisoning.

2 *Acute digoxin overdose* in adults is usually intentional. Clinical manifestations include:
   (i) Nausea and vomiting.

(ii) Hyperkalaemia.

(iii) Bradycardia and ventricular arrhythmias.

3   *Chronic digoxin toxicity* occurs particularly in the elderly and may be precipitated by renal impairment, hypokalaemia, hypercalcaemia and drugs such as amiodarone and quinidine. Clinical manifestations include:

(i) Nausea, vomiting, diarrhoea.

(ii) Sedation, confusion, delirium.

(iii) Visual disturbances, such as yellow haloes (xanthopsia).

(iv) Cardiac automaticity and a wide range of ventricular and supraventricular arrhythmias.

4   Gain i.v. access and send bloods for U&Es and a serum digoxin level.

(i) Therapeutic range for digoxin is 0.5–2.0 ng/mL.

(ii) Take serum levels early to confirm poisoning, and repeat in 4 h if acute ingestion is suspected.

(iii) The serum digoxin level is most predictive after 6 h post-ingestion.

5   Perform an ECG:

(i) Any cardiac arrhythmia may be seen in both acute and chronic ingestions.

(ii) The most common arrhythmias are bradycardia, heart block, paroxysmal atrial tachycardia, ventricular ectopics and ventricular tachycardia.

MANAGEMENT

1   Treatment depends on haemodynamic stability, conscious state, and whether it is an acute or chronic intoxication.

2   Gain i.v. access in all patients and start fluid resuscitation for hypotension, continuous cardiac monitoring, and perform regular ECGs.

3   **Acute digoxin intoxication**

(i) Administer oral activated charcoal if presentation is within 1 h of significant overdose. This may be impossible if the patient is vomiting continuously. Repeated administration should not delay other interventions.

(ii) Treat hyperkalaemia with a dextrose–insulin infusion (see p. 134)

(a) do **not** use i.v. calcium as this may precipitate asystole.

(iii) Administer digoxin-specific antibody fragments (Digibind™) for:

(a) cardiac arrest

(b) haemodynamic instability with cardiac arrhythmia

(c) serum potassium >5.5 mmol/L

(d) serum digoxin level >15 nmol/L (11.7 ng/mL)

(e) ingested digoxin dose >10 mg (4 mg in a child).

(iv) Calculate the number of vials of Digibind™ required from the estimated ingested dose or the serum digoxin concentration, if obtained at least 6 h post acute poisoning

(a) give empiric dosing starting with 5–10 vials of Digibind™ if the acutely ingested dose is unknown.

(v) Admit all acute poisonings for cardiac monitoring and close observation for a minimum of 12 h.

4 Chronic digoxin intoxication

(i) Cease the digoxin medication.

(ii) Correct any hypokalaemia with potassium chloride 10 mmol/h i.v., and hypomagnesaemia with magnesium sulphate 10 mmol in 100 mL normal saline i.v. over 30 min.

(iii) Administer two vials of digoxin-specific antibody fragments (Digibind™) i.v. over 30 min to symptomatic patients with an altered mental state, cardiac arrhythmia or gastrointestinal symptoms.

(iv) Patients usually recover quickly. Admit under the medical team for treatment of any ongoing cardiac instability, renal impairment and electrolyte disturbances.

LITHIUM

DIAGNOSIS

1 Lithium toxicity may be acute or chronic. Toxicity is associated with significant morbidity and mortality particularly in the presence of renal impairment, or an acute overdose of >250 mg/kg (25 g).

2 Acute overdose

(i) Clinical manifestations of acute overdose include:

(a) gastrointestinal: nausea, vomiting, diarrhoea

(b) CNS: similar to chronic intoxication, but features rarely develop with adequate treatment with i.v. crystalloid therapy, providing there is no renal impairment.

3 Chronic toxicity

(i) This is commonly associated with renal impairment, dehydration, diuretic or NSAID use and congestive cardiac failure.

(ii) Clinical manifestations of chronic toxicity include:

(a) CNS:

  – mild: tremor, hyper-reflexia, ataxia, muscle weakness
  – moderate: rigidity, hypotension, stupor
  – severe: myoclonus, coma and convulsions

(b) gastrointestinal symptoms are not prominent in chronic toxicity.

4 Gain i.v. access and send bloods for U&Es, blood sugar and serum lithium level.

5 Perform an ECG.

MANAGEMENT

1 *Acute overdose*

    (i)   Do not administer activated charcoal.

    (ii) Commence normal saline to correct hypotension, salt and water deficits, and to maintain a urine output >1 mL/kg per h.

    (iii) Most patients recover quickly with adequate fluid resuscitation. Observe until they have a normal mental status, the serum lithium level is falling and is <2.5 mmol/L.

    (iv) Consider haemodialysis in a patient with impaired renal function, late presentation, a serum lithium level that is not falling, or progressive neurological signs. Contact the ICU.

2 *Chronic toxicity*

    (i)   Discontinue lithium medications. Commence normal saline to correct hypotension, salt and water deficits, and to maintain a high urine output.

    (ii) Refer the following patient to ICU for consideration of haemodialysis:

        (a) neurological abnormalities such as an altered mental state, coma or convulsions

        (b) serum lithium level of >2.5 mmol/L

        (c) persistent renal impairment.

THEOPHYLLINE

DIAGNOSIS

1 Theophylline toxicity may result from acute ingestion >10 mg/kg or chronic use. Both are associated with significant morbidity and mortality.

    (i)   Chronic toxicity is exacerbated by intercurrent illness or the concomitant administration of drugs that interfere with hepatic metabolism such as sulphonamides and erythromycin.

2 Clinical manifestations include:

    (i)   Gastrointestinal tract: nausea, abdominal pain, intractable vomiting.

    (ii) Cardiovascular: sinus tachycardia, hypotension and cardiac arrhythmias.

    (iii) CNS: anxiety, agitation and insomnia.

    (iv) Tachypnoea, hypokalaemia, metabolic acidosis, convulsions, coma and ventricular tachycardia in severe toxicity.

3 Clinical signs of significant toxicity may be delayed by up to 12 h in acute overdose, when sustained-release tablets have been ingested.

4 Gain i.v. access and send bloods for U&Es, LFTs, blood sugar and a theophylline level.

    (i)   Look for hypokalaemia, hypomagnesaemia, hyperglycaemia and metabolic acidosis, particularly in severe acute ingestions.

5 Determine the serum theophylline level.
  (i) Acute poisoning:
     (a) toxic symptoms occur with a theophylline level over 25 mg/L
     (b) levels of 40–80 mg/L are serious, and a level >100 mg/L is potentially fatal.
  (ii) Chronic toxicity:
     (a) levels over 20 mg/L cause symptoms, and over 40 mg/L may be life-threatening.

6 Perform an ECG and cardiac monitoring. Cardiac arrhythmias are common and include sinus tachycardia, supraventricular tachycardia, atrial flutter and VT.

MANAGEMENT

1 Ensure the airway is secure and administer high-flow oxygen. Correct fluid depletion and hypokalaemia with normal saline and potassium under ECG monitoring.

2 Administer oral activated charcoal in acute overdose, even if presentation is delayed. Give repeat doses at 4-h intervals.

3 Give high-dose metoclopramide 10–40 mg i.v. for intractable vomiting, or give ondansetron 8 mg i.v. if this fails.

4 Give midazolam 0.05–0.1 mg/kg, diazepam 0.1–0.2 mg/kg i.v., or lorazepam 0.07 mg/kg i.v. up to 4 mg for seizures, although endotracheal intubation may be required.

5 Administer a β-blocker such as propranolol 1 mg i.v. over 1 min, repeated up to a maximum of 10 mg **only** in the non-asthmatic patient for supraventricular tachycardia.

6 Admit all patients with signs of toxicity for cardiac monitoring.
  (i) Refer patients with severe toxicity, obtundation and seizures to ICU for haemodialysis or charcoal haemoperfusion.

β-BLOCKERS

DIAGNOSIS

1 Significant β-blocker toxicity is associated particularly with propranolol ingestion, coexistent cardiac disease, and in polypharmacy overdose with calcium-channel blockers and TCAs.

2 Clinical evidence of toxicity usually presents within the first 6 h of overdose. Toxicity is associated with:
  (i) Bradycardia, arrhythmias, hypotension and cardiogenic shock.
  (ii) Sedation, altered mental status, convulsions and coma.

3 Gain i.v. access and send blood for U&Es and a blood sugar level, as hypoglycaemia may occur, especially with atenolol. Attach a cardiac monitor and pulse oximeter to the patient.

4 Perform an ECG. Look for toxic conduction defects such as atrioventricular block, right bundle branch block, ventricular arrhythmias from prolongation of the QRS (propranolol) and QTc (sotalol).

MANAGEMENT

1 Ensure the airway is secure and administer high-flow oxygen. Commence i.v. fluid administration for hypotension.

2 Administer oral activated charcoal as soon as possible.

3 Give atropine 0.6–1.2 mg i.v. for bradycardia, up to a maximum of 0.04 mg/kg.

4 Give glucagon 50–150 μg/kg i.v. bolus followed by an infusion at 1–5 mg/h.

5 Titrate an adrenaline (epinephrine) or isoprenaline infusion to maintain organ perfusion in resistant cases. Cardiac pacing may be necessary.

    (i) Give 8.4% sodium bicarbonate 1–2 mmol/kg (1–2 mL/kg) for QRS widening in severe propranolol toxicity.

6 Admit all symptomatic patients to coronary care or ICU.

CALCIUM-CHANNEL BLOCKING DRUGS

DIAGNOSIS

1 Toxicity is related to underlying cardiac disease, co-ingestants, delay to treatment, increased age, and the specific calcium-channel blocker (CCB) ingested.

    (i) Sustained-release (SR) verapamil or diltiazem are associated with the majority of significant poisonings.

2 Clinical signs of toxicity usually present within 2 h, but may be delayed up to 8 h with sustained-release preparations. Features include:

    (i) Gastrointestinal: nausea and vomiting.

    (ii) Cardiovascular: hypotension, sinus bradycardia and complex cardiac arrhythmias.

    (iii) CNS: lethargy, slurred speech, confusion, coma and convulsions.

3 Gain i.v. access and send blood for U&Es, LFTs and a blood sugar level. Take an arterial or venous blood gas.

    (i) Hyperglycaemia and lactic acidosis are common with significant toxicity.

4 Perform an ECG. Look for toxic conduction defects such as high-grade AV block, complete heart block, and accelerated atrioventricular nodal rhythms.

MANAGEMENT

1 Ensure the airway is secure and administer high-flow oxygen. Commence i.v. fluid administration.

2 Administer oral activated charcoal to all patients as soon as possible. More aggressive decontamination, such as whole bowel irrigation, may be required with large ingestions of SR tablets.

3   Give 10% calcium chloride 10 mL i.v. bolus, and repeat up to 30 mL i.v. followed by an infusion. Calcium increases cardiac output and restores perfusion to vital organs.

4   If hypotension and reduced myocardial contractility persist:

  (i)   Commence an adrenaline (epinephrine) infusion at up to 0.5–1.0 μg/kg per min, titrated to maintain organ perfusion.

  (ii) Give high-dose insulin therapy (0.5–1.0 IU/kg/h), in combination with 50% dextrose infusion to maintain euglycaemia for severe CCB poisoning.

  (iii) Discuss management **early** with a poisons centre clinical toxicologist.

5   Admit the patient to ICU for cardiorespiratory monitoring.

CARBON MONOXIDE

DIAGNOSIS

1   Carbon monoxide poisoning is usually associated with the combustion of fuel with an inadequate flue, e.g. a blocked domestic heater, or from the fumes of a car exhaust. It is a colourless odourless gas and the most common poison used for successful suicide in the UK and Australia.

2   Clinical manifestations are directly related to early ABG carboxyhaemoglobin (COHb) concentration levels around the time of exposure. Later COHb levels lack prognostic value:

  (i)   0–10%: asymptomatic (may be seen in smokers).

  (ii) 10–25%: throbbing frontal headache, nausea, shortness of breath.

  (iii) 25–40%: cognitive impairment, auditory and visual disturbances, dizziness, ataxia and confusion.

  (iv) 40–50%: collapse, coma and seizures.

  (v)   50–70%: hypotension, respiratory failure, cardiac arrhythmias and cardiac arrest.

  (vi) >70%: death.

3   A strong clinical suspicion is important in making the diagnosis. Suspect carbon monoxide toxicity if several members of one household present in a similar fashion.

4   Remember that a pulse oximeter does not distinguish between carboxyhaemoglobin and oxyhaemoglobin, and so will record misleadingly normal oxygen saturations.

  (i)   Therefore send an ABG or VBG sample in all cases. Look for evidence of metabolic acidosis and an elevated carboxyhaemoglobin level.

5   Gain i.v. access and send blood for FBC, U&Es, LFTs, troponin, serum lactate and blood sugar level. Check a β-human chorionic gonadotrophin (hCG) pregnancy test in women.

6 Perform an ECG. Look for evidence of cardiac arrhythmias or myocardial ischaemia.

7 Request a CXR and arrange a CT brain scan in a comatose patient.

MANAGEMENT

1 Secure the airway and give 100% oxygen by tight-fitting mask with reservoir bag.
  (i) Call the senior ED doctor and prepare for endotracheal intubation in comatose patients, to protect and maintain the airway and to optimize ventilation with 100% oxygen.

2 Commence fluid resuscitation for hypotension and to correct acid–base disturbances. Hypotension usually responds to fluids, but may require inotropic support.

3 Give 20% mannitol 0.5–1.0 g/kg (2.5–5 mL/kg) for clinical or radiographic evidence of cerebral oedema.

4 Refer the patient to a hyperbaric oxygen (HBO) unit if the patient was found unconscious, has significant neurological symptoms, or is pregnant.
  (i) Local referral practices will vary, as the efficacy of HBO is controversial.

CYANIDE

DIAGNOSIS

1 Cyanide is used industrially and in agriculture, but most poisonings follow smoke inhalation. It is a rapid potent cellular toxin.

2 Features of toxicity include:
  (i) Cardiovascular: initial hypertension followed by profound hypotension, bradycardia, arrhythmias, cardiovascular collapse and cardiorespiratory arrest.
  (ii) CNS: headache, anxiety, sedation, respiratory depression, seizures and coma.

3 Gain i.v. access and send blood for a serum lactate level and ABG analysis.

4 A raised anion gap metabolic acidosis with a raised lactate level >10 mmol/L relate closely to clinical signs of intoxication. A serum cyanide level is not available acutely.

MANAGEMENT

1 Assess and secure the airway immediately. Give 100% oxygen and commence fluid resuscitation.

2 Call for immediate senior ED doctor help, and/or advice from a clinical toxicologist if time allows. Give the following:
  (i) Hydroxocobalamin 70 mg/kg up to 5 g i.v. over 30 min or as a bolus in critical cases. Although unlicensed, it is preferred to dicobalt edetate.

(ii)   Plus 25% sodium thiosulphate 12.5 g (50 mL) i.v. at a rate of 2–5 mL/min. Do not mix in the same infusion as the hydroxocobalamin.

(iii) Repeat the above within 15 min, if there is no or only partial improvement.

3   Refer a patient with significant toxicity to ICU.

CHLOROQUINE

DIAGNOSIS

1   Overdose with quinine, chloroquine and hydroxychloroquine is potentially fatal with as little as 2.5–5 g ingested, and is associated with significant morbidity.

2   Clinical manifestations from quinine ('cinchonism') are dose related and include:

(i)   Mild: flushed and sweaty skin, tinnitus, blurred vision, confusion, reversible high-frequency hearing loss, abdominal pain, vertigo, nausea and vomiting.

(ii) Severe: hypotension, deafness, blindness, cardiac arrhythmias and cardiac arrest.

3   Gain i.v. access and send blood for FBC, U&Es, LFTs, blood sugar level and β-hCG in females. Attach a cardiac monitor and pulse oximeter to the patient.

4   Perform an ECG. Look for QRS widening, QT prolongation and ventricular arrhythmias.

MANAGEMENT

1   Assess and secure the airway and give high-flow oxygen. Commence i.v. fluid resuscitation for hypotension.

2   Give oral activated charcoal to patients presenting within 1 h of overdose.

3   Administer midazolam 0.05–0.1 mg/kg i.v., diazepam 0.1–0.2 mg/kg i.v. or lorazepam 0.07 mg/kg up to 4 mg to treat seizures and agitation, and to reduce the tachycardia.

4   Commence an isoprenaline infusion for torsades de pointes, or arrange for overdrive cardiac pacing for the QT prolongation, because magnesium is contraindicated.

(i)   Give 8.4% sodium bicarbonate 1–2 mmol/kg (1–2 mL/kg) for QRS widening.

5   There are no specific treatment modalities to reverse blindness and deafness in severe toxicity, other than supportive care.

6   Admit the patient to CCU or ICU.

COCAINE

DIAGNOSIS

1 Cocaine hydrochloride is a fine white powder, which may be mixed with baking soda to make 'crack' (free base cocaine) and smoked. It rapidly reaches the cerebral circulation and has a half-life of 90 min.

2 Complications following cocaine abuse include:
   (i) Respiratory: dyspnoea, pneumothorax, pneumonitis and thermal airway injury.
   (ii) Cardiovascular: palpitations, hypertension, aortic dissection, myocardial ischaemia, arrhythmias and cardiac arrest.
   (iii) Nervous system: agitation, altered mental state, psychosis, syncope, seizures, focal neurological signs, intracranial haemorrhage and coma.
   (iv) Hyperthermia.

3 Base the diagnosis on history and clinical suspicion. Monitor the core temperature for hyperthermia.

4 Gain i.v. access and send blood for FBC, U&Es, LFTs, blood sugar level and troponin as indicated clinically. Attach a cardiac monitor and pulse oximeter to the patient.

5 Perform an ECG and look for signs of myocardial ischaemia, infarction and cardiac arrhythmias.

6 Request a CXR.

MANAGEMENT

1 Assess and secure the airway and give high-flow oxygen.

2 Give midazolam 0.05–0.1 mg/kg i.v., diazepam 0.1–0.2 mg/kg i.v. or lorazepam 0.07 mg/kg up to 4 mg to treat seizures, agitation and to reduce the tachycardia, hypertension and hyperthermia.

3 Treat myocardial ischaemia with sublingual or i.v. nitrates and benzodiazepine sedation.
   (i) Ideally arrange for percutaneous coronary intervention (angioplasty) if myocardial infarction occurs.
   (ii) Further i.v. nitrates or sodium nitroprusside may be required to treat hypertension.
   (iii) Give 8.4% sodium bicarbonate 1–2 mmol/kg (1–2 mL/kg) for QRS widening.
   (iv) Avoid β-blockers, which exacerbate the effects of α-adrenergic mediated vasoconstriction.

4 Admit all patients requiring high-dose benzodiazepine therapy and patients with evidence of cardiovascular instability for cardiac monitoring and observation.

ORGANOPHOSPHATES

DIAGNOSIS

1   Organophosphates are toxic pesticides, which produce acetylcholine excess with muscarinic, nicotinic and CNS effects.

2   They are rapidly absorbed through the skin, bronchi and small intestine if ingested orally.

3   Patients present with degrees of cholinergic crisis, usually within 4 h of ingestion or exposure. Specific manifestations include:
   (i)   *Muscarinic*:
         (a) bronchorrhoea, bronchospasm, vomiting, pinpoint pupils, bradycardia and hypotension
         (b) excessive sweating, lacrimation, salivation, profuse diarrhoea and urination.
   (ii) *Nicotinic*: fasciculation, tremor, weakness, muscle paralysis, tachycardia and hypertension.
   (iii) *CNS*: initial agitation followed by sedation and altered mental status leading to convulsions and coma.

4   Gain i.v. access and send blood for FBC, U&Es, LFTs and a plasma cholinesterase level, which is a marker of exposure, but a poor indicator of severity.

5   Perform an ECG to evaluate cardiac arrhythmias.

6   Request a CXR as aspiration pneumonitis is common.

MANAGEMENT

1   Instruct all staff to wear a gown and gloves when removing soiled clothing or washing the skin.

2   Give oxygen, and call an airway-skilled doctor to pass an endotracheal tube for severe bronchorrhoea and respiratory failure.

3   Commence a normal saline infusion to manage hypotension and replace losses.

4   Treat seizures with midazolam 0.05–0.1 mg/kg i.v., diazepam 0.1–0.2 mg/kg i.v. or lorazepam 0.07 mg/kg up to 4 mg i.v.

5   Give atropine 1.2 mg i.v. in rapidly escalating doses until the skin becomes dry, and bronchial secretions are minimal.
   (i)   Massive doses (50–100 mg) may be necessary; do not rely on pupillary dilatation and tachycardia as indicative end points, as they may not reflect adequate atropinization.

6   Give pralidoxime 2 g (30 mg/kg) i.v. over 15 min and then 500 mg/h for at least 24 h, in all moderate-to-severe cases (except for carbamate poisoning).
   (i)   Monitor serial plasma or red cell cholinesterase levels and look for signs of clinical improvement before ceasing treatment.

7 Admit the patient to ICU. Delayed paralysis 'intermediate syndrome' occurs with some agents such as fenthion.

> **Warning:** staff treating patients exposed to organophosphates may develop mild headache, eye irritation and pulmonary symptoms secondary to the hydrocarbon solvent and *not* the organophosphate itself. These resolve with simple analgesia and by removing the staff from the exposure source.

PARAQUAT

DIAGNOSIS

1 Paraquat is a highly toxic herbicide. Significant oral ingestion is associated with fulminant multi-organ failure. If patients survive this, they develop progressive pulmonary fibrosis, and may die 4–6 weeks later from hypoxaemia.

2 Clinical effects depend on the route of exposure:
  (i) Skin: localized irritation, erythema, blistering, ulceration.
  (ii) Eyes: corneal inflammation, oedema, ulceration.
  (iii) Systemic from oral ingestion:
    (a) <15 mL of 20% solution: nausea, vomiting and diarrhoea with reversible pulmonary irritation
    (b) >15 mL of 20% solution: pharyngeal necrosis, hypersalivation, pneumonitis, intractable vomiting, haematemesis, severe abdominal pain and bowel perforation.

3 Gain i.v. access and send blood for FBC, U&Es, LFT, coagulation profile and blood sugar level. Request a serum paraquat level.
  (i) A serum level of >5 mg/L is invariably fatal.

4 A qualitative urine test may be performed by adding 1 mL of 1% sodium dithionite solution to 10 mL of urine. Paraquat ingestion is confirmed if the urine turns blue.

5 Perform an ECG.

6 Request a CXR to look for evidence of mediastinitis, aspiration, pulmonary opacities and abdominal viscus perforation.

MANAGEMENT

1 Early gastrointestinal decontamination is paramount. Give activated charcoal 50–100 g **immediately** orally or via a nasogastric tube.
  (i) The traditional alternative adsorbing agent 15% aqueous suspension Fuller's earth (bentonite) 1000 mL is rarely available now.

2 Administer oxygen only if the SaO_2 is <90%, as otherwise oxygen enhances pulmonary toxicity.

3 Refer the patient immediately for admission to ICU. Early haemodialysis may benefit.

CHEMICAL BURNS

DIAGNOSIS

1 These occur at home, in schools, in laboratories and in industrial accidents.

2 Most agents are strong acids or alkalis, although occasionally phosphorus and phenol are responsible.

3 Alkali burns are generally more serious than acid as they penetrate deeper.

MANAGEMENT

1 Wear gloves to remove any contaminated clothing. Treat by copious irrigation with running water. Continue irrigating for at least 30 min.

2 Do **not** attempt to neutralize the chemical, as many resultant reactions produce heat and will exacerbate the injury, *except* in the case of hydrofluoric acid.

3 *Hydrofluoric acid burns*
   (i) Neutralize these as follows:
      (a) convert hydrofluoric acid to the calcium salt by covering the affected area with dressings soaked in 10% calcium gluconate solution, or by rubbing in 2.5% calcium gluconate gel
      (b) inject s.c. 10% calcium gluconate if the pain and burning persist
      (c) give i.v. regional treatment with 10% calcium gluconate (similar to a Bier's block technique) for an extensive limb burn.
   (ii) Dermal absorption of fluoride ions may result in systemic fluorosis causing hypocalcaemia, hypomagnesaemia, hyperkalaemia and cardiac arrest
      (a) *systemic fluorosis* may follow burns affecting as little as 2–5% of body surface area from concentrated 70% hydrofluoric acid
      (b) seek immediate senior ED doctor help, and give large amounts of i.v. calcium chloride and magnesium sulphate as indicated clinically, from serum levels and ECG monitoring for QTc prolongation.

4 Refer all patients to the surgical team unless the area burnt is minimal and the patient is pain free.

5 Refer patients with systemic fluorosis to ICU. The hyperkalaemia may require haemodialysis.

FURTHER READING

American Heart Association (2015) Part 10: Special circumstances of resuscitation: 2015 American Heart Association guidelines update for cardiopulmonary resuscitation and emergency cardiovascular care. *Circulation* **132**: S501–S518.

European Resuscitation Council (2015). European Resuscitation Council Guidelines for Resuscitation 2015 Section 4. Cardiac arrest in special circumstances. *Resuscitation* **95**: 148–201.

Murray L, Little M, Pascu O, Hoggett K (2015). *Toxicology Handbook*, 3rd edition. Elsevier, Sydney.

National Poisons Information Service TOXBASE®. http://www.toxbase.org/ (poisons information).

Therapeutic Guidelines. eTG complete 2015. http://www.tg.org.au/

Toxinz. http://www.toxinz.com/ (toxicology first aid and management).

TOXINOLOGY EMERGENCIES

SNAKE BITES

Australian snakebite management advice is available from the Poisons Information Centre (24 h) on **13 11 26**. There are no endemic venomous snakes in New Zealand, although poisons prevention and education including toxinology advice is available from the National Poisons Centre on 03 479 7248 (or **0800 764 766** (24 h) within New Zealand).

Snake bite is exceedingly rare in the UK, but may present in zookeepers and herpetologists, or following a mishap with an exotic pet. Advice on management is always available from the National Poisons Information Service (24 h) TOXBASE® on **0844 892 0111** in the UK.

ELAPID SNAKE BITES

DIAGNOSIS

1 Some of the most venomous snakes in the world are elapid snakes found in Australia.
   - (i) Elapids have small, permanently erect front fangs and produce venom containing haemotoxins, neurotoxins and myotoxins
     - (a) major species include brown snake, black snake, taipan, tiger snake and death adder
     - (b) however, only 5–10% snake bites by a venomous snake lead to severe envenomation, with just 1–5 deaths annually in Australia
     - (c) the rest are non-envenoming 'dry bites'.

2 Bites such as from the tiger snake and black snake may cause immediate local pain, bruising or swelling within hours, although local signs following a snakebite are usually minimal, with fine scratches or small puncture marks only.

3 Look for the following signs that indicate systemic envenomation, although these may be subtle or fluctuate:
   - (i) Non-specific findings such as headache, sweating, nausea, vomiting, abdominal pain, diarrhoea and transient hypotension.
   - (ii) Tissue-specific findings indicating severe envenomation (any one of):
     - (a) *haemotoxic* effects including asymptomatic venom-induced consumptive coagulopathy (VICC) with undetectable fibrinogen/raised international normalized ratio (INR) >3.0/ raised D-dimer (10 times assay cut-off) on laboratory testing, or causing bite- or venepuncture-site oozing, haematemesis, melaena or collapse
     - (b) *thrombotic microangiopathy* with raised creatinine with or without renal failure, thrombocytopenia and intravascular haemolysis on blood film

      (c) *neurotoxic* effects including ptosis, diplopia, dysphagia and respiratory or distal paralysis

      (d) *myotoxic* effects including muscle pain or tenderness with creatine kinase (CK) >1000 U/L, myoglobinuria and renal failure.

    (iii) Sudden collapse, convulsions and cardiac arrest (especially brown snake).

4 Gain i.v. access and send blood for full blood count (FBC), urea and electrolytes (U&Es), CK and coagulation profile including INR, activated partial thromboplastin time (aPTT) and fibrinogen. Attach a cardiac monitor and pulse oximeter to the patient.

5 Send urine for protein, haemoglobin and myoglobin estimation.

6 Attempt to identify the snake species with a venom detection kit (VDK) analysis from a bite-site swab (carefully taken from a window cut in the pressure bandage), or on the urine.

    (i) Visual inspection and an amateur 'guess' at the species is unreliable and misleading, and is a waste of time unless you are a trained herpetologist.

7 Perform an electrocardiogram (ECG), chest radiograph (CXR) and spirometry in significant envenoming.

MANAGEMENT

1 Make sure that first aid has been applied to impede the spread of venom through local lymphatics, using a pressure bandage with immobilization (PBI) technique:

    (i) Apply a broad firm bandage around the bite site and extend proximally up the limb to cover it completely, as tight as one would bandage a sprained ankle.

    (ii) Splint the dependent limb and organize for transport to be brought to the patient.

    (iii) Keep the pressure bandage with immobilization in place until the first set of bloods are negative and the patient is asymptomatic, or if envenomed until definitive treatment has been instituted and the patient is systemically improved.

2 Give high-flow oxygen via face mask and watch for any signs of airway compromise.

3 Give antivenom for definite systemic envenomation. Do **not** give antivenom for a positive VDK result alone, if no other abnormal clinical or laboratory features are present:

    (i) Indications for antivenom therefore include the presence of clinical signs particularly impending respiratory arrest, refractory hypotension, cardiac arrhythmias and renal failure, and/or for abnormal laboratory findings, including consumption coagulopathy.

(ii) Give the appropriate species-specific monovalent antivenom if the snake species has been positively identified on VDK (or by an expert herpetologist).

    (a) start with one vial (1000 units) in brown snake envenoming whilst awaiting resynthesis of clotting factors over the next 12–18 h

    (b) likewise give one vial (3000 units) for tiger snake envenoming; one vial (12000 units) for taipan; and start with one vial for envenoming by black snake (18000 units) and death adder (6000 units).

(iii) Get expert advice urgently if the snake species is still unknown in an envenomed patient

    (a) give one vial of monovalent tiger snake antivenom in Tasmania, as tiger snakes are the only terrestrial venomous snake native to that state

    (b) give one vial each of tiger and brown snake monovalent antivenom in Victoria which cover all medically important species

    (c) in the other Australian states, give one vial of polyvalent antivenom i.v. This is more expensive and carries a greater risk of anaphylaxis.

(iv) Give antivenom slowly by i.v. infusion over 30 min after 1 in 10 dilution with normal saline

    (a) give an undiluted neat bolus of antivenom as a life-saving measure if the patient is in cardiac arrest or has circulatory collapse.

(v) Pre-treatment with adrenaline (epinephrine) is unhelpful, but adrenaline must be available as there is the possibility of anaphylaxis to the horse-serum derived antivenom:

    (a) although up to one-third of antivenom administrations cause a hypersensitivity reaction, <5% are anaphylaxis.

4   Give tetanus prophylaxis according to the patient's immune status.

5   Refer all patients with signs of systemic envenomation to ICU or the local toxicology unit.

6   Remove the pressure bandage and observe carefully those patients who remain systemically well, with no clinical signs of envenomation and who have normal initial laboratory blood tests.

(i) Repeat the laboratory tests 1 h after bandage removal, including INR, aPTT and CK

    (a) treat with antivenom if they become abnormal, of if the patient develops any clinical signs of envenoming.

(ii) Observe the patient for a further 12 h prior to discharge, with careful clinical examination looking particularly for delayed neurotoxicity or myotoxicity

(a) repeat the same laboratory tests including INR, aPTT and CK at 6 h and again at 12 h after bandage removal. If these remain normal and the patient is well, discharge.

VIPER (ADDER) SNAKE BITES

DIAGNOSIS

1 Snakes of the viper species include the North American rattlesnake, the African rhinoceros viper and the adder, which is the only naturally occurring venomous snake in the UK.

2 Local effects of an adder bite from the relatively long, foldable fangs include pain, bruising, swelling and local tender lymphadenopathy within hours of the bite.

(i) However, fewer than 50% of bites are associated with envenomation, and occasionally systemic poisoning may occur with no local reaction.

3 Systemic envenomation causes:

(i) Early features including non-allergic anaphylaxis with transient syncope and hypotension, angioedema, urticaria, abdominal pain, vomiting and diarrhoea.

(ii) Late features including recurrent or persistent hypotension, ECG changes, spontaneous bleeding, coagulopathy, adult respiratory distress syndrome and acute renal failure.

4 Gain i.v. access, and send blood for FBC, clotting screen, lactate, U&Es and liver function tests (LFTs).

5 Perform an ECG and a CXR in severe cases.

MANAGEMENT

1 Reassure the patient, apply a firm bandage proximal to the bite, immobilize the dependent limb and transport the patient rapidly to hospital.

2 Treat non-allergic anaphylaxis reactions with oxygen, adrenaline (epinephrine) and fluids (see p. 27).

3 Give European viper venom antiserum for significant adder envenomation:

(i) Indications for viper venom antiserum include:

(a) hypotension/acidosis

(b) ECG changes

(c) peripheral neutrophil leucocytosis

(d) bleeding

(e) extending limb swelling within 4 h of the bite.

    (ii)   Add one 10 mL vial to normal saline 5 mL/kg diluent and infuse over 30 min, repeated as indicated.

    (iii) Have adrenaline (epinephrine) immediately available for anaphylactic reactions to the antivenom.

4 Give tetanus prophylaxis, and refer all patients to the medical team for admission, even in the absence of initial symptoms or signs.

SPIDER BITES

The majority of spider bites are associated with local symptoms of pain and erythema. Certain species are associated with significant envenomation, and may be fatal.

DIAGNOSIS

1 *Latrodectus* species includes the red-back (Australia), the black widow (America), and the katipo (New Zealand) spiders. Envenomation is by the female. Clinical features of latrodectism include:

    (i)   Local pain, erythema, sweating, lymphadenopathy and piloerection.

    (ii) Systemic features such as headache, nausea, vomiting, abdominal pain, generalized sweating and hypotension.

2 Over 40 species of funnel-web spider occur in Australia, with the most significant envenomation by the male Sydney funnel-web spider. Clinical features of funnel-web spider envenomation include:

    (i)   Severe localized pain, with erythema.

    (ii) Generalized muscle fasciculations, nausea, vomiting, abdominal pain, sweating, lacrimation and salivation.

    (iii) Initial tachycardia and hypertension progressing to hypotension, pulmonary oedema and finally convulsions and coma.

3 Base the diagnosis on history and clinical examination, as no laboratory tests are helpful.

4 Perform an ECG and request a CXR if funnel-web spider bite is suspected.

MANAGEMENT

1 Apply a pressure-immobilization bandage immediately after a funnel-web spider bite to retard the spread of the venom. **Never** use this in red-back spider envenomation.

2 Otherwise, give general first-aid treatment by applying ice or heat and giving oral analgesia as symptomatic relief.

3   Observe all sick patients in a monitored resuscitation area, assess and secure the airway, and administer oxygen. Gain i.v. access only if antivenom is indicated.

4   Antivenom administration:
  (i)   **Red-back spider antivenom**
     (a)   administer red-back spider antivenom to patients with clinical manifestations of systemic toxicity or severe uncontrolled local pain
     (b)   give two vials (1000 units) by slow i.v. infusion over 20 min diluted in 100 mL normal saline.
  (ii)   **Funnel-web spider antivenom**
     (a)   administer funnel-web spider antivenom to patients with clinical manifestations of systemic toxicity or severe uncontrolled local symptoms
     (b)   give two vials (250 units) i.v. slowly and repeat every 15 min until symptoms have resolved
     (c)   refer all patients with persistent local symptoms or significant systemic envenomation to the intensive care unit (ICU)
     (d)   discharge other patients who remain systemically well, with absence of signs of envenoming by 4 h after removal of any first-aid pressure bandage applied.

MARINE ENVENOMATION

Several hazardous marine animals are found in coastal waters around the world. Warm water immersion is useful symptomatic treatment for injuries from many species of spiny fish, with antivenom therapy available for only a few specific instances.

DIAGNOSIS

1   *Jellyfish*
  (i)   *Irukandji syndrome* (Australia). This causes mild local pain followed 30–40 min later by severe generalized muscle cramps, back and abdominal pain, hypertension, and pulmonary oedema. It is potentially fatal.
  (ii)   *Box jellyfish* (Australia). This causes severe local pain and cross-hatched erythematous dermal lesions, associated with cardiovascular and respiratory collapse. It is also potentially fatal.
  (iii)   *Bluebottle or Portuguese man-of-war* (worldwide). These cause severe local stinging pain, erythema, and elliptical blanched

wheals, rarely associated with a muscle pain syndrome and/or abdominal pain with vomiting.

2 **Poisonous fish** such as the stonefish, lionfish, bullrout (Australia) or lesser weever (UK):
    (i) These fish have venomous spines that can cause extreme local pain and oedema.
    (ii) Systemic effects include diarrhoea, respiratory depression and hypotension.

3 **Sea urchins, fire coral** (worldwide)
    (i) Sea urchins cause local erythema and pain from the many tiny spines which may break off and enter a joint cavity or the deep palmar or plantar spaces.
    (ii) Fire coral causes local burning similar to a jellyfish sting.

MANAGEMENT

1 Assess and secure the airway first and provide basic life support to patients with cardiovascular collapse and systemic toxicity.

2 **Jellyfish first aid**
    (i) Box jellyfish and Irukandji (tropical regions): rinse jellyfish wounds with seawater, remove adherent tentacles, and prevent further nematocyst discharge with 5% acetic acid (vinegar).
    (ii) Bluebottle (non-tropical regions): rinse with seawater (**not** vinegar), remove adherent tentacles, and immerse the affected area in warm water at 40–45°C without scalding.

3 **Jellyfish systemic envenomation**
    (i) *Irukandji*
        (a) administer oxygen and give opiate analgesia, e.g. with fentanyl 5 µg/kg i.v. every 10 min until pain is controlled
        (b) commence a glyceryl trinitrate (GTN) infusion if severe hypertension is not controlled with pain management.
    (ii) *Box jellyfish*
        (a) administer oxygen and commence i.v. fluid resuscitation for hypotension. Give morphine 5–10 mg i.v. for severe local pain
        (b) administer box jellyfish antivenom if the pain is refractory to opiates, the patient is shocked, or in cardiac arrest:
            – give one vial (20 000 units) diluted 1 in 10 with normal saline i.v. over 30 min or up to six vials as a bolus in cardiac arrest
            – give 0.1 mL/kg up to 5 mL of 49.3% magnesium sulphate i.v. bolus over 15 min as well, particularly for cardiovascular collapse

4 *Poisonous fish*

    (i)   Immerse the affected area in warm water at 40–45°C without scalding. If pain persists, perform a regional block with 2% lignocaine (lidocaine) and give morphine 5–10 mg i.v.

    (ii)   Debride the wound, remove spines and give tetanus prophylaxis according to the patient's immune status.

    (iii) Systemic stonefish envenomation: give one vial (2000 units) of stonefish antivenom i.m. for every two puncture marks visible.

5 *Sea urchins and fire coral*

    (i)   Relieve pain by immersion in warm water at 40–45°C without scalding or by using a local anaesthetic block, followed by exploration, irrigation and debridement as necessary, and give tetanus prophylaxis.

    (ii)   Give an antibiotic such as doxycycline 100 mg orally b.d. for 5 days (not in children or pregnant patients), for deep or necrotic wounds.

BEE AND WASP STINGS

DIAGNOSIS

1 There are more deaths from anaphylaxis following bee or wasp stings than from all the other venomous bites and stings combined.

2 Local pain predominates and may be followed by a severe anaphylactic reaction causing laryngeal oedema, bronchospasm, hypotension and collapse (see p. 27).

MANAGEMENT

1 Remove a bee sting by scraping the sting out with a knife, without squeezing.

2 Anaphylaxis:

    (i)   Assess and secure the airway, give oxygen, gain i.v. access and commence fluid resuscitation for shock.

    (ii)   Give 1 in 1000 adrenaline (epinephrine) 0.3–0.5 mg (0.3–0.5 mL) i.m. early.

    (ii)   Give 1 in 10 000 adrenaline (epinephrine) or 1 in 100 000 adrenaline (epinephrine) 0.75–1.5 µg/kg, i.e. 50–100 µg slowly i.v. if circulatory collapse occurs, with a bolus of normal saline 20–40 mL/kg.

3 Arrange for patients prone to anaphylaxis from bee or wasp stings to carry a pre-filled adrenaline (epinephrine) syringe (EpiPen® or Anapen®) at all times.

Murray L, Little M, Pascu O, Hoggett K (2015) *Toxicology Handbook*, 3rd edition, Elsevier, Sydney.

National Poisons Information Service TOXBASE®. http://www.toxbase.org/ (poisons information).

Therapeutic Guidelines. eTG complete 2015. http://www.tg.org.au/

Toxinz. http://www.toxinz.com/ (toxicology first aid and management).

University of Adelaide. *Clinical Toxinology Resources.* http://www.toxinology. com/(global toxinology database).

Section XVI

ENVIRONMENTAL EMERGENCIES

HEAT, COLD AND DROWNING

HEAT ILLNESS

Heat illness occurs when the body's capacity to dissipate heat is exceeded by internal heat production and/or by heat stress from an external source.

Heat illness is predisposed to by hot weather, exercise, obesity, fever, lack of physical fitness or acclimatization, skin disease such as psoriasis or eczema, alcohol intake, and drugs such as anticholinergic agents, cocaine and amphetamines.

DIAGNOSIS

1   **Mild to moderate heat illness**

Thermoregulatory mechanisms remain intact.
   - (i)   *Heat cramps*
      - (a) pain develops in heavily exercising muscles in hot weather secondary to sodium depletion and dehydration.
   - (ii)   *Heat exhaustion*
      - (a) thirst, cramps, headache, vertigo, anorexia, nausea and vomiting occur
      - (b) the patient is flushed and sweating, with rectal temperature of 38–39°C
      - (c) tachycardia and orthostatic hypotension occur secondary to dehydration.

2   **Severe heat illness: Heat stroke**

Thermoregulatory mechanisms fail and the rectal temperature is over 40°C.
   - (i)   *Classic (non-exertional) heat stroke* (CHS):
      CHS usually occurs in the elderly or very young during a heat wave secondary to high environmental temperatures.
   - (ii)   *Exertional heat stroke* (EHS):
      EHS is associated with young adults exercising in high temperatures.
   - (iii)   Symptoms include headache, vomiting and diarrhoea associated with mental state change progressing to aggressive or bizarre behaviour, collapse, seizures and coma.
   - (iv)   Hot dry skin is usual, but profuse sweating occurs in up to 50% of patients with exertional heat stroke.
   - (v)   The patient is flushed, tachypnoeic, tachycardic and hypotensive. Muscle rigidity, rhabdomyolysis, transient hemiplegia, dilated pupils, disseminated intravascular coagulation (DIC) and multi-organ failure may all occur.

(vi) Gain i.v. access and send blood for full blood count (FBC), coagulation profile, urea and electrolytes (U&Es), blood sugar, liver function tests (LFTs), creatinine kinase (CK) and lactate.

(vii) Check an arterial blood gas (ABG). Attach an electrocardiographic (ECG) monitor and pulse oximeter to the patient.

MANAGEMENT

1 *Heat cramps*

(i) Rest in a cool environment, and replace fluid orally with added salt or give 1 L normal saline iv.

(ii) The patient is usually able to go home.

2 *Heat exhaustion*

(i) Rest in a cool environment and give up to 3 L cooled normal saline i.v.

(ii) Cool the patient with tepid sponging and fanning.

(iii) Admit for observation, particularly when elderly or if orthostatic hypotension persists.

3 *Heat stroke*

(i) Give oxygen and aim for an oxygen saturation above 94%. Call the senior emergency department (ED) doctor for help, and arrange for endotracheal intubation for airway protection.

(ii) Commence urgent cooling by tepid sponging, fans, cooling mattress and cold packs to the groin and axillae until the temperature is <38.5°C

  (a) avoid excessive shivering, but do not use chlorpromazine 25 mg i.v. to suppress this due to its multiple side effects

  (b) antipyretics such as aspirin and paracetamol are also *not* indicated.

(iii) Give 1 L cooled normal saline over 20 min, then give fluid according to the blood pressure, serum sodium level and urine output.

(iv) Give midazolam 0.05–0.1 mg/kg up to 10 mg i.v., diazepam 0.1–0.2 mg/kg up to 20 mg i.v., or lorazepam 0.07 mg/kg up to 4 mg i.v. for seizures and/or agitation.

(v) Monitor for complications such as hypoglycaemia and give 50% dextrose 50 mL.

(vi) Give 8.4% sodium bicarbonate 50 mL plus 20% mannitol 0.5–1.0 g/kg (2.5–5 mL/kg) for rhabdomyolysis, and maintain a urinary output of 1–2 mL/kg per h.

(vii) Admit the patient to the intensive care unit (ICU) for sedation, intubation and ongoing cooling, plus exclusion of infection and other hyperthermia syndrome causes.

OTHER HYPERTHERMIA-RELATED ILLNESS

Hyperthermia-related syndromes may be associated with specific drug administration such as anticholinergic agents, serotonin agonists, dopamine antagonists and inhalational anaesthetics. Sepsis must be excluded as part of the diagnosis.

DIAGNOSIS

1 Neuroleptic malignant syndrome
> (i)   Rare but potentially lethal syndrome complicating the use of dopamine receptor-blocking drugs such as antipsychotic agents (e.g. chlorpromazine, haloperidol) and some antiemetics (metoclopramide).
> (ii) Or the patient may have had a dopaminergic drug such as levodopa or bromocriptine suddenly withdrawn.
> (iii) It is associated with development of muscle rigidity, bradyreflexia, bradykinesia, altered mental status, extrapyramidal symptoms and hyperthermia.

2 Serotonin syndrome
> (i)   This is a clinical manifestation of excessive stimulation of serotonin receptors in the central nervous system (CNS).
> (ii) It follows drug combinations with selective serotonin reuptake inhibitors (SSRIs), monoamine-uptake inhibitors, lithium, analgesics such as fentanyl or tramadol, antiemetics such as ondansetron, and illicit drugs such as amphetamine or cocaine.
> (iii) It has a spectrum of severity ranging from agitation and hyperreflexia through to generalized rigidity worse in the legs, myoclonus, autonomic instability, mental status changes and hyperthermia.

3 Malignant hyperthermia syndrome
> (i)   A rare autosomal dominant disorder that develops during or after receiving an inhalational anaesthetic or suxamethonium.
> (ii) Characterized by muscular rigidity, hypercapnoea, tachycardia, hypertension, mottled diaphoretic skin and cardiac arrhythmias.

4 Gain i.v. access and send urgent bloods including FBC, coagulation profile, electrolyte and liver function tests (ELFTs), CK and lactate. Add two sets of blood cultures if sepsis is suspected.

5 Check an ABG, perform an ECG, and send a midstream urine (MSU) sample.

MANAGEMENT

1 Give high flow oxygen and commence i.v. normal saline.

2 Check the temperature, begin supportive care and admit under the medical team, or to ICU.

    (i) Temperature >38.5° is an indication for continuous core-temperature monitoring.

    (ii) Temperature >39.5° with an altered mental status is an emergency:

        (a) arrange a senior doctor to perform endotracheal intubation and ventilation with muscle paralysis, to protect the airway and prevent further muscle-generated heat production leading to multiple organ failure, neurological injury and death.

3 *Neuroleptic malignant syndrome*

    (i) Give bromocriptine (a dopamine agonist) orally or via a nasogastric tube. Start at 2.5 mg 8-hourly, increasing to 5 mg every 4 h (maximum 30 mg/day) in moderate to severe cases.

4 *Serotonin syndrome*

    (i) Give cyproheptadine 8 mg orally or via nasogastric tube, repeated 8-hourly in mild to moderate cases.

    (ii) Add midazolam 0.05–0.1 mg/kg i.v., or diazepam 0.1–0.2 mg/kg i.v. titrated to achieve gentle sedation.

5 *Malignant hyperthermia syndrome*

    (i) Administer dantrolene 1 mg/kg i.v. for severe muscle rigidity and hyperthermia. Further doses of 1–2.5 mg/kg (up to a maximum of 10 mg/kg/24 h) may be required.

HYPOTHERMIA

This is present when the core temperature drops to <35°C (95°F), and occurs when heat loss exceeds the body's ability to produce and conserve heat.

Mild hypothermia is classified as 32–35°C (89.6–95°F), moderate hypothermia as 29–32°C (84.2–89.6°F), and severe hypothermia as <29°C (84.2°F).

DIAGNOSIS

1 Hypothermia is predisposed by the following:

    (i) Exposure to low air temperatures, particularly with wind and rain.

    (ii) Exposure in cold water.

    (iii) Unconscious patient, or patients who have taken sedative drugs, especially alcohol.

    (iv) Infants or the elderly with intercurrent illness, e.g. stroke, sepsis, diabetic ketoacidosis (DKA).

    (v) Endocrine disorders, such as myxoedema or hypopituitary coma (rare).

2 Clinical manifestations include:

    (i) *Mild hypothermia:* poor judgement, lethargy, ataxia, shivering and tachypnoea.

    (ii) *Moderate hypothermia:* bradycardia, hypotension, bradypnoea, and confusion. Shivering ceases.

(iii) *Severe hypothermia:* the patient is comatose and may appear dead with an undetectable pulse, absent reflexes, unrecordable blood pressure and fixed pupils.

3   Record the core temperature rectally with a low-reading thermometer. This is more accurate than any tympanic membrane device.

4   Send blood for FBC, U&Es, CK, coagulation profile and blood sugar level. Check serum lipase/amylase, as pancreatitis may be associated. Send ABGs.

5   Perform an ECG.
    (i)   Look for evidence of bradycardia, low-voltage complexes, atrial fibrillation and prolongation of the QT interval.
    (ii) Osborn 'J' waves (a slurred notching of the terminal portion of the QRS complex) may be present at core temperatures of <32°C
          (a) Osborn waves are not pathognomic and are seen in other conditions such as subarachnoid haemorrhage, head trauma and hypercalcaemia.

6   Request a CXR.

MANAGEMENT

1   **Mild hypothermia**
    (i)   Remove wet clothing and cover the patient in warm blankets and layers of polythene to minimize evaporative, convective and conductive heat loss.
    (ii) Rehydrate the alert but shivering patient, and give high-energy food and warm drinks.

2   **Moderate and severe hypothermia** (core temperature ≤32°C)
    (i)   Remove wet clothing and cover the patient in warm blankets and layers of polythene to minimize evaporative, convective and conductive heat loss.
    (ii) Give high-flow, warmed 42–46°C (108–115°F), humidified oxygen.
    (iii) Use a forced-air re-warming blanket, e.g. Bair Hugger®, and aim for a core temperature rise of at least 1°C/h in younger patients and 0.5°C per h in the elderly.
    (iv) Give i.v. fluids cautiously through a warming device at 43°C (109°F). Pulmonary oedema may be precipitated by excessive fluid administration.
    (v)   Take extreme care with any airway manoeuvres such as endotracheal intubation, as this may precipitate ventricular fibrillation (VF) in severe hypothermia. Call the senior ED doctor for help.

3   **Cardiac arrest in a hypothermic patient**
    (i)   *Severe hypothermia* (core temperature <29°C)
          (a) attempt defibrillation once for VF, delivering 150–200 J biphasic

      (b) standard resuscitation drugs are usually ineffective as the efficacy of adrenaline (epinephrine) and amiodarone are reduced, with an increased circulation time

      (c) provide aggressive active internal re-warming with warmed 40°C pleural, gastric or peritoneal lavage, aiming for a core temperature rise to at least 33°C

      (d) extracorporeal blood re-warming is ideal, when available.

  (ii) **Moderate hypothermia** (core temperature 29–32°C)

      (a) attempt defibrillation with one direct current (DC) shock

      (b) administer standard resuscitation medications, but double the time between doses.

  (iii) Apply usual resuscitation protocols with core temperatures of ≥33°C.

  (iv) Continue resuscitation attempts in hypothermic cardiac arrest until the core temperature rises to at least 33°C, or until a senior doctor advises to the contrary

      (a) this may involve a prolonged period of resuscitation and aggressive measures as outlined.

DROWNING

DIAGNOSIS

1 Drowning is a common cause of accidental death in Australasia and Europe. It is defined as any process that results in primary respiratory impairment following immersion (face and upper airway), or submersion (whole body) in a liquid medium.

2 Duration of hypoxia is the most important factor that determines outcome and a full neurological recovery. Victims with spontaneous circulation and breathing on arrival at hospital usually have a good outcome.

3 The presence of lung crackles indicates likely inhalation of water, with the risk of hypoxaemia. The initial difference between sea water (hypertonic) and fresh water (hypotonic) drowning is of little clinical significance. However, contaminated water such as sewage will require antibiotic prophylaxis.

  (i) About 15% of drowned victims experience 'dry drowning', likely due to laryngospasm, where little or no fluid is found in the lungs.

4 Consider other more relevant factors:

  (i) Preceding injury, especially to the cervical spine in a diving accident.

  (ii) Sudden preceding illness, such as an arrhythmia, hypoglycaemia or epileptic seizure that may have led to the drowning.

  (iii) Alcohol or drug use (a contributing factor in up to 50% of drownings).

  (iv) Hypothermia depending on water temperature and exposure.

5 Check FBC, U&Es, blood sugar, lactate and ABGs. Attach a cardiac monitor and pulse oximeter to the patient.

6 Perform an ECG and request a CXR.

MANAGEMENT

1 Record the rectal temperature and re-warm the patient if the core temperature is low.

2 Commence cardiopulmonary resuscitation if the patient has no detectable cardiac output or is not breathing.
  (i) Be careful to control the cervical spine if a neck injury is suspected.
  (ii) Insert a nasogastric tube early to decompress the stomach. Gastric regurgitation is common in patients requiring basic life support.
  (iii) Continue prolonged resuscitation efforts, which may be successful particularly with drowning in cold water associated with sudden hypothermia.

3 Otherwise, give high-flow oxygen and aim for an oxygen saturation above 94%.

4 Call an airway-skilled doctor to intubate the patient if unconscious or he or she develops respiratory failure with a PaO_2 of <75 mmHg (10 kPa) on 50% oxygen, or a rising $PaCO_2$ >56 mmHg (7.5 kPa).

5 Refer all patients to the medical team or ICU for admission.
  (i) Delayed adult respiratory distress syndrome (ARDS) may develop 6–72 h after submersion, previously referred to as 'secondary drowning'.
  (ii) Initiate cerebral protection measures in the comatose patient. Prevent and treat hypoglycaemia, hypotension, seizures and intracranial hypertension. Maintain normocarbia.

SPORTS-DIVING ACCIDENTS

Dysbarism is the medical complication of exposure to gases at higher than normal atmospheric pressure. It manifests clinically as decompression illness (DCI), which may be further classified by the acuity, evolution, presence or absence of barotrauma and the organs involved.

It is most commonly associated with sports-diving accidents such as scuba (self-contained underwater breathing apparatus) diving.

DECOMPRESSION ILLNESS

Decompression illness (DCI) occurs when inert nitrogen gas forms bubbles within the venous and lymphatic systems, or body tissues, rather than being eliminated by the lungs.

DIAGNOSIS

1 Symptoms may occur within minutes of surfacing or up to 48 hours after diving. It is important to look for and treat any patient who presents within hours of a dive as DCI until proven otherwise.

2 Clinical manifestations include:

(i) *Mild*

(a) joint pain, ranging from a dull ache to the crippling 'bends'. Pain usually commences in large joints such as the elbow or shoulder and may migrate

(b) unusual fatigue and malaise

(c) skin itching, marbling (*cutis marmorata*), scarlatiniform rashes, painful lymphadenopathy and local oedema.

(ii) *Serious*

(a) cardiopulmonary:

– '*the chokes*': retrosternal or pleuritic chest pain, dyspnoea, cough and haemoptysis

– may be associated with myocardial infarction, hypotension and cardiac arrhythmia, and progress to respiratory failure

(b) central nervous system:

– '*the staggers*': labyrinthine damage with deafness, tinnitus, nystagmus, vertigo and nausea

– motor and sensory loss with hemiplegia and paraplegia

– personality disorder, seizures and urinary retention.

3 Gain i.v. access and take blood for FBC, U&Es, LFTs, blood sugar level, troponin and CK. The peak CK can be a marker for the severity of acute gas embolism, although does not directly influence management.

4 Perform an ECG and request a CXR in patients with cardiopulmonary symptoms.

MANAGEMENT

1 Give the patient 100% oxygen by tight-fitting face mask with reservoir bag. Manage the patient in the supine or left lateral position.

2 Commence normal saline rehydration, avoiding glucose-containing solutions as they may exacerbate CNS injury.

3 Give midazolam 0.05–0.1 mg/kg i.v., diazepam 0.1–0.2 mg/kg i.v. or lorazepam 0.07 mg/kg up to 4 mg i.v. for seizures.

(i) These drugs may also be used for severe labyrinthine disturbance after discussion with a hyperbaric medicine unit.

4 Minimize strong analgesics, particularly opiates, as they mask symptoms.

5 Fill the endotracheal tube cuff with saline to avoid changes in volume on recompression if mechanical ventilation is required.

6 Refer every patient, however strange their symptoms, to a hyperbaric medicine unit:

    (i)   Provide information about any dive in the preceding 48 h, including the depth and duration, gas mix, time and duration of symptoms.

    (ii) Advice on diagnosis and arrangements for treatment are available by telephoning local or national hyperbaric medicine units

        (a) in a dire emergency ring the police or coastguard, who will have the relevant contact details.

    (iii) Long-distance retrievals require air transport pressurized to 1 atmosphere.

DECOMPRESSION ILLNESS WITH BAROTRAUMA

DIAGNOSIS

1   *Middle ear barotrauma*

    (i)   This is the most common medical disorder associated with diving, almost always occurring on descent.

    (ii) Symptoms include local pain, tinnitus and conductive hearing loss.

    (iii) The tympanic membrane appears reddened or may rupture with sudden relief of pain and minor bleeding.

2   *Inner ear barotrauma*

    (i)   This is associated with too rapid descent without equalising.

    (ii) Vertigo, tinnitus and sensorineural deafness occur secondary to rupture of the round or oval windows and an associated perilymph fistula.

    (iii) It mimics labyrinthine CNS decompression illness.

3   *Sinus barotrauma*

Local pain occurs over the maxillary and frontal sinus, sometimes associated with epistaxis.

4   *Dental barotrauma*

Pain occurs in or around fillings or carious teeth and percussion of the involved tooth is painful.

5   *Pulmonary barotrauma*

This is the most serious form of barotrauma on ascending that causes:

    (i)   Surgical emphysema, pneumothorax or pneumomediastinum associated with chest pain and dyspnoea.

    (ii) Arterial gas embolus affecting the:

        (a) coronary circulation, with cardiac pain, arrhythmia and cardiac arrest

        (b) cerebral circulation, with sudden onset of neurological symptoms just before or within 5 min of surfacing (without the delay seen in CNS decompression illness)

           – any neurological symptom or sign from confusion to seizures or coma may occur, and may fluctuate.

6 Gain i.v. access and take blood for FBC, U&Es, LFTs, blood sugar level and cardiac biomarkers.

7 Perform an ECG in patients with cardiopulmonary symptoms, and request a CXR to exclude pneumothorax or pneumomediastinum.

MANAGEMENT

1 *Middle ear barotrauma*
   (i) Give an analgesic such as paracetamol 500 mg and codeine phosphate 8 mg.
   (ii) Give amoxicillin 500 mg orally t.d.s. for 5 days if tympanic membrane rupture is present, and refer the patient to the next ENT clinic.
   (iii) The patient should not dive again until the drum is fully healed.

2 *Inner ear barotrauma*
   Discuss immediately with a hyperbaric medicine unit, as labyrinthine CNS decompression illness is possible.

3 *Sinus and dental barotrauma*
   Give an analgesic such as paracetamol 500 mg and codeine phosphate 8 mg.

4 *Pulmonary barotrauma*
   (i) Give oxygen and insert an intercostal drain if a significant pneumothorax is present (see p. 473)
      (a) manage a pneumomediastinum and surgical emphysema conservatively.
   (ii) If arterial gas embolus is suspected:
      (a) keep the patient horizontal on their left side (not head-down, as this raises intracranial pressure)
      (b) give 100% oxygen by tight-fitting face mask with reservoir bag
      (c) commence normal saline rehydration
      (d) give midazolam 0.05–0.1 mg/kg i.v., diazepam 0.1–0.2 mg/kg, or lorazepam 0.07 mg/kg up to 4 mg i.v. for seizures
      (e) refer the patient immediately to a hyperbaric medicine unit, even after apparent recovery, as delayed deterioration can occur and recompression may still be required.

ELECTROCUTION AND LIGHTNING STRIKE

Factors influencing the severity of electrical injury include whether the current is alternating or direct, the resistance to current flow, voltage, the pathway of current through the patient and the area and duration of skin contact.

Skin resistance is decreased by moisture which increases the current and the likelihood of injury.

Electrical injury may be considered in four groups:
- Low-voltage electrocution.
- High-voltage electrocution.
- Electrical flash burns.
- Lightning strike.

LOW-VOLTAGE ELECTROCUTION

DIAGNOSIS

1 Injury primarily occurs in the home through faulty electrical equipment or carelessness. Household voltage supply is usually 240 V alternating current (AC).

2 AC is more dangerous than DC and may induce tetanic muscle spasm. The longer the duration of contact, the greater the potential for injury.
    (i) Gripping the electrical source by hand will prevent release and worsens the injury, particularly if sweating occurs.

3 Low-voltage electrical injury causes local tissue necrosis with a contact surface burn that is often full-thickness. The underlying thermal tissue damage may be extensive and include blood vessels and muscle. There may be a similar exit (earthing) burn.

4 Arrhythmias (including VF) and unconsciousness may occur if the charge crosses the heart or brain.

5 Attach a cardiac monitor and pulse oximeter to the patient. Perform a 12-lead ECG.

6 Request a computed tomography (CT) head scan if there is coma, confusion or focal neurological signs.

MANAGEMENT

1 Manage cardiac or respiratory arrest as for cardiopulmonary resuscitation (see p. 2).

2 Otherwise, give oxygen and aim for an oxygen saturation over 94%.

3 Give i.v. normal saline for any hypotension, aiming for a urine output of 100 mL/h if there is evidence of myoglobinuria (tea-coloured urine with a false-positive urine dipstick test for blood).

4 Treat muscle pain with simple analgesia such as paracetamol 500 mg and codeine phosphate 8 mg.

5 Admit patients with an abnormal ECG or history of arrhythmias for cardiac monitoring.

6 Discharge the patient if there is no history of altered consciousness or cardiac arrhythmia, and the neurological state and ECG are normal, provided there is no significant thermal soft-tissue burn.
    (i) A lethal delayed cardiac arrhythmia is exceptionally rare in a patient with no initial history of an arrhythmia.

> **Warning:** electrical burns may look deceptively innocent. A white blister or small area of broken skin can cover extensive deep-tissue damage requiring admission to hospital. Always look for the entry and exit wound.

HIGH-VOLTAGE ELECTROCUTION

DIAGNOSIS

1 These injuries occur from electric shocks sustained from sources >1000 V such as electrical cables and power stations. These are serious injuries, and often fatal.

2 Injuries are associated with:

   (i) Electrical flash burns with full-thickness injury at points of electricity entry and exit, or flame burns secondary to clothing ignition.

   (ii) Extensive tissue damage, deep muscle necrosis, and compartment syndrome requiring fasciotomy and potentially limb amputation.

   (iii) Tetanic muscle spasm causing long-bone fracture, vertebral crush fracture, muscle tears and joint dislocations.

   (iv) Indirect injury from a resultant fall.

3 According to the pathway the charge follows, other effects include:

   (i) Lungs: asphyxia from respiratory paralysis and lung parenchyma burns.

   (ii) Heart: cardiac arrest or arrhythmia. The most common cardiac arrest rhythm is VF.

   (iii) Brain and CNS: confusion, coma, cerebral haemorrhage, spinal cord damage and peripheral nerve damage.

   (iv) Gastrointestinal tract: bowel perforation and intestinal ileus.

   (v) Kidneys: acute kidney injury secondary to tubular deposition of myoglobin and haemoglobin.

   (vi) Visceral and connective tissue: immediate damage to nerves, muscle and bone from heat, vascular thrombosis or delayed secondary haemorrhage.

   (vii) Eyes and ears: dilated pupils, uveitis, vitreous haemorrhage, ruptured eardrum, deafness and the late development of cataracts.

4 Gain i.v. access and send blood for FBC, U&Es, blood sugar, CK, lactate, group and save (G&S) and ABGs. Attach a cardiac monitor and pulse oximeter to the patient.

5 Perform an ECG.

6 Request a CXR, pelvic or limb X-rays, and/or a CT head and neck scan according to the suspected additional injuries.

MANAGEMENT

1 Assess the airway, give oxygen and commence an i.v. infusion ensuring adequate volume replacement guided by the blood pressure and urine output.

    (i) Fluid requirements are higher than they appear from assessment of the burnt areas alone. Aim for a urine output of 100 mL/h if there is myoglobinuria.

2 Examine for major injuries secondary to falls and treat accordingly.

3 Refer patients to the specialist burns unit or surgical team for admission. Escharotomy, fasciotomy, surgical debridement and limb amputation may all become necessary.

ELECTRICAL FLASH BURNS

DIAGNOSIS

1 The external passage of current from the point of contact to the ground is associated with arcing. Electrical energy is converted to heat as electricity traverses the skin associated with brief high temperatures that may ignite clothing.

2 Burns are usually superficial partial-thickness, but they may be deep dermal or even full-thickness. Secondary flame burns may occur if clothing ignites.

MANAGEMENT

1 Assess the depth and extent of the burn (see p. 200).

2 Check the eyes for evidence of corneal injury using fluorescein.

3 Dress the areas as for a thermal burn and treat accordingly.

LIGHTNING STRIKE

DIAGNOSIS

1 Lightning strike can deliver from 300 000 to over 100 000 000 V DC in a few milliseconds, most of which passes over the surface of the body as 'external flashover'.

2 Death is secondary to cardiac or respiratory arrest (as in industrial and domestic electrical injuries).

    (i) The most common rhythm in cardiac arrest is asystole, as opposed to VF with a high-voltage injury.

    (ii) Overall mortality is up to 30%, with 70% of survivors sustaining significant morbidity.

3 Lightning strike can produce a wide range of clinical effects:

    (i) Full-thickness contact burns usually to the head, neck and shoulders, which may follow flashover burning of clothing.

    (ii) Respiratory arrest secondary to thoracic muscle spasm and depressed respiratory drive

(a) this may persist even after return of spontaneous circulation, and may lead to secondary hypoxic arrest.

(iii) Cardiac arrest secondary to depolarization of the entire myocardium.

(iv) Massive autonomic stimulation with hypertension, tachycardia and myocardial necrosis.

(v) Neurological deficits ranging from initial loss of consciousness, sensorineural deafness and vestibular dysfunction to peripheral nerve damage, intracerebral haemorrhage, cerebral oedema and transient total body or limb paralysis (keraunoparalysis).

(vi) Arborescent, feathery cutaneous burns presenting within the first 6 h post injury, known as Lichtenberg figures or lightning flowers.

(vii) Miscellaneous injuries including tympanic membrane rupture, corneal defects, retinal detachment and optic nerve damage.

4   Send bloods for FBC, U&Es, LFTs, CK, blood sugar, lactate and G&S.

5   Perform an ECG and request trauma X-rays such as chest and pelvis, and CT scan of the head and cervical spine as indicated clinically.

(i) Non-specific ECG changes include QT prolongation and T wave inversion.

Warning: do not take fixed dilated pupils as an indicator of death after lightning strike. Full recovery is possible.

MANAGEMENT

1   Use standard protocols for VF and asystolic cardiac arrest if there is no pulse or absent respirations (see p. 2).

2   Assess the airway and give high-flow oxygen. Remove smouldering clothing to prevent secondary thermal injury to skin.

3   Perform early endotracheal intubation to prevent airway obstruction secondary to soft tissue oedema associated with head and neck burns. Call for urgent senior ED doctor help.

(i) Ventilatory support is also essential to prevent hypoxic cardiac arrest secondary to thoracic muscle paralysis.

(ii) Maintain spinal precautions and inline cervical immobilization during endotracheal intubation and physical examination, as there is a risk of unrecognized spinal trauma.

4   Commence an i.v. infusion with normal saline.

(i) Ensure adequate volume replacement guided by blood pressure, urine output and the degree of metabolic and respiratory acidosis.

    (ii)   Give vigorous fluid resuscitation to maintain urine output >1.5 mL/kg per hour to enhance excretion of tissue necrosis by-products such as myoglobin and potassium from extensive rhabdomyolysis.

5   Examine for major injuries secondary to a fall and treat accordingly.

6   Admit all patients. Survivors of the initial lightning strike have an excellent prognosis provided secondary hypoxia or other trauma have not occurred.

Tip: resuscitate those patients at the scene in cardiac arrest *first*, the opposite to a mass casualty disaster, where they would be left for dead while other patients with survivable injuries are treated as the priority.

FURTHER READING

American Heart Association (2015) Part 10: Special circumstances of resuscitation: 2015 American Heart Association guidelines update for cardiopulmonary resuscitation and emergency cardiovascular care. *Circulation* **132**: S501–S518.

European Resuscitation Council (2015) European Resuscitation Council Guidelines for Resuscitation 2015 Section 4. Cardiac arrest in special circumstances. *Resuscitation* **95**: 148–201.

Therapeutic Guidelines. eTG complete 2015. http://www.tg.org.au/

Section XVII

ADMINISTRATIVE AND LEGAL ISSUES

HABITS OF A GOOD EMERGENCY DEPARTMENT DOCTOR

EXCELLENCE IN EMERGENCY DEPARTMENT CARE

Provide excellence in emergency department (ED) care by exhibiting the following traits:

- Communicate clearly in a caring and compassionate manner.
- Listen to the patient, find out what he or she has to say and answer any questions.
- Aim to exclude the differential diagnoses ('rule out') and refine the possible diagnosis ('rule in') when assessing a patient, starting with potentially the most life-or limb-threatening conditions.
- Seek advice and avoid getting out of depth by asking for help early.
- Make sure the patient and relatives know at all times what is happening and why, and what any wait is for.
- Maintain a sense of teamwork. Consider all ED colleagues as equals whether medical, nursing, allied health, administrative or support services.
- Keep exemplary ED medical records (see below).
- Communicate whenever possible with the general practitioner (GP) (see p. 447).
- Know how to break bad news with empathy (see p. 448).
- Adopt effective risk management techniques (see p. 449).

EMERGENCY DEPARTMENT MEDICAL RECORDS

Record accurate and concise information for every patient examined in the department. Details will vary according to the nature and layout of each department's records. Computerization of the medical record mandates the same high standards of recording.

1   Ensure all the boxes at the top of the page have been filled in (usually by the reception staff) to identify the patient fully.

2   Start by printing your own name and designation, and the date and time you commenced seeing the patient.

3   Write legibly throughout. Other members of staff will be reading your notes, which will be valueless if they are illegible.

4   Record all the positive clinical findings in the history and examination, and relevant negative findings.
    (i)   Avoid the use of abbreviations, except for unambiguous, approved examples, such as BP. Digits should be named not numbered, and 'left' and 'right' should be written in full.

5   Make particular notes in assault or motor vehicle crash attendances from the patient's recall of events, or from a witness. Document the exact size of bruises or lacerations measured with a ruler.
    (i)   Statements may subsequently be required by the police or a solicitor, and could be requested months or even years later, so you cannot rely on your memory.

6 Record your impression and differential diagnosis.

7 Record any investigations performed, and put down the results, including your own interpretation of the electrocardiogram (ECG) or X-ray.

8 Record whether you discussed the case with a senior ED doctor, their name and grade, the time, and exactly what they advised.

9 Detail your proposed management plan.

10 Document any verbal or written instructions or advice given to the patient.

11 Record the disposition of the patient.
- (i) Record on the notes to whom clinical responsibility has been transferred, if you hand the patient over to another ED doctor at the end of your shift.
- (ii) Record the name and seniority of the doctor concerned, if you refer to an inpatient team, and the time the patient was referred.
- (iii) Write the ward and the consultant under whom the patient was admitted, when a patient is admitted.
- (iv) Record the clinic name and the consultant if possible, when a patient is referred to outpatients.
- (v) Attach a copy to the ED record of any discharge letter to the GP, when the patient is referred back to their own doctor
  - (a) computerization of the medical record now enables a printed letter to be generated for every patient discharged home.

12 Sign your name clearly at the end of the record, and print your name and initials underneath for future identification.

Tip: the above points may appear obvious, but are essential to the quality and continuity of the medical care of patients, and underpin good risk management practice.

COMMUNICATING WITH THE GENERAL PRACTITIONER

Communicate whenever possible with the GP.

1 Ring the GP to clarify current management, including medications and allergies when the patient is unsure, or for a recent past history in complex or atypical presentations.

2 Write or generate a computerised ED discharge letter if:
- (i) The GP writes a referral letter to you.
- (ii) You do any tests, including bloods, urinalysis, ECG or X-ray, even if they are normal.
- (iii) You make a new diagnosis.
- (iv) You start new medication, or change or stop an existing treatment regimen.
- (v) You refer the patient back to the GP for further care and review, including removing sutures or changing dressings.

    (vi) You refer the patient to outpatients.

    (vii) The patient is admitted, or a patient is brought in dead (or dies in the department).

3   Fax or email the letter. If you give the patient a copy to deliver by hand

    (i)   Assume it is likely to be opened and read, so fax, post or email **only** letters containing sensitive information, and when you have any doubt about the reliability or capacity of the patient to transfer the letter on.

BREAKING BAD NEWS

1   Breaking bad news to a relative concerning critical illness, injury or sudden death, especially when unexpected after trauma or cardiac arrest, must be done in the privacy of a quiet relatives' room.

2   Be accompanied by an experienced nurse and/or social worker. Introduce yourself, identify the patient's nearest relative, and sit by them.

3   Come to the point avoiding preamble or euphemisms. Use the words 'dead' or 'death' or 'critically ill' early on, followed by a brief account of events.

4   Be prepared to touch or hold the relative's hand and do not be afraid to show concern or empathy yourself. Allow a period of silence, avoiding platitudes or false sympathy, but encourage and answer any questions.

5   Understand that the relative's reaction may vary from numbed silence, disbelief, acute distress to anger, denial and guilt.

6   Encourage the relative, when ready to do so, to see and touch the body in cases involving death, and to say goodbye to their loved one alone.

7   Indicate that the nurse or social worker can stay with them.

8   Ask whether the relative wishes the hospital chaplain or bereavement counsellor to be contacted. Avoid giving sedative drugs, which will only postpone acceptance of what has happened.

9   Telephone or email the GP and inform the coroner if appropriate.

10 Retain the property of the patient, whatever its condition, for collection by the next of kin in accordance with his or her wishes. Avoid then presenting the property in a plastic bin bag.

11 Finally, appreciate the stress and anxiety caused to yourself and the nursing team following an unsuccessful or critical resuscitation.

    (i)   Try to meet together briefly to talk over events and express your own feelings and emotions, rather than simply debriefing the medical aspects of the care.

    (ii) Thank everyone for their efforts, particularly the nurse who dealt with the relatives and the nurses who were left to lay out the body in the case of sudden death.

RISK MANAGEMENT AND INCIDENT REPORTING

Mainstays of effective risk management include the credentialling of medical staff in infection control practices such as handwashing, incident monitoring and tracking, complaints monitoring and tracking, detailed medical records, and in risk education such as e-learning resources.

1   Recognize the types of ED situations that lead to incidents and claims, or to an ED doctor requiring medicolegal assistance from a medical defence organization (MDO). These include:

  (i)   Failure to correctly diagnose the patient's medical condition.
  (ii)   Delay in diagnosis.
  (iii) Failure to treat the patient.
  (iv)   Dissatisfaction with treatment.
  (v)   Dissatisfaction with the medical practitioner's conduct.
  (vi)   Medicolegal assistance:
     (a) regarding death of a patient
     (b) for a medical report including a coronial statement.

2   Some of the more common reasons ED presentations are reported as incidents to an MDO are for the following:

  (i)   *Misdiagnosis*
     (a) myocardial infarction
     (b) cerebral haemorrhage, particularly subarachnoid
     (c) appendicitis
     (d) torsion of the testis
     (e) fractures, e.g. scaphoid, phalanx, neck of femur, talus, calcaneus, etc.
  (ii)   *Failure to diagnose or treat appropriately*
     (a) tendon/nerve injury, particularly lacerations to the hand or foot
     (b) wounds/wound infections, particularly inadequate debridement and cleaning
     (c) foreign body, including glass and intraocular
     (d) spinal fracture.
  (iii) *Prescribing error*

3   Adopt the following strategies to minimize risk:

  (i)   Never stereotype a patient, trivialize his or her complaint, or jump to an early conclusion.
  (ii)   Use checklists or protocols, reflect on what you have decided, and always ask more senior ED staff for advice when you are unsure.
  (iii) Follow the guidelines above for clear ED record keeping.
  (iv)   Be an excellent communicator – with the patient, your medical colleagues, nursing staff and with the GP.

4   Notify the senior ED doctor and contact your MDO immediately if an incident occurs that you believe could turn into a complaint or claim. Include the following situations:

    (i)   Missed or delayed diagnosis.

    (ii)   Adverse outcome.

    (iii) Communication breakdown.

    (iv) Angry or disgruntled patient.

    (v)   'Gut feeling' that something is not quite right.

5   Your initial reaction to an incident can help ameliorate the likelihood of a claim subsequently being lodged or pursued. Make sure you:

    (i)   Are honest, open and concerned – *never* defensive, evasive or dismissive.

    (ii)   Talk the problem through with the patient in lay-person's language.

    (iii) Express regret and empathy for an adverse outcome, including saying sorry.

    (iv) Liaise with medical colleagues to ensure proper follow-up.

    (v)   Document meticulously – **never** backdate, alter or delete a medical record.

    (vi) Contact your MDO early, while events are fresh in your mind.

TRIAGE

1   Patients presenting to an ED are sorted or triaged on arrival, usually by an experienced, specially trained ED nurse in order to direct resources to the more seriously ill first.

    (i)   The triage nurse allocates an acuity category from the relevant National Triage Scale following assessment of current physiological disturbance and the risk of serious underlying illness or injury.

2   The triage category answers the question: 'This patient should wait for medical assessment and treatment no longer than …', an ideal time period embodied in the treatment acuity (see Tables 17.1 and 17.2).

3   Children and patients who are in pain may be up-triaged to a more acute category to facilitate expeditious care. Psychiatric patients are triaged according to a Mental Health Triage Scale.

4   A patient's triage category underpins sentinel ED performance indicators, such as waiting time (by triage category), admission rate, and 'did not wait' (DNW) rate, and aids the prediction of optimal staffing levels, resources, space and budget requirements.

Table 17.1 Australasian triage scale

Designation	Treatment acuity	Numeric code
Resuscitation	Immediately	1
Emergency	Within 10 min	2
Urgent	Within 30 min	3
Semi-urgent	Within 60 min	4
Non-urgent	Within 120 min	5

Table 17.2 UK national triage scale

Designation	Treatment acuity	Numeric code
Immediate resuscitation	Immediately	1
Very urgent	Within 10 min	2
Urgent	Within 60 min	3
Standard	Within 120 min	4
Non-urgent	Within 240 min	5

CONSENT, COMPETENCE AND REFUSAL OF TREATMENT

CONSENT AND COMPETENCE

1 *Consent* may be implied, verbal or written. However, to be valid it must be informed, specific, freely given and cover what is actually done, and the patient should be mentally and legally capable of giving it.

2 Patients >16 years in many circumstances, and 18 years in most, may sign or withhold their own informed consent. This may be done under common law principles or as set out in local legislation, provided they are deemed competent to do so.

3 *Competence* requires capacity to understand what is proposed, the options involved, the treatment and the risks of treatment or lack of it, the possible outcomes, and to be able to maintain and communicate a choice.

   (i)   Thus competence incorporates the elements of comprehension, appreciation, reasoning and choice.

4 Explain the details of any proposed procedure, and warn of possible complications. The patient must understand the implications and nature of the treatment proposed, or of not accepting the treatment.

5   Patients who are not deemed competent, that is with conditions that preclude comprehension of the nature and implications of the treatment proposed, may be given emergency treatment without consent to save life or to prevent serious damage to health.

6   The doctor should also proceed in cases of emergency to save life, even if consent was not obtained in a competent patient.

7   Patients under the age of 16 years may be able to consent for minor treatment provided they have the ability to understand what is proposed, although for major treatment it is more appropriate to seek consent from the parent or guardian (or teacher in an emergency).

    (i)   Importantly, medical information should not then be supplied to others, including parents, without permission.

    (ii) It is appropriate to proceed to life-saving treatment of a minor even if the parent or guardian refuses, including a blood transfusion in a Jehovah's Witness minor.

    (iii) Contact the hospital administration, the paediatric team and at least commence application for a court order as necessary.

REFUSAL OF TREATMENT AND DISCHARGE AGAINST MEDICAL ADVICE

1   Patients who refuse admission to hospital and/or a recommended treatment plan may be permitted to discharge themselves against advice, provided they are competent and well informed – that is, they understand fully the consequences of their actions.

2   Make meticulous notes of exactly what was said to the patient, and his or her response, demonstrating that they clearly understood the issues.

    (i)   The patient may sign the appropriate form, accepting responsibility for his or her own action.

    (ii) However, it is much more important to document details in the medical notes of exactly what was discussed, and what the patient understood and decided.

3   Record if the patient refuses to sign any form, or disappears before a form is signed, and have this countersigned by a witness, such as a senior nurse or a second doctor.

4   A patient suffering from a mental illness may be involuntarily detained against his or her will under the relevant Mental Health Act, if he or she is a danger to themselves or others (see p. 391).

    (i)   They may receive treatment under common law if there is the overriding principle of best care by the treating doctor.

5   Similarly a patient deemed not competent due to alcohol, drugs or medical illness causing acute confusion may be advised to stay against his or her will under common law, if there is an overriding medical precedent to continue care, such as following a head injury in an intoxicated patient.

The police are involved within the ED in a number of ways.

POLICE REQUEST FOR PATIENT INFORMATION

1 Medical information concerning the care of a patient in the ED is confidential and must not be divulged without the patient's written consent, except on behalf of a coroner (or procurator fiscal in Scotland).

2 Traffic police investigating a crash may be told the name, address and age of any patient involved, and a brief description of the injury, and in particular whether the crash is likely to prove fatal or whether the patient is to be admitted or sent home.

3 A doctor may disclose information to a senior police officer concerning a patient suspected of being involved in a serious arrestable offence, such as murder, rape, child abuse, armed robbery or terrorist activity, thereby acting in the public interest for the safety of the lives of others.
   (i) Obtain the advice of the senior ED doctor or hospital administration whenever there is any doubt as to the appropriateness of releasing information to the police.

POLICE REQUEST TO INTERVIEW A PATIENT

1 Grant permission if the patient is medically in a fit state to be seen, after informing the patient.

2 The doctor may suggest a time limit.

POLICE REQUEST FOR AN ALCOHOL BREATH TEST OR BLOOD SAMPLE

1 The doctor should first give the police permission to perform this, provided the patient's clinical condition will not be adversely affected.

2 Permission cannot be granted in certain circumstances: if the patient is unconscious, critically ill, or incapable of cooperating, possibly due to a facial injury. Local legislation may still permit a blood alcohol sample to be drawn.

3 Inform the patient that you have allowed the police to be involved if permission is granted, and write in the ED record that in your opinion the patient was fit to be seen at the time.

4 A police medical officer or police surgeon may then take the sample, using all their own equipment that does not involve the hospital facilities at any stage.
   (i) Usually, local legislation dictates that the ED doctor draws the blood sample.

REQUEST FOR A POLICE MEDICAL STATEMENT

1   The purpose of this statement is to act as a record to be read out in court without necessitating the doctor being present.

(i)   The patient must first provide written consent **before** you may disclose confidential medical information.

(ii)   Use any pre-printed forms supplied by the police.

(iii) State your full name, age, contact address and telephone number, medical qualifications, job status, your employing health authority and duration of that employment.

(iv)   State the date you were on duty in the ED, the hospital's name and the time you examined the patient.

(v)   Continue with the full name, age, sex, occupation and address of the patient. Record the time and date of any subsequent attendances in the ED.

(vi)   Recount the history (as told to you) without making personal inferences.

(vii) Record the physical findings noted using language a non-medical person can understand

(a) state the actual size of any abrasions, bruises and lacerations, including whether the true skin was broken

(b) make a comment as to whether the injuries found were consistent with the use of a particular weapon or implement as suggested by the patient's history.

(viii) List all the investigations performed, such as X-rays and laboratory tests, and their results, including relevant negatives.

(ix)   State the treatment given, including sutures and their number, and record the time the patient spent in hospital or attending outpatients.

(x)   Finally, end the report where possible with a rough prognosis.

(xi)   Sign the report where indicated on each separate page.

2   Keep a photocopy of your report, and note the name and number of the police officer requesting the statement, and his or her police station.

CORONER

1   Inform the coroner (procurator fiscal in Scotland) of all sudden or unexpected deaths, and deaths involving homicide, suicide, an accident or injury, drowning, poisoning, surgery, abortion, infancy, neglect, negligence, or patients in police custody or held in a mental hospital.

2   Thus, virtually all patients brought in dead are reported to the coroner.

3   Any patient actually dying in the ED is also usually reported.

(i)   This should be done whatever the time of day or night if there were any suspicious circumstances, by contacting the local police station (the police are very often involved anyway).

4   Therefore, the ED doctor is rarely in a position to sign a death certificate.

    (i)   However, try to contact the patient's own doctor when death has clearly occurred as a direct result of a known illness, to see if that doctor is able to sign the certificate.

ATTENDING AN INQUEST OR COURT

1   An inquest takes place in the coroner's court. Although it is essentially a fact-finding inquiry, not a trial, there is usually a mix of 'inquisitorial' and 'adversarial' legal approaches. It is held in public, and the press may be present.

    (i)   The coroner's office will inform you of the date, time and place of the inquest. Make sure you tell your MDO that you have been asked to attend

       (a) legal representation may be arranged for you by your MDO if, on discussion with them, they consider it appropriate.

    (ii)   Arrive punctually and dress suitably.

    (iii) Take the medical notes and a copy of your statement with you. Read both thoroughly beforehand several times so you have the facts readily available.

    (iv)   Take the oath or affirmation, then the coroner will go through your statement with you and ask questions.

    (v)   Your replies should be concise, clear and factual. Indicate whether they are based on hearsay.

    (vi)   You may be examined following this, by any 'properly interested persons' or usually their lawyer. You are not obliged to answer any questions that may incriminate you.

    (vii) The coroner's officer will pay you the appropriate witness fee and expenses after the inquest.

2   Follow the same sort of preparation for a civil court negligence trial, where although using hearsay is admissible, the rules of evidence are based on the 'balance of probabilities'.

    (i)   Make absolutely sure your MDO has been involved throughout.

3   Attending a criminal trial is exceedingly rare. Evidence must be 'beyond all reasonable doubt'. MDO and legal representation are essential.

RETRIEVAL AND INTER-HOSPITAL TRANSFER

1   Retrieval is the transport of a sick or injured patient by specially trained staff from a lesser-equipped (sending) hospital to a higher-level (receiving) hospital for further care.

2   The sending doctor should speak directly to the receiving hospital doctor or retrieval specialist using a dedicated, single-point-contact coordinated communication system.

3 The decision to transfer, the risks involved, the benefits expected and the patient preparation are agreed on.

    (i) The sending doctor commences usual required care, such as two i.v. cannulae, nasogastric tube, indwelling catheter, fracture splinting, and advanced airway/respiratory/cardiovascular procedures, according to their ability.

4 A transfer letter, photocopy of notes and forms, lab results, X-rays, ECGs, etc. are prepared for the retrieval team/receiving hospital.

5 Road transport is suitable for short distances, and helicopters for longer ones. Light aircraft are used when helicopter flying time exceeds 90–120 minutes.

    (i) Helicopters and small aircraft require expert crew and landing areas, incur high costs, need dedicated equipment, and involve flight physiology considerations such as altitude hypoxia and trapped gas expansion (e.g. in a pneumothorax).

6 Retrieval equipment must be compact, portable, light, robust and reliable, and have adequate battery capacity. Special ventilators, monitors, suction equipment, alarms, defibrillator, mattress and an equipment frame 'bridge' are essential.

7 Retrieval staff will spend time assessing, stabilizing and packaging the patient at the sending hospital, pre-empting any potential complications prior to transfer. It is not a time to rush.

8 The aim is to maintain or improve the level of care, particularly during high-risk times such as loading and unloading during the inter-hospital travel.

MAJOR INCIDENT

EXTERNAL DISASTER

1 A sudden influx of a large number of casualties is variously known as an External Disaster, Code Brown, Major Incident or Mass Casualty Disaster.

2 This is defined locally by the facility or facilities involved as 'any external health incident which requires an extraordinary response from the health-care system'.

3 Prior planning is an essential component of major incident management, utilizing an 'all hazards' approach.

    (i) Involves adopting a flexible, generic plan that can be adapted to suit any potential major incident.

    (ii) The underlying principle is to do the 'most good for the most people' with the resources available.

(iii) Certain types of incident will require a special response such as incidents involving chemicals, infectious diseases or large numbers of children.

4 Each hospital's local plan should be linked to the regional and state plans for mass casualty, as well as integrating with the plans of the other emergency services involved.

(i) A copy of the plan should be available for viewing in all key areas of the hospital.

5 The principles governing any hospital major incident response are Command and Control; Safety and Staffing; Communication; Assessment; Triage; Treatment; Transportation (CSCATTT).

(i) *Command and Control*
   (a) adopts a vertical model, with questions and decisions passed directly to the clinicians and managers coordinating the hospital response
   (b) an overall impression of the hospital's activity and capabilities is thus maintained at all times.

(ii) *Safety and Staffing*
   (a) safety of hospital staff is paramount
   (b) protecting clinicians and their working environment from hazards optimizes the delivery of care.

(iii) *Communication*
   (a) communications frequently break down when overstretched by a major incident
   (b) include the use of radios or runners to carry messages to maintain maximum flexibility, as an alternative form of communication to land or mobile telephones.

(iv) *Assessment*
   (a) a major incident is a dynamic evolving situation
   (b) continuous, rapid assessment and reassessment of the situation enable available resources to be most efficiently matched to demand.

(v) *Triage*
   (a) most ambulance or site medical services utilize some form of standardized triage that divides patients into certain categories
      - *red*: severely injured but salvageable; in need of urgent care
      - *yellow*: non-ambulant significant injuries, but stable
      - *green*: walking wounded; hospital admission unlikely
      - *black*: not expected to survive
   (b) a colour-coded and numbered priority tag is attached to the patient

(c) triage remains a dynamic process repeated after any significant intervention at each stage of patient care

(d) however, patients may still make their own way to hospital without utilizing the ambulance and thus arrive untriaged.

(vi) *Treatment*

(a) key principle is to do 'the most for the most'

(b) can involve delivering minimum acceptable care at certain stages to facilitate enhanced flow through the system

(c) definitive care may be delayed until the surge in patients is abating and the major incident is resolving

(d) this time period can vary from hours to days.

(vii) *Transport*

Flow through the system is vital to prevent the ED becoming blocked to further patients

(a) efficient, rapid but safe transfer of patients from the ED to theatre, intensive care unit (ICU), inpatient wards or home is vital.

6 Portions of the external disaster plan pertinent to individual members of staff are summarized on action cards.

(i) Those concerned with the medical and nursing roles within the ED should be distributed to, and read by, all members of staff.

7 New ED doctors must also make certain that the switchboard has a reliable contact telephone number for the purpose of an emergency call-out. In addition, make sure you:

(i) Know the call-out procedure, the different states of alert, and the significance of being the designated hospital or the supporting hospital.

(ii) Understand your role within the department, which senior doctor you are responsible to, and from whom you should receive advice.

(iii) Can operate any equipment reserved for a major incident, including that used by the Mobile Medical Team.

(iv) Are familiar with the special stationery and records used in a major incident, including the significance of the triage tags and where to find details of any pre-hospital care given, particularly drugs and fluids.

(v) Know where to obtain social and psychological support following the incident to minimize the potential for post-traumatic stress.

SPECIALIZED HAZARDOUS MATERIALS RESPONSES

A chemical, biological and radiological (CBR) hazardous materials (HAZMAT) incident requires a specialized response, necessitating staff to wear specific personal protective equipment (PPE) and patients to be decontaminated.

1 *Personal protective equipment*

Get advice as to what constitutes appropriate PPE for the incident, as it is essential for the safety of staff that appropriate PPE is worn.

(i) PPE may at one extreme require self-contained breathing apparatus with a full face mask and a protective suit with boots and gloves for a hazard which presents a significant vapour and contact threat, or

(ii) A simple face mask, eye protection, gloves, cap, gown and shoe covers for a relatively minor contact hazard.

(iii) Practice in both donning and removing PPE is essential, as well as in the process of patient decontamination, for instance during a mass casualty disaster exercise.

(iv) Staff must be aware of the threat of hyperthermia while using protective equipment. Any staff member experiencing symptoms suggestive of heat stress should immediately self-decontaminate, remove their PPE in a safe area and rehydrate.

2 *Decontamination*

(i) Decontamination is the reduction or removal of substances such that they are no longer a hazard.

(ii) The fire service is responsible for the decontamination of patients at the scene of a CBR incident.

(iii) As patients may self-present to hospital, staff must have the equipment, facilities, and training to decontaminate a patient locally

(a) set up a designated decontamination area in a discrete, outdoor, well-ventilated space

(b) create a 'Clean-Dirty line' between the decontamination area and the ED

(c) only allow staff wearing appropriate PPE to cross this line into the decontamination area

(d) conversely, no staff, patients or equipment may cross back from the decontamination area across this line, unless they have been decontaminated

– patients from the incident are only allowed to enter the ED once they have been decontaminated

(e) ambulant patients should be capable of self-decontamination, having received instruction

(f) non-ambulant patients are decontaminated by staff.

(iv) The decontamination process is best determined by the process: 'wet, strip, wash, redress'

(a) *wet* – the patient is wetted down with water to prevent any powder residue from being disturbed and potentially spreading when clothing is removed

(b) *strip* – the patient's clothes are removed by cutting longitudinally on the anterior aspect of the body. Clothing is then folded back on itself and tucked under the patient's body, leaving the relatively clean inner surface on the outside. The patient can then be log rolled, and the contaminated clothing removed, bagged, sealed and labelled with identifying details

(c) *wash* – the patient's entire body is gently washed down with warm, soapy water taking care to avoid dermal abrasion and thus enhancing absorption of any toxic agents. Ears and eyes may require irrigation with saline

(d) *redress* – patients are dressed in appropriate clean clothing.

(v) The patient is then ready to be transported across the 'Clean-Dirty line' by staff on the clean side of the line sliding him or her off the dirty trolley onto a clean trolley.

CHEMICAL INCIDENT

An incident involving an industrial chemical or weaponized chemical agent has the potential for large numbers of casualties following accidental or deliberate release.

1 Appropriate PPE and patient decontamination are essential. Most patients will require admission for a period of observation, even if apparently asymptomatic.

2 Chemicals are broadly categorized into four groups based on their injury pathophysiology including blood agents, nerve agents, vesicants and choking agents.

(i) *Blood agents*

(a) volatile agents that evaporate quickly, which are hazardous by both inhalation and ingestion

(b) largely composed of the cyanogens, which bind to cellular cytochrome oxidase to stop cellular aerobic metabolism despite adequate blood oxygenation

(c) quick acting, with casualties showing rapid onset of symptoms that consist of dyspnoea, gasping, confusion, convulsions, collapse, coma and ultimately respiratory arrest

(d) the skin may be cherry pink and cyanosis is unusual. The pupils are normal or dilated and secretions are minimal

(e) mouth-to-mouth ventilation poses a risk to the rescuer and should not be performed

(f) antidotes are unnecessary in a patient who is conscious and breathing normally within 5 min after removal from source. Give simple oxygen therapy

(g) patients with respiratory depression or impaired consciousness should receive assisted ventilation and an intravenous cyanide antidote as soon as possible (see p. 412).

(ii) *Nerve agents*

    (a) highly toxic chemicals which are hazardous by contact to skin or eyes, inhalation and ingestion

    (b) organophosphate compounds can be easily weaponized to form agents such as sarin, tabun, soman and VX

    (c) clinical effects depend on dose, duration and exposure route, and may be local or systemic, with death occurring from respiratory arrest due to central nervous system (CNS) depression and/or muscle paralysis

    (d) cholinergic effects include diarrhoea, urination, miosis and muscle weakness, bronchorrhoea, and bradycardia, emesis, lacrimation, salivation and sweating (DUMBELS)

    (e) rapid decontamination is essential

    (f) patients with isolated eye symptoms should be observed for a minimum of 2 h post exposure, and may be treated with atropine or tropicamide 0.5% eye drops

    (g) treatment for more severely affected patients includes high-doses of atropine i.v. to dry secretions and increase heart rate, pralidoxime i.v. and seizure management (see p. 415).

(iii) *Vesicants*

    (a) agents, such as mustard gas, which are irritant and cause blistering of the skin, eyes and respiratory system. They are hazardous by contact, inhalation and ingestion, and are rapidly absorbed with clinical effects that are often delayed by a latent period from 1–24 h

    (b) exposure results in gritty, painful eyes with periorbital oedema, blepharospasm, corneal ulceration and blindness, which is usually temporary

    (c) skin blistering occurs, with hoarseness, cough and dyspnoea followed by a chemical pneumonitis and acute respiratory distress syndrome (ARDS)

    (d) treatment includes decontamination and supportive care similar to that of thermal burns.

(iv) *Choking or pulmonary agents*

    (a) agents such as chlorine and phosgene are both irritant, and corrosive due to dissolving in tissue water to form hydrochloric acid

    (b) skin or eye effects are seen as well as following inhalation, with individuals with pre-existing lung disease particularly vulnerable

    (c) symptoms include watering eyes, blepharospasm, skin erythema, dyspnoea, cough and wheeze, with pneumonitis and non-cardiogenic pulmonary oedema

(d) death may follow high concentrations with mass displacement of air/oxygen

(e) treatment includes decontamination and supportive care with inhaled bronchodilators and steroids, and if required, mechanical ventilation until resolution of the acute lung injury.

BIOLOGICAL INCIDENT

Biological incidents take two distinct forms: natural phenomena such as an influenza pandemic or dengue epidemic, and deliberate release or a 'white powder'-type incident.

1   Naturally occurring incidents are managed in accordance with current infectious disease isolation and treatment procedures.

2   A range of biological pathogens could potentially be used in a deliberate release incident. These include:

   (i)   Bacteria such as the plague, viruses such as smallpox, spores such as anthrax, fungi such as *Fusarium* or toxins such as ricin

      (a) some have also been genetically engineered to produce resistance to usual recognized treatments.

3   As effects from contamination with a biological agent may take days or even weeks to manifest, a major challenge in any deliberate release incident is to recognize it and to initiate the appropriate systems response.

   (i)   ED staff must be alert to an unusual pattern of infectious disease and should liaise closely with infectious disease and population health specialists.

   (ii) Patterns that *may* indicate possible deliberate release include:

      (a) unusual illness, e.g. sudden unexplained febrile death, critical illness or pneumonia death in a previously healthy young adult

      (b) unexpected number of patients with the same symptoms

      (c) unusual illness for that time of year, e.g. influenza in summer

      (d) unusual illness for the patient's age group, e.g. chickenpox in a middle-aged adult

      (e) illness in an uncommon patient category, e.g. cutaneous anthrax in a patient with no history of contact with animals, animal hides or products

      (f) illness acquired in a non-endemic area

      (g) unusual clinical signs, e.g. mediastinal widening on chest radiograph (CXR), sudden onset of symmetrical flaccid paralysis

      (h) atypical progression of an illness, e.g. lack of response to usually effective antibiotics.

4 A 'white powder'-type incident should be dealt with by external decontamination in an outdoor area by staff wearing full PPE.

  (i) All patients after decontamination and initial management must be observed until the nature of the threat is established by the appropriate forensic scientific services involved.

RADIOLOGICAL INCIDENT

The two forms of radioactivity most likely to be encountered in a radiological incident are α and β particles.

1 α particles consist of two neutrons and two protons, are able to travel short distances and are unable to penetrate human skin.

  (i) α emitters are thus only harmful when inhaled, ingested or absorbed (e.g. through an open wound).

2 β particles are high speed electrons or positrons, and are able to penetrate human tissue to the level of the dermis.

  (i) Prolonged exposure to bare skin may result in a 'beta burn', but clothing and/or PPE provide some degree of protection.

  (ii) Similarly, β emitters are thus only harmful when inhaled, ingested or absorbed.

3 Two types of radiation-induced injury can occur:

  (i) External irradiation, where the patient has been exposed to radiation from an external source, such as a nuclear blast. Patients who have been externally irradiated are not radioactive and do not require decontamination.

  (ii) Contact with radiological materials, where the patient has become contaminated externally, internally, or both, with radioactive particles. These particles continue to emit α or β ionizing radiation leading to cellular radiation injury if not removed.

4 Patients requiring urgent treatment are taken to the nearest major ED.

  (i) Decontamination is required for any patient from a radiological incident with contact with radiological material.

  (ii) Patients must be quarantined to an appropriate outdoor area for assessment and decontamination.

  (iii) Minimum PPE consists of a cap, eye protection, facemask, gown and shoe covering.

  (iv) External decontamination is only required for patients who have radioactive matter deposited on their skin or clothing.

  (v) Management of internal decontamination is highly specialized. Expert advice should be sought from the from:

    (a) Poisons Information Centre on 13 11 26 (Australia), and in New Zealand on 03 479 7248 (or 0800 764 766 within New Zealand)

    (b) National Poisons Information Service (NPIS) in the UK.

(vi) Even if the patient is externally contaminated, the risk to a caregiver wearing a surgical facemask, gloves, eye protection, gown and shoe covers is extremely small
   (a) triage and treatment of life-threatening conditions in such patients can be done prior to full decontamination
   (b) if the patient's condition is not life-threatening, then decontamination is completed before starting treatment.
(vii) Advice on the management of radiological incidents should also be sought from the Hospital Radiation Safety Officer, Medical Physics Department or by contacting the local National Arrangements for Incidents involving Radioactivity (NAIR) staff or police.

FURTHER READING

Avant Mutual Group Ltd. http://www.avant.org.au/home/ (risk management, medicolegal).

Emergency Medicine Clinics of North America (2015) Vol 33 (1) (management of hazardous materials emergencies).

MDA National. http://www.mdanational.com.au/ (risk management, medico-legal).

Medical Indemnity Protection Society (MIPS). http://www.mips.com.au/ (risk management, medicolegal).

Medical Protection Society. http://www.medicalprotection.org/uk (risk management, medicolegal).

Parker R, Terris J (2015) The Coroner: The Australasian and UK perspectives. In: Cameron P, Jelinek G, Kelly A-M *et al. Textbook of Adult Emergency Medicine*, 4th edn. Churchill Livingstone, Edinburgh, pp. 817–24.

Public Health England. https://www.gov.uk/government/organisations/public-health-england (CBR hazards).

Terris J, Brentnall E (2015) Consent and competence: The Australasian and UK perspectives. In: Cameron P, Jelinek G, Kelly A-M *et al. Textbook of Adult Emergency Medicine*, 4th edn. Churchill Livingstone, Edinburgh, pp. 825–9.

The MDU. http://www.themdu.com/ (risk management, medicolegal).

The Medical Insurance Group. http://www.miga.com.au (risk management, medicolegal).

Section XVIII

PRACTICAL PROCEDURES

ENDOTRACHEAL INTUBATION

INDICATIONS
Endotracheal intubation creates, maintains and/or protects the airway, plus facilitates ventilation.

CONTRAINDICATIONS
1 Unskilled operator.
2 Awake patient, jaw clenching.

TECHNIQUE
1 Pre-oxygenate with 100% non-rebreather or bag-valve mask and position patient in the 'sniffing position' with neck flexed and head extended on a pillow.
2 Remove poorly fitting dentures and suction oropharynx.
3 Standing at the patient's head, hold the laryngoscope in the left hand and gently insert the laryngoscope blade over the right side of the tongue.
4 Advance the curved blade of the laryngoscope until the tip of the blade sits within the vallecula. Lift the blade forwards and upwards (taking care not to use the upper teeth as a fulcrum) to visualize the vocal cords.
5 Use the BURP (backward, upward, rightward pressure) manoeuvre on the thyroid cartilage as necessary to improve the view of the vocal cords.
6 Pass the endotracheal tube (size 8.5–9.5 mm internal diameter in adult males, and a 7.5–8.5 mm diameter in adult females) through the cords under direct vision, to a distance of 20–22 cm at the lips.
   (i) Insert an introducer first to 'stiffen' the tube to facilitate placement, if problematic.
   (ii) Or pass an airway bougie through the cords and then railroad the endotracheal tube over the bougie into the trachea.
7 Inflate the cuff, connect the oxygen supply, and check correct position of the tube by exhaled carbon dioxide detection, and by observing tube fogging, bilateral chest expansion and auscultation. Tie the tube in place.
8 Ventilate the lungs at 10 breaths/min.

COMPLICATIONS
1 Failure to intubate, with hypoxia.
2 Misplaced tube, e.g. oesophagus, or right main bronchus.
3 Airway trauma.
4 Aspiration.
5 Raised intracranial pressure.

The objective of rapid sequence induction (RSI) intubation is to secure the airway as rapidly as possible and assumes that the patient has a full stomach and is at risk of aspiration of gastric contents. Pre-determined doses of i.v. anaesthetic and a rapid-acting paralysing drug are given to enable the intubation.

INDICATIONS

1   Failure of airway maintenance or protection:
   (i)   Loss of protective reflexes (e.g. severe head injury or drug overdose).
   (ii) Prophylaxis (e.g. airway burns, laryngeal oedema, pre-transfer).
   (iii) Prevention of aspiration of blood, mucus or gastric contents in the comatose patient with reduced gag reflex.

2   Failure of oxygenation or ventilation:
   (i)   Treatment of inadequate oxygenation (hypoxaemic respiratory failure).
   (ii) Treatment of inadequate ventilation (hypercapnoeic respiratory failure).

3   Therapeutic intervention:
   (i)   Provision of controlled mechanical ventilation.
   (ii) Hyperventilation.
   (iii) Pulmonary toilet, bronchoscopy.

CONTRAINDICATIONS

1   Unskilled or untrained operator.

2   Pre-arrest/moribund – proceed without drugs (see Endotracheal Intubation above).

3   Obstructed airway, unless operator absolutely confident of success.

4   Difficult airway, unless operator absolutely confident of success, and/or is able to bag-mask ventilate.

TECHNIQUE

1   *Preparation*
   (i)   Resuscitation area with comprehensive non-invasive monitoring, pre-checked intubation trolley with drugs drawn up, trained personnel
      (a) requires up to five people in a trauma intubation (intubator, assistant, in-line manual stabilization, cricoid pressure, drug administrator).
   (ii) Two functioning laryngoscopes with choice of blades, introducer, test endotracheal tube cuff inflation.
   (iii) Use a checklist to optimise role delineation, teamwork and crisis planning.

2 Pre-oxygenation

   (i)   Provide high concentration oxygen via bag-valve-mask for 3–5 min prior to RSI, to maximize oxygen reserve in the lungs by washing out nitrogen, to compensate for the impending period of apnoea.

   (ii) Change to continuous, high-flow nasal cannulae oxygen at 15 L/min to provide ongoing apnoeic oxygenation once paralysis occurs.

3 Pre-treatment

   (i)   Option to administer fluid bolus in hypotension, or additional drugs such as atropine 10–20 µg/kg in children.

4 Paralysis and induction

   (i)   Use an i.v. induction agent such as thiopentone (thiopental) 0.5–5 mg/kg, etomidate 0.3 mg/kg, ketamine 0.75–2 mg/kg, propofol 0.5–2 mg/kg, or midazolam 0.1 mg/kg plus fentanyl 2.5–5 µg/kg.

   (ii) Follow with muscle relaxant suxamethonium 1.5 mg/kg, or rocuronium 1 mg/kg, if suxamethonium contraindicated by hyperkalaemia, neuromuscular disease.

5 Protection and positioning

   (i)   Provide in-line stabilization in trauma where a cervical spine injury is possible.

   (ii) Apply cricoid pressure (2 kg or 4.5 lb force) from the moment the patient loses muscle tone and maintain pressure until the endotracheal tube has been correctly placed, position verified and the cuff inflated.

      (a) request some relaxation of cricoid pressure if the glottic view is worsened.

   (iii) Use the BURP manoeuvre on the thyroid cartilage as necessary to improve the view of the vocal cords.

6 Placement with proof

   (i)   Confirm tube placement by:

      (a) capnography to measure end-tidal carbon dioxide ($ETCO_2$) – most reliable

      (b) direct visualization of endotracheal tube passing through the cords

      (c) auscultation over the lung fields and stomach.

   (ii) Release cricoid pressure once placement is confirmed.

7 Post-intubation management

   (i)   Tie the tube in place and watch for cardiorespiratory changes, as a chest radiograph (CXR) is arranged.

COMPLICATIONS

1 Failure or delay to intubate, with critical hypoxia.

2 Misplaced tube, e.g. oesophagus, or right main bronchus.

3 Airway trauma.

4 Drug reaction such as anaphylaxis.

5 Aspiration.

 Warning: never attempt rapid sequence induction (RSI) unless you have been trained. Use a bag-valve mask technique instead, while waiting for help.

CRICOTHYROTOMY

INDICATIONS

1 'Can't intubate, can't ventilate'.

2 Tracheal intubation considered impossible, or unacceptably high risk:
  (i) Severe maxillofacial trauma.
  (ii) Massive oedema of the throat tissues (e.g. angioedema, airway burns).
  (iii) Severe trismus or clenched teeth; masseter spasm after suxamethonium.
  (iv) Foreign body/tumour blocking upper airway.

CONTRAINDICATIONS

1 Children <12 years of age (use needle cricothyrotomy only).

2 Acute or pre-existing laryngeal pathology (e.g. laryngeal fracture).

3 Inability to identify landmarks (e.g. surgical emphysema/haemorrhage/inflammation).

TECHNIQUE

1 Extend the patient's neck and identify the cricothyroid membrane between the lower border of the thyroid cartilage and the upper border of the cricoid cartilage (see Fig. 18.1).

2 *Surgical cricothyroidotomy*
  (i) Make a transverse incision through the skin and cricothyroid membrane with a scalpel blade.
  (ii) Rotate the scalpel blade and pass a bougie caudally through the hole into the trachea.
  (iii) Insert (railroad) a 6 mm endotracheal tube (or small tracheostomy tube) over the bougie and into the trachea.
  (iv) Remove the bougie, inflate the cuff and connect the tube to an Ambu or Laerdal bag and oxygen supply.

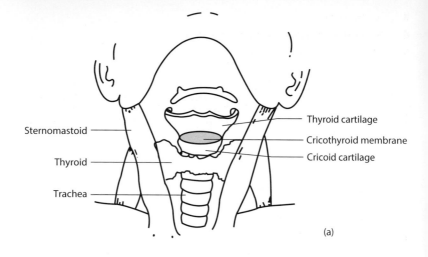

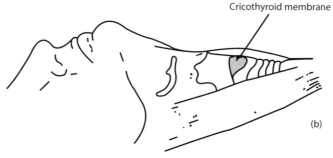

Figure 18.1 Cricothyrotomy.
The anatomical relationships of the cricothyroid membrane **(a)** anteroposterior view, and **(b)** oblique lateral view.

3 *Needle cricothyroidotomy*
  (i)   Insert a large-bore 14-gauge i.v. cannula with syringe at 45°
         caudally through the cricothyroid membrane, and aspirate air to
         confirm correct placement.
  (ii) Remove the needle and attach the cannula to wall oxygen at
         15 L/min using a Y-connector.
  (iii) Insufflate oxygen by intermittent occlusion of the open end of the
         Y-connector for 1 s in every 5.

COMPLICATIONS

1   Failure, with malposition outside trachea.

2   Haemorrhage.

3 Tracheal tear.

4 Mediastinal emphysema or pneumothorax.

5 Dysphonia/hoarseness.

NEEDLE THORACENTESIS

INDICATIONS

1 Therapeutic:
- (i) Tension pneumothorax.
- (ii) Aspiration of pneumothorax.
- (iii) Aspiration of an effusion.

2 Diagnostic:
- (i) Determine cause of pleural effusion.

CONTRAINDICATIONS

1 Uncooperative patient.

2 Uncorrected bleeding diathesis (in particular platelets <50 or international normalized ratio [INR] >1.5).

3 Local skin infection.

4 Bullous lung disease, small effusion or single functioning lung (special care).

TECHNIQUE

1 *Therapeutic tap (air)*
- (i) Lie the patient on a bed at 45° and infiltrate local anaesthetic down to the pleura in the second intercostal space in the mid-clavicular line.
- (ii) Insert a 16-gauge cannula along the anaesthetized track into the pleural cavity, bevel up, at 90° to the surface of the skin, working 'just above the rib below'
    - (a) alternatively use a proprietary chest aspiration kit, with special fenestrated cannula and one-way valve.
- (iii) Withdraw the needle, and connect to a 50 mL syringe with three-way tap.
- (iv) Aspirate air until resistance is felt, the patient coughs excessively, or >2500 mL is aspirated.

2 *Diagnostic tap*
- (i) Sit the patient on the edge of the bed, arms folded in front of the body and leaning forward over a bedside tray table. Expose the whole of the back.

(ii) Percuss down the chest to confirm the upper border of the effusion (stony dull percussion), then auscultate (decreased breath sounds, and decreased vocal resonance).

(iii) Infiltrate local anaesthetic down to the pleura on the posterolateral aspect of the chest wall (mid-scapular or posterior axillary line), one to two intercostal spaces below the percussed upper border of the effusion (but no lower than the 8th intercostal space).

(iv) Attach a 21-gauge needle to a 20 mL syringe and insert along the anaesthetized track, bevel up, at 90° to the surface of the skin, working 'just above the rib below'.

(v) Maintain constant negative pressure on the syringe by drawing back on the plunger as the needle is advanced.

(vi) Aspirate 10–20 mL sample. Remove the needle and press firmly over the site with a gauze swab, then apply an occlusive dressing.

(vii) Send fluid for biochemistry (protein, glucose, lactate dehydrogenase [LDH], pH and amylase), microbiology (M,C&S and Gram stain) and for cytology.

3 Therapeutic tap (fluid)

(i) Position and infiltrate local anaesthetic as for a diagnostic tap.

(ii) Insert a 16-gauge cannula along the anaesthetized track, bevel up, at 90° to the surface of the skin, working 'just above the rib below'.

(iii) When flashback is seen, hold the stylet steady and advance the plastic cannula as far into the thorax as it will go. Remove the stylet while the patient holds a breath in expiration, and place your gloved thumb over the cannula.

(iv) Secure the cannula with tape and attach the three-way tap and 50 mL syringe, again with the patient holding a breath in expiration (reduces the risk of a pneumothorax).

(v) Once 1000–1500 mL of fluid have been drained, remove the cannula and press firmly over the site with a gauze swab. Apply an occlusive dressing.

COMPLICATIONS

1 Pneumothorax.

2 Haemothorax.

3 Hypotension due to a vasovagal response.

4 Re-expansion pulmonary oedema (large volume aspirated).

5 Infection at the skin site.

6 Spleen or liver injury.

7 Air embolism.

8 Empyema.

INTERCOSTAL CATHETER INSERTION

INDICATIONS

1 Drainage of a significant pneumothorax, haemothorax, large pleural effusion or empyema.

2 Prophylactic insertion prior to positive-pressure ventilation or aeromedical transport, in a patient with a chest injury and rib fractures or flail chest, or even a small pneumothorax.

CONTRAINDICATIONS

1 Infection over insertion site.

2 Uncorrected bleeding diathesis (in particular platelets <50 or INR >1.5).

TECHNIQUE

1 Review recent CXR and confirm the side, position and size of the pneumothorax/fluid.

2 Give analgesia 0.05–0.1 mg/kg morphine i.v., and/or 0.05 mg/kg midazolam i.v., titrated to effect in the haemodynamically stable patient, as the procedure is painful and potentially distressing.

3 Select appropriate size of chest tube:
 (i) Adult 16–22 F for pneumothorax, or 28–32 F for effusion, haemothorax or empyema.
 (ii) Child 12–20 F, or newborn 10–12 F.

4 Infiltrate generously with local anaesthetic down to the pleura in the fifth intercostal space in the mid-axillary line.

5 Use a scalpel blade to incise the skin and subcutaneous fat, then blunt dissect down to and through the parietal pleura.

6 Slide the drain in gently with a pair of curved artery forceps having **removed** the trocar. Connect the drain to an underwater seal, and confirm it swings with respiration.

7 Secure the chest tube in place and check position of chest tube with a post-procedure CXR.

COMPLICATIONS

1 Malposition: extrathoracic (obvious on CXR as it runs up external to chest wall), or intrathoracic but extrapleural (not obvious on CXR, but exceedingly painful!).

2 Haemothorax (may even require thoracotomy if does not settle).

3 Subcutaneous emphysema.

4 Re-expansion pulmonary oedema.

5   Trauma to heart, liver, lung or spleen.
6   Local nerve injury (e.g. long thoracic nerve).
7   Infection, either skin site or empyema.

DC CARDIOVERSION

INDICATIONS

1   Emergency treatment of a haemodynamically 'unstable' patient (chest pain, confusion, hypotension, heart failure) with a tachyarrhythmia.
2   Elective treatment of a stable patient with a tachyarrhythmia (e.g. atrial fibrillation [AF]) with onset within previous 24–48 h.

CONTRAINDICATIONS

1   Sinus tachycardia.
2   Multifocal atrial tachycardia.
3   Arrhythmias due to enhanced automaticity in digoxin toxicity (risk of resistant ventricular fibrillation [VF]).
4   Reversion of AF of >48 h duration (risk of embolism).

TECHNIQUE

1   Use procedural sedation such as low-dose propofol 0.5–1.0 mg/kg, or fentanyl 0.5 μg/kg plus midazolam 0.05 mg/kg titrated to effect for a conscious patient undergoing elective cardioversion (less if shocked).
2   Set the defibrillator to 'synchronous' mode so that the shock is delivered with the R wave of the ECG to reduce the risk of precipitating VF.
3   Energy requirements are generally less than those for defibrillating VF.
    (i)   Atrial flutter (and paroxysmal supraventricular tachycardia [SVT] other than AF): start with 50–100 J biphasic.
    (ii) Monomorphic VT and AF: use 120–150 J biphasic.

COMPLICATIONS

1   Pain (inadequate sedation), thermal burn to skin (inadequate conduction).
2   Myocardial injury to epicardial and subepicardial tissue (repeated shocks).
3   Pacemaker malfunction (avoid area).
4   Post-cardioversion arrhythmia.
5   Excessive sedation with respiratory depression or hypotension.

PERICARDIAL ASPIRATION

INDICATIONS

1 Cardiac tamponade.

CONTRAINDICATIONS

1 Absolute: none in the critically unstable patient.

2 Relative: uncontrolled bleeding diathesis, lack of experience, delaying emergency thoracotomy in traumatic tamponade (preferred option).

TECHNIQUE

1 Insert a 14-gauge i.v. cannula connected to a 20 mL syringe just below the xiphisternum to the left of the mid-line.

2 Place at 30–45° angle, aiming for the tip of the left scapula, aspirating as the needle is advanced (see Fig. 18.2).

3 Monitor the ECG looking for ectopic beats or change in morphology suggesting the needle has contacted the myocardium. If this occurs, withdraw slightly until the injury pattern resolves.

4 Advance slowly until the pericardial sac is reached. A 'giving' sensation suggests penetration of the pericardium.

5 Aspirate fluid or blood from the pericardial space. Withdrawal of just 20–30 mL can dramatically improve the patient's haemodynamic status.

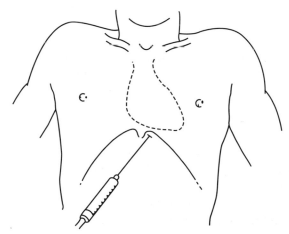

Figure 18.2 Pericardial aspiration.

6 Use of the Seldinger technique allows a pig-tail catheter to be inserted for further fluid removal.

7 Monitor the patient for recurrent tamponade, which may result from catheter blockage or fluid reaccumulation.

COMPLICATIONS

1 Myocardial damage, coronary artery laceration and cardiac arrhythmias.

2 Pneumothorax.

3 Hepatic injury.

CENTRAL LINE INSERTION

INDICATIONS

1 Inability to obtain timely/adequate peripheral IV access in critically unwell patient.

2 Intravenous administration of certain drugs (e.g. adrenaline [epinephrine], noradrenaline [norepinephrine]).

3 Central venous pressure monitoring in critically unwell patient.

4 Large-bore i.v. access for rapid volume resuscitation (or haemodialysis/plasmapheresis).

5 Hyperalimentation such as total parenteral nutrition (TPN) administration.

6 Long-term chemotherapy/antibiotics (e.g. Hickman's line).

CONTRAINDICATIONS

1 Uncooperative patient.

2 Less invasive form of i.v. access possible and adequate.

3 Overlying skin cellulitis or burn.

4 Pneumothorax on opposite side (particularly subclavian insertion – use same side).

5 Uncorrected bleeding diathesis (particularly subclavian line, as not able to compress).

TECHNIQUE

1 Common sites are the internal jugular vein (IJV), subclavian vein (SCV) and femoral vein. All are all located close to arteries and nerves that may be damaged by a misplaced needle.

    (i) In addition the SCV lies near the pleura of the lung with a greater risk of pneumothorax.

2 Similar basic principles, techniques and equipment are required for each site. Specific anatomical considerations and complications for each site are described below (see Fig. 18.3).

3 Position the patient for the route chosen and identify the anatomical landmarks, then use ultrasound guidance to direct needle insertion and direction.

4 Wash hands well and wear sterile gown and gloves. Use strict aseptic technique to prepare and check central line equipment, in particular that the guidewire passes through the large-bore needle.

5 Draw up 10 mL normal saline and prime the central line ports and tubing.

6 Clean a wide area of skin around the insertion site with chlorhexidine and cover the sterile area with a large fenestrated drape.

7 Infiltrate the skin and deeper tissues with 5 mL 1% lignocaine (lidocaine). Work around the site and towards the vein drawing back on the syringe plunger prior to injecting each time, to ensure that the vein has not been penetrated.

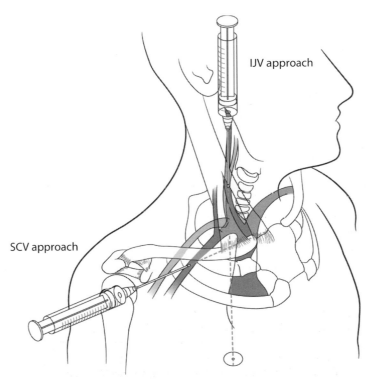

Figure 18.3 Central line insertion.

8   IJV insertion

   (i)   Turn the patient's head 30–60° to the contralateral side to improve access to the IJV, but avoid turning the head too far laterally, as this increases the risk of arterial puncture.

   (ii)   Stand at the head of the patient and palpate the carotid artery at the level of the cricoid cartilage, at the apex of the triangle formed by the heads of the sternocleidomastoid.

   (iii) Keeping a finger over the artery, insert the needle bevel up at an angle of 30–40° one finger-breadth lateral to the artery. Aim for the ipsilateral nipple in men and the ipsilateral anterior superior iliac spine in women.

   (iv)   Always direct the needle away from the artery and keep the artery guarded under your finger. The vein is usually only 2–3 cm under the skin, so if the vein is not entered, re-direct the needle tip more laterally under ultrasound guidance.

9   SCV insertion

   (i)   Turn the head away from the side to be cannulated. Normally, the right subclavian is cannulated, as the thoracic duct is on the left and may occasionally be damaged during cannulation, resulting in a chylothorax.

   (ii)   Improve access to the vein by caudal traction on the ipsilateral arm, or by placing a roll under the ipsilateral shoulder.

   (iii) Stand beside the patient on the side to be cannulated. Identify the mid-clavicular point and the sternal notch. Insert the needle through the skin 1 cm below and lateral to the mid-clavicular point.

   (iv)   Keeping the needle horizontal, advance just under the clavicle aiming for the sternal notch. If the needle hits the clavicle 'walk off the bone' moving inferiorly, and direct slightly deeper to pass beneath it under ultrasound guidance.

   (v)   Do not pass the needle further than the sternal head of the clavicle.

10   Femoral vein insertion

   (i)   Palpate the femoral artery two finger-breadths below the inguinal ligament using the non-dominant hand.

   (ii)   Insert the needle, bevel up, one finger-breadth medial to the femoral pulse and aim towards the umbilicus at an angle of 20–30° to the skin. In adults, the vein is normally found 2–4 cm beneath the skin

          (a) reduce the elevation on the needle to 10–15° in small children as the vein lies more superficial.

   (iii) Keep a finger over the artery during the procedure to reduce the risk of arterial puncture. The right leg is therefore easier to access for the right-handed operator.

11 Use a 10 mL syringe with large-bore insertion needle attached and aspirate gently until the vein is entered.

12 Once blood is aspirated, remove the syringe and thread guidewire through the needle and into the vein. The wire should advance easily and needs no force.

    (i) Do not over-insert or force the wire, as it may cause cardiac arrhythmias (with SCV and IJV), kink or even perforate the vessel wall.

13 Use one hand to secure the guidewire and remove the needle. Make a 2–3 mm skin incision where the wire penetrates the skin and thread the dilator over the wire and into the vein with a light twisting motion. Push it firmly through the skin as far as it will go.

14 Remove the dilator, being careful not to dislodge the guidewire, and thread the central venous catheter (CVC) over the guidewire towards the skin. Hold the catheter steady when the tip is 2 cm above the surface of the skin, and slowly reverse the guidewire up the catheter tube away from the patient, until the wire tip appears from the line port (i.e. the central port).

15 Holding the proximal portion of the wire protruding from the catheter port, advance the catheter through the skin, over the wire and into the vein. Do not allow the wire to be pushed further into the vein while advancing the catheter.

16 Withdraw the wire and close off the insertion port. Check that blood can be aspirated freely from all lumens of the catheter and then flush with saline.

17 Secure the catheter in place with sutures and cover with a sterile dressing. Tape any redundant tubing, carefully avoiding kinking or loops that may snag and pull the catheter out.

18 With IJV and subclavian lines, order a CXR to confirm the position of the catheter tip and to exclude a pneumo- or haemothorax.

    (i) The tip of the central venous pressure (CVP) line should lie in the superior vena cava just above its junction with the right atrium, around the level of the carina.

COMPLICATIONS

1 *Immediate (early)*

    (i) Arterial dissection, laceration or false aneurysm:
        (a) less likely with subclavian route than IJV or femoral route
        (b) but haemorrhage from the femoral or carotid much easier to control than from the subclavian artery.

    (ii) Route-specific injury:
        (a) pneumothorax, haemothorax and cardiac arrhythmia (SCV, IJV)
        (b) malposition of subclavian vein catheter, which may ascend into the IJV or cross the midline horizontally.

    (iii) Air embolism.

    (iv) Loss of guidewire.

2 Delayed (late)

   (i)   Local infection – more common with femoral access than with SCV and IJV.
   (ii) Systemic infection – bacteremia, endocarditis. More common with femoral than IJV and SCV.
   (iii) Venous thrombosis – incidence up to 10–25% for femoral catheter left *in situ* >24 h.
   (iv) Cardiac tamponade and hydrothorax.

INTRAOSSEOUS LINE INSERTION

INDICATIONS

1 Alternative access in emergent or resuscitative situation, when peripheral i.v. access fails or will take over 60 s in child.

2 Immediate venous access for administering drugs, fluids or blood products, particularly in child aged 0–7 years, including neonates.

3 Access in adults when i.v. insertion is impossible, or delayed.

CONTRAINDICATIONS

1 Open fracture, local skin infection or osteomyelitis at proposed insertion site.

2 Femoral fracture on ipsilateral side.

TECHNIQUE

1 Infiltrate the skin surface and periosteum with 1 mL of 1% lignocaine (lidocaine) using a 25-gauge needle if time permits (not necessary in coma).

2 Position the limb:
   (i)   Flex the knee to 45° and support with a sandbag or pillow.
   (ii) Locate the tibial tuberosity.
   (iii) Palpate the insertion site 2 cm distal on the anteromedial side in children >1 year of age, 1 cm distal aged 6–12 months, and just distal to the tibial tubercle in neonates (see Fig. 18.4).
   (iv) Fix the limb in position by holding the knee.

3 Grip the stylet ball of the intraosseous needle in the palm of your hand, and place the tip of your index finger 1–1.5 cm from the tip of the needle.

4 Insert the needle at 90° to the skin and in a slightly caudal direction (away from the epiphyseal plate).

5 Advance the needle with a gentle twisting or boring motion, until it gives on entering the marrow cavity, and remove the stylet.

6 Aspirate blood and marrow contents to confirm correct placement, attach IV tubing and secure the needle with sterile gauze and strapping.

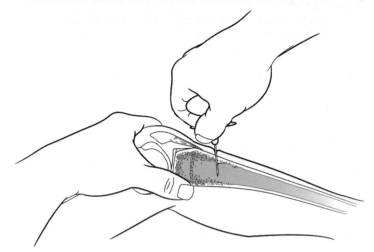

Figure 18.4 Intraosseous line insertion.

7 Alternatively use a semi-automatic, hand-held, intraosseous drill device, available with different age and size-related catheter lengths.

8 Flush each drug with a bolus of normal saline to ensure dispersal beyond the marrow cavity, and to achieve faster central circulation distribution.

COMPLICATIONS

1 Failure – malposition (slips off bone).

2 Through-and-through penetration.

3 Local haematoma.

4 Extravasation, if opposite cortex broached or multiple attempts.

5 Cellulitis at insertion site, or osteomyelitis (rare).

LUMBAR PUNCTURE

INDICATIONS

1 *Diagnostic*
    (i) Analyse cerebrospinal fluid (CSF) in suspected meningitis, subarachnoid haemorrhage (SAH), syndromes such as Guillain–Barré, multiple sclerosis and carcinomatosis.
    (ii) Measure CSF pressure.

2 Therapeutic
    (i)   Removal of CSF in benign intracranial hypertension (pseudotumour cerebri).
    (ii) Blood patch (post-lumbar puncture [LP] headache).
    (iii) Intrathecal administration of medications.

CONTRAINDICATIONS

1   Indicators of raised intracranial pressure (ICP) with or without mass effect such as focal neurological signs, papilloedema, altered conscious level, bradycardia, hypertension and abnormal respiratory pattern (irrespective of what the computed tomography (CT) scan shows).

2   Space-occupying lesion on CT, particularly posterior fossa.

3   Uncorrected bleeding diathesis (in particular platelets <50 or INR >1.5).

4   Local skin infection.

5   Uncooperative patient.

TECHNIQUE

1   Explain the procedure and gain verbal consent. Give 0.05 mg/kg midazolam i.v. if the patient is anxious or unable to lie still for up to 15–30 min.

2   Position the patient. Take your time with this:
    (i)   Lie the patient on a bed/trolley on their left side as close as possible to the right edge of the bed.
    (ii) Ask the patient to flex the hips, knees and neck as much as they can (i.e. fetal position).
    (iii) Keep the back straight with the vertebral column parallel to the edge of the bed, the shoulders square to the hips, and vertical. Place a pillow between the knees to prevent rotation of the pelvis by the upper leg.

3   Determine the site of needle insertion:
    (i)   Palpate the iliac crest and locate the vertebra lying on an imaginary line dropped from it (L4 vertebra).
    (ii) Mark the two spaces above (L 3–4 space) and (L 2–3 space) with a pen cap, or fingernail indent.

4   Use a no-touch, sterile gown-and-glove technique to prepare and drape the site.

5   Anaesthetize the skin using the 25-gauge needle and s.c. infiltration. Then use a 21-gauge needle for deeper infiltration down to the interspinous ligament. Wait 2–3 min for full local anaesthetic effect.

6   Confirm that the stylet releases freely from within the LP needle, then orientate bevel up and at 90° to the skin in all planes, and 5–10° cephalad (i.e. needle tip pointing up to the head). Enter just above the lower vertebral process in the intervertebral space (see Fig. 18.5).

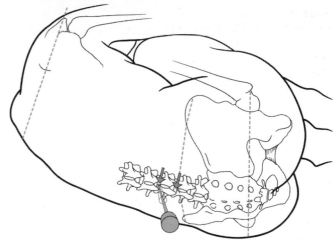

Figure 18.5 Lumbar puncture.

7 Advance the needle through the skin, between the spinous processes aiming towards the patient's umbilicus.

    (i) Stop if bone is contacted, withdraw and re-advance the needle.

    (ii) Feel for increased resistance and then a 'give' as the needle passes through the interspinous ligament then ligamentum flavum.

    (iii) Withdraw the stylet and watch for a 'flashback' of CSF.

    (iv) If there is none, replace the stylet and advance the needle another few millimetres, checking for evidence of CSF return each time.

8 Once in the subarachnoid space and CSF is draining, remove the stylet fully and attach the manometer.

    (i) Measure the CSF pressure (normal opening pressure is 6–18 cm H_2O).

9 Disconnect the manometer and catch CSF from the open end of the spinal needle.

    (i) Collect 10–20 drops into each of three specimen containers. Label them 1, 2, and 3.

10 Send CSF to laboratory for cell count with differential, Gram stain plus culture for bacteriology, sugar and protein content, polymerase chain reaction (PCR) testing (meningitis/encephalitis), xanthochromia (subarachnoid haemorrhage) and cytology (carcinoma suspected).

11 Re-insert the stylet to reduce post-LP headache risk, then slowly remove the entire spinal needle.

    (i) Place a small dressing or plaster over the puncture site.

12 Advise the patient to initially lie prone (on his or her stomach) to reduce CSF leak by gravity.

COMPLICATIONS

1 Post-LP headache (up to 20% or more).
2 Failure (may need CT or fluoroscopy guidance).
3 Bloody tap.
4 Epidural haematoma, with signs of acute spinal cord compression.
5 Local skin haemorrhage, pain.
6 Infection (rare): meningitis, epidural abscess.

INDWELLING URETHRAL CATHETER INSERTION

INDICATIONS

1 *Continuous*
    (i) Acute or chronic urinary retention.
    (ii) Measurement of urine output (e.g. volume resuscitation, shock therapy, fluid balance).
    (iii) Short term (e.g. post-operatively) or long term (e.g. when transurethral resection of the prostate [TURP] is medically contraindicated).

2 *Intermittent*
    (i) Obtaining uncontaminated urine for microscopy and culture (especially in females or young children).
    (ii) Facilitating adequate bladder emptying (e.g. in conditions associated with atonic bladder).
    (iii) Intravesical installation of contrast or drugs (e.g. in suspected bladder trauma).

CONTRAINDICATIONS

1 Traumatic urethral rupture suggested by penile, scrotal or perineal haematoma, blood at the urethral meatus and a high-riding prostate on rectal examination.
2 Postoperative urological patient or patient with known urethral stricture.
    (i) Consult the urologist first if the patient has had bladder neck or prostate surgery.

TECHNIQUE

1 Perform thorough aseptic hand wash and put on sterile gloves. Draw up sterile water for balloon inflation and place fenestrated drape over the patient's perineum.

2   Open the catheter wrapping at the distal (tip) end and, holding the proximal portion (still in the wrapping), lubricate the catheter tip with lignocaine (lidocaine) gel 2%.

  (i) *Male catheterization*

    (a) retract the patient's foreskin and swab the urethral meatus and glans with sterile gauze soaked in saline. Hold the penis firmly and in an upright position and instil lignocaine (lidocaine) gel 2% into the urethra

    (b) gently squeeze the tip of the glans to close off the urethra to retain the gel for 90 s to allow the anaesthetic time to work

    (c) insert the catheter gently and slowly into the urethra, withdrawing the plastic covering in stages

    (d) advance catheter to the hilt and wait for urine to flow

    (e) replace the foreskin.

  (ii) *Female catheterization*

    (a) position the patient as for a vaginal examination, supine with knees and hips flexed and ankles together. Allow the legs to rest gently in full abduction

    (b) use non-dominant gloved hand to gently separate labia minora and clean the area with saline. The hand holding the labia must be kept in place until catheter is successfully inserted and urine flows

    (c) locate the urethral opening (inferior to the clitoris, but may still be difficult to define), and swab anterior to posterior with cleaning solution

    (d) instil a small amount of lignocaine (lidocaine) gel into the tip of the urethral meatus and introduce well-lubricated catheter along urethra until urine flows.

3   Inflate the balloon with 10 mL sterile water (or as indicated on the catheter). Stop immediately if the patient experiences pain, as catheter may have become malpositioned within urethra (particularly in a male).

4   Once balloon is inflated, gently retract the catheter until resistance is felt.

5   Connect bag aseptically to catheter.

COMPLICATIONS

1   Inability to pass catheter. Do not persist with multiple attempts at catheterization, but consult urology early for consideration of suprapubic catheterization.

2   Urethral trauma, e.g. creation of a false passage.

3   Paraphimosis from failure to replace foreskin.

4   Introduction of infection, bacteraemia.

NASOGASTRIC TUBE INSERTION

INDICATIONS

1 Aspiration of stomach contents to decompress the stomach of fluid, air or occasionally blood.

2 Reduce risk of vomiting or aspiration, such as in bowel obstruction or acute gastric dilatation.

3 Introducing liquids to the stomach such as charcoal, oral contrast media or enteral feed.

CONTRAINDICATIONS

1 Base of skull fracture or severe mid-face trauma.

2 Caustic ingestion or known oesophageal stricture (risk of perforation).

TECHNIQUE

1 Explain to the patient exactly what you are about to do, and why.

2 Assess the patient's ability to swallow and the patency of either nostril and sit the patient upright with neck slightly flexed.

3 Measure the required length of tube: from nose to earlobe, then earlobe to xiphoid process and add 15 cm.

4 Cover the tip of the nasogastric tube with lubricating jelly and insert into the largest patent nostril horizontally and backwards, at a right angle to the face (under the inferior turbinate). Do **not** pass upwards towards the nasal bridge.

5 Gently advance the tube past the naso- and oropharynx to the pre-selected distance. Ask the patient to swallow when the tube is felt at the back of the mouth and, as the patient swallows, carefully push the tube down further.
    (i) A sip of water may assist the patient in swallowing.

6 Check that the tube is positioned correctly:
    (i) Aspirate slowly on the tube using a 50 mL syringe. Then test syringe contents with blue litmus paper (as gastric contents are acid they will turn blue litmus paper red).
    (ii) Rapidly inject 20 mL of air into the tube while auscultating over the left hypochondrium. Listen for 'bubbling' over the stomach (correct position).
    (iii) Request a CXR. Look for the path of the tube and trace its course below the diaphragm, and deviation to the left into the gastric area. Make sure it is **not** entering the chest or coiled up in the oesophagus.

7 Attach the drainage bag and secure the nasogastric tube to the tip of the nose with non-allergenic tape, taking care to avoid pressure on the medial or lateral nares.

COMPLICATIONS

1 Failure to pass – can be distressing for patient who may not wish to continue.

2 Misplacement, such as inadvertent tracheal placement, or curled back on itself in the oesophagus or hypopharynx.

3 Epistaxis (turbinate trauma).

4 Oesophageal trauma or penetration.

5 Intracranial penetration – should never happen if the procedure is avoided in midface or basal skull trauma.

BIER'S INTRAVENOUS REGIONAL BLOCK

INDICATIONS

1 Anaesthesia for the reduction of distal forearm fractures.

CONTRAINDICATIONS

1 Inability to site i.v. cannula in injured-side hand (cannot proceed).

2 Peripheral vascular disease, Raynaud's phenomenon or local sepsis.

3 Hypertension with systolic blood pressure >200 mmHg, uncooperative patient (including children who will not tolerate cuff pressure).

4 Local anaesthetic sensitivity (rare), homozygous sickle cell disease (also rare).

5 Relative: patients who have sustained a crush injury of the limb, as potentially viable tissue will be subjected to a further period of hypoxia.

TECHNIQUE

1 Two doctors are required, one with anaesthetic experience and previous training in the procedure to perform the block, and the other to perform the manipulation.

    (i)   At least one nurse attends to the patient, checks the blood pressure and assists the doctors.

2 Explain the technique to the patient, who should sign a written consent form.

3 ECG and blood pressure monitoring must be available in an area with full resuscitation facilities and a tipping trolley. Ideally the patient should be starved for 4 h before the procedure.

4   Use a specifically designed and properly maintained Bier's block cuff, and check first for leaks or malfunction. Apply the cuff to the upper arm over cotton-wool padding.

5   Insert a small i.v. cannula into the dorsum of the hand on the affected side and a second cannula into the other hand or wrist.

6   Elevate the affected arm for 2–3 min to empty the veins in preference to using an Esmarch bandage, which is generally too painful.

7   Inflate the cuff to 100 mmHg above systolic blood pressure, keeping the arm elevated, but to no more than 300 mmHg. The radial pulse should no longer be palpable and the veins should remain empty.

8   Lower the arm and slowly inject 0.5% prilocaine 2.5 mg/kg (0.5 mL/kg) and make a note of the time of injection.

9   Continuously monitor the cuff pressure for leakage. Keep the cuff inflated for a minimum of 20 min to ensure the prilocaine is fully tissue bound, and for a maximum of 45 min (usually not tolerated longer).

10   Wait at least 5 min before performing the manipulation after confirming the adequacy of the block. Request a check X-ray and repeat the manipulation immediately if reduction is unsatisfactory.

11   If satisfactory, deflate the cuff then re-inflate for 2 min observing for signs of local anaesthetic toxicity, although, as the maximum safe dosage of prilocaine is 6 mg/kg (over double the amount used in the block), toxicity is rare.

COMPLICATIONS

1   Local anaesthetic toxicity from cuff failure – **never** use bupivacaine.

2   Transient peripheral nerve neurapraxia.

FEMORAL NERVE BLOCK

INDICATIONS

1   Analgesia for femoral shaft fracture, particularly prior to dynamic splintage.

2   Analgesia for femoral neck fracture, particularly if significant quadriceps spasm.

3   Analgesia for surgery on the anterior thigh, knee, quadriceps.

4   Postoperative pain management after femur and knee surgery.

CONTRAINDICATIONS

1   Local infection.

2   Femoral vascular graft (relative).

TECHNIQUE

1 Use either 0.5% bupivacaine 10 mL (total of 50 mg: maximum safe dosage 2 mg/kg), or 1% lignocaine (lidocaine) 10 mL (total of 100 mg: maximum safe dosage 3 mg/kg).

2 Palpate the femoral artery and insert a 21-gauge needle with syringe perpendicular to the skin, lateral to the artery and just below the inguinal ligament (see Fig. 18.6).

3 Withdraw slightly if paraesthesiae are elicited down the leg, indicating proximity of the needle to the femoral nerve.

    (i) Aspirate to exclude vessel puncture, and inject 10 mL of the local anaesthetic.

4 Alternatively, a characteristic loss of resistance may be felt as the needle passes through the fascia lata then fascia iliaca:

    (i) Aspirate to exclude vessel puncture.

    (ii) Inject 10 mL of local anaesthetic solution fan-wise, moving outwards up to 3 cm lateral to the artery.

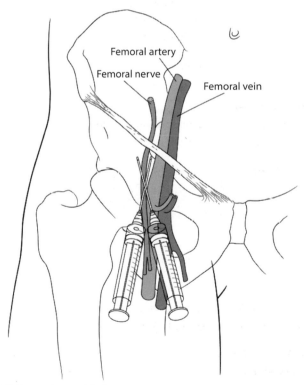

Figure 18.6 Femoral nerve block.

COMPLICATIONS

1 Femoral artery puncture – avoid by never redirecting the needle medially.

2 Injury to the femoral nerve.

3 Infection.

DIGITAL NERVE RING BLOCK

INDICATIONS

1 Laceration of digit (fingers, thumb or toes).

2 Dislocation or fracture relocation.

3 Management of nail injury/removal.

CONTRAINDICATIONS

1 Peripheral vascular disease.

2 Raynaud's phenomenon.

3 Local sepsis at the base of the digit.

TECHNIQUE

1 Document a neurological examination *prior* to the procedure.

2 Use 2% plain lignocaine (lidocaine) without adrenaline (epinephrine).

    (i) Do not use a tourniquet due to the risk of creating high pressures locally and occluding the digital vessels.

    (ii) Clean the base of the finger first with antiseptic.

    (iii) Insert a 25-gauge orange needle into the side of the base of the digit, and angle at 45° from the vertical injecting up to 1.5 mL of 2% plain lignocaine (lidocaine) without adrenaline (epinephrine) into the lateral palmar (plantar) aspect of the digit (see Fig. 18.7).

    (iv) Remove the needle until subcutaneous, and rotate until it is pointing to the extensor surface of the digit. Inject 0.5 mL into the lateral extensor (dorsal) aspect of the digit.

    (v) Perform the same procedure on the other side of the digit.

    (vi) Allow at least 5–10 min for the ring block to take effect.

COMPLICATIONS

1 Infection.

2 Digital nerve injury.

3 Haematoma or vascular insufficiency/gangrene of the digit.

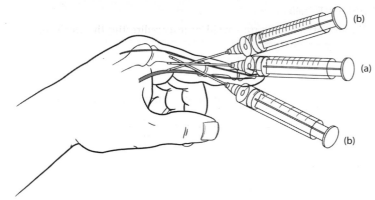

Figure 18.7 Digital nerve block.
(a) Site of needle insertion. **(b)** Sites of anaesthetic injection.

KNEE ASPIRATION

INDICATIONS

1 *Diagnostic*

    (i)   Remove joint fluid for biochemical testing including microbiology, cytology and polarizing light microscopy, to differentiate a septic arthritis from an inflammatory (gouty) or bloody (haemarthrosis) effusion.

2 *Therapeutic*

    (i)   Remove excess fluid or blood from the joint to provide symptomatic relief, increase mobility and decrease pain in a large effusion, crystal-induced arthropathy or haemarthrosis.

    (ii) Intra-articular steroid injection (first discuss with orthopaedics or rheumatology consultant).

CONTRAINDICATIONS

1   Local skin cellulitis/infection.

2   Acute fracture or joint prosthesis (may introduce infection).

3   Uncorrected bleeding diathesis (in particular platelets <50 or INR >1.5).

4   Uncooperative patient.

TECHNIQUE

1   Explain the procedure to the patient and position the patient comfortably on the bed, with the affected joint fully exposed.

2   Use a strict aseptic technique. Clean the skin with chlorhexidine and inject 2% lignocaine (lidocaine) 2–3 mL into the skin, subcutaneous tissue and synovium.

3   Insert a large-bore, 14-gauge cannula at the mid-point of the superior portion of the patella 1 cm lateral to the anterolateral edge (see Fig. 18.8).

4   Aim the cannula between the posterior surface of the patella and the intercondylar femoral notch.

5   **Diagnostic tap**
    (i)   Aspirate 15–20 mL fluid from the joint, and then withdraw the syringe and needle.
    (ii) Transfer 5 mL of fluid into each of the three sterile containers, and label for biochemical testing including polarizing light microscopy, microbiology and cytology.

6   **Therapeutic tap**
    (i)   Withdraw the needle and attach a 20 mL syringe with three-way tap to the remaining catheter.
    (ii) Do not apply too great a negative pressure on the syringe, as it will cause the local tissues to occlude the cannula.
    (iii) Remove all available fluid – this may be up to 70 mL or more
          (a) gently squeeze the suprapatellar region to 'milk' any residual fluid.
    (iv) Look for evidence of fat globules floating on the surface of blood dispelled into a kidney dish from a haemarthrosis, which would indicate an intra-articular fracture.

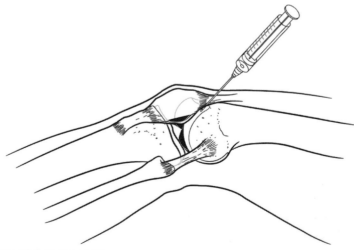

Figure 18.8 Knee aspiration.

COMPLICATIONS

1 Joint infection — poor aseptic technique may rarely result in septic arthritis.

2 Local haematoma, haemarthrosis.

3 Synovial fistula.

FURTHER READING

Roberts JR (2014) *Roberts & Hedges' Clinical Procedures in Emergency Medicine*, 6th edn. Elsevier, New York.

GLOSSARY

AAA	abdominal aortic aneurysm
ABG	arterial blood gas
AC	alternating current
ACE	angiotensin-converting enzyme
ACL	anterior cruciate ligament
ACS	acute coronary syndrome
ACTH	adrenocorticotrophic hormone
ADT	adsorbed diphtheria and tetanus toxoid
AED	automatic external defibrillator
AF	atrial fibrillation
AIDS	acquired immune deficiency syndrome
AION	anterior ischaemic optic neuropathy
ALP	alkaline phosphatase
ALS	advanced life support
ALT	alanine aminotransferase
AMPLE	allergies, medications, past history, last meal, events preceding present injury
ANA	antinuclear antibody
anti-CCP	anticyclic citrullinated peptide
AP	anteroposterior
APTT	activated partial thromboplastin time
ARDS	acute respiratory distress syndrome
AST	aspartate aminotransferase
ATLS	Advanced Trauma Life Support
ATN	acute tubular necrosis
AV	atrioventricular
b.d.	*bis die* (twice daily)
BLS	basic life support
BNF	*British National Formulary*
BP	blood pressure
BSA	body surface area
BURP	backwards upwards rightward pressure
C1/C7	first and seventh cervical vertebrae
C7/T1	seventh cervical and first thoracic vertebrae
CABG	coronary artery bypass graft
CAD	coronary artery disease

CAGE	cut down, annoyed, guilty, eye-opener
CAP	community-acquired pneumonia
CBR	chemical, biological, radiological
CCB	calcium-channel blocker
CCU	coronary care unit
CD4+	cluster designation (of antigen) 4+
CDAD	*Clostridium difficile* antibiotic-related diarrhoea
CDC	Centers for Disease Control and Prevention
CHS	classic heat stroke
CK	creatine kinase
CK-MB	creatine kinase MB isoenzymes
Cl	chloride
CLD	chronic lung disease
CLL	chronic lymphatic leukaemia
CMV	cytomegalovirus
CNS	central nervous system
CO_2	carbon dioxide
COPD	chronic obstructive pulmonary disease
CPAP	continuous positive airways pressure
CPR	cardiopulmonary resuscitation
CPU	chest pain unit
CRF	chronic renal failure
CRP	C-reactive protein
CSF	cerebrospinal fluid
CSM	carotid sinus massage
CSU	catheter specimen of urine
CT	computed (axial) tomography
CTG	cardiotocograph
cTnI	cardiac troponin I
cTnT	cardiac troponin T
CTPA	computed tomography pulmonary angiogram
CVA	cerebrovascular accident
CVC	central venous catheter
CVP	central venous pressure
CXR	chest X-ray
D&C	dilation and curettage
DBP	diastolic blood pressure
DC	direct current
DCI	decompression illness
DHF	dengue haemorrhagic fever
DIC	disseminated intravascular coagulation
DKA	diabetic ketoacidosis
DNA	deoxyribonucleic acid
DNW	did not wait

DPL	diagnostic peritoneal lavage
DU	duodenal ulcer
DVT	deep vein thrombosis
EBV	Epstein–Barr virus
ECC	Emergency Cardiovascular Care
ECG	electrocardiogram
ED	emergency department
EEG	electroencephalograph
EHS	exertion heat stroke
ELFTs	electrolytes and liver function tests
ELISA	enzyme-linked immunosorbent assay
EMD	electromechanical dissociation
EMST	Early Management of Severe Trauma
ENT	ear, nose and throat
EPEU	early pregnancy evaluation unit
ERC	European Resuscitation Council
ERCP	endoscopic retrograde cholangiopancreatography
ERPC	evacuation of retained products of conception
ESR	erythrocyte sedimentation rate
EST	exercise stress test
ET	endotracheal
FAST	focused assessment by sonography for trauma/focused abdominal sonogram for trauma
FBC	full blood count
FEV_1	forced expiratory volume in 1 second
FiO_2	fractional inspired oxygen concentration
G&S	group and save (blood)
GA	general anaesthesia
GCS	Glasgow Coma Scale
GFR	glomerular filtration rate
GI	gastrointestinal
GP	general practitioner
GTN	glyceryl trinitrate
GU	gastric ulcer
h	hour
H_1/H_2	histamine type 1 and type 2
HAART	highly active anti-retroviral therapy
HAZMAT	hazardous materials
Hb	haemoglobin
HBIG	hepatitis B immune globulin
HBO	hyperbaric oxygen
HBsAg	hepatitis B surface antigen
HCG	human chorionic gonadotrophin
HCO_3	bicarbonate

Hct	haematocrit
HDL	high density lipoprotein
HDU	high-dependency unit
HELLP	haemolysis, elevated liver enzymes, low platelets
HHS	hyperosmolar, hyperglycaemic state
HIV	human immunodeficiency virus
HLA	human leucocyte antigen
HRIG	human rabies immunoglobulin
HSV	herpes simplex virus
HTIG	human tetanus immunoglobulin
HUS	haemolytic-uraemic syndrome
i.m.	intramuscular
i.o.	intraosseous
i.v.	intravenous
ICC	intercostal catheter
ICS	intercostal space
ICU	intensive care unit
IDC	indwelling catheter
Ig	immunoglobulin
ILCOR	International Liaison Committee on Resuscitation
INR	international normalized ratio (of prothrombin time)
ITP	idiopathic thrombocytopenic purpura
IU	international units
IUCD	intrauterine contraceptive device
IVP	intravenous pyelogram
J	joule
JVP	jugular venous pressure
K	potassium
KCl	potassium chloride
kPa	kilopascal
KUB	kidneys, ureters, bladder
LBBB	left bundle branch block
LDL	low-density lipoprotein
LFT	liver function test
LMW	low-molecular-weight
LP	lumbar puncture
MAP	mean arterial pressure
M,C&S	microscopy, culture and sensitivity
MCP	metacarpophalangeal
MDAC	multiple-dose activated charcoal
MDI	metered-dose inhaler
MDO	medical defence organization
mEq/L	milliequivalents per litre
MHA	Mental Health Act

MHS	malignant hyperthermia syndrome
MI	myocardial infarction
min	minute
mmHg	millimetres of mercury
MMSE	Mini-Mental State Examination
MOF	multi-organ failure
MRSA	methicillin (meticillin)-resistant *Staphylococcus aureus*
MSA	multiple systems atrophy
MSU	midstream urine
mth	month
MTP	metatarsophalangeal
Mu	megaunit
Na	sodium
NAA	nucleic acid amplification
NAC	*N*-acetylcysteine
NAI	non-accidental injury
NAIR	National Arrangements for Incidents involving Radioactivity
NAPCAN	National Association for Prevention of Child Abuse and Neglect
NGT	nasogastric tube
NIH	National Institutes of Health
NIV	non-invasive ventilation
NMS	neuroleptic malignant syndrome
NOAC	new oral anticoagulant/novel oral anticoagulant
NPA	nasopharyngeal aspirate
NSAID	non-steroidal anti-inflammatory drug
NSPCC	National Society for the Prevention of Cruelty to Children
NSTEMI	non-ST elevation myocardial infarction
NTS	nose/throat swab
NZ	New Zealand
O&G	obstetrics and gynaecology
OM	occipitomental
OPG	orthopantomogram
ORS	oral rehydration solution
p.r.	per rectum
$PaCO_2$	partial pressure of carbon dioxide (arterial)
PaO_2	partial pressure of oxygen (arterial)
PBI	pressure bandage with immobilization
PCI	percutaneous coronary intervention (coronary angioplasty)
PCP	*Pneumocystis carinii* pneumonia
PCR	polymerase chain reaction
PCV	packed cell volume
PE	pulmonary embolus
PEA	pulseless electrical activity
PEF	peak expiratory flow

PEP	post-exposure prophylaxis
PGL	persistent generalized lymphadenopathy
pH	negative logarithm of the hydrogen ion concentration
PID	pelvic inflammatory disease
PMR	polymyalgia rheumatica
PND	paroxysmal nocturnal dyspnoea
PPE	personal protective equipment
PTA	post-traumatic amnesia
PTI	prothrombin index
q.d.s.	*quater in die sumendus* (four times daily)
RAPD	relative afferent pupil defect (Marcus Gunn pupil)
RBBB	right bundle branch block
RhD	rhesus blood group D antigen
RNA	ribonucleic acid
ROSC	return of spontaneous circulation
r-PA	recombinant plasminogen activator
RSI	rapid sequence induction
rt-PA	recombinant tissue-type plasminogen activator
RV	right ventricular
s	second
s.c.	subcutaneous
SAH	subarachnoid haemorrhage
SaO_2	arterial oxygen saturation
SARS	severe acute respiratory syndrome
SBP	systolic blood pressure
SCBU	special care baby unit
SCIWORA	spinal cord injury without radiological abnormality
SIADH	syndrome of inappropriate antidiuretic hormone secretion
SIDS	sudden infant death syndrome
SIRS	systemic inflammatory response syndrome
SJS	Stevens–Johnson syndrome
SLE	systemic lupus erythematosus
SLR	straight-leg raising
SNP	sodium nitroprusside
SOMANZ	Society of Obstetric Medicine of Australia and New Zealand
SPA	suprapubic aspirate (urine)
SR	sustained release
SS	serotonin syndrome
SSRI	selective serotonin reuptake inhibitor
STD	sexually transmitted disease
STEMI	ST elevation myocardial infarction
SUDI	sudden unexpected death in infancy
SUFE	slipped upper femoral epiphysis
SVT	supraventricular tachycardia

t.d.s.	*ter in die sumendus* (three times daily)
TA	transabdominal
TB	tuberculosis
TCA	tricyclic antidepressant
TEN	toxic epidermal necrolysis
TIA	transient ischaemic attack
TNK	tenecteplase
TTP	thrombotic thrombocytopenic purpura
TURP	transurethral resection of the prostate
TV	transvaginal
u	unit
U&Es	urea and electrolytes
UA	unstable angina
UF	unfractionated (heparin)
UTI	urinary tract infection
V/Q	ventilation perfusion (lung scan)
VBG	venous blood gas
VDK	venom detection kit
VEB	ventricular ectopic beat (extrasystole)
VF	ventricular fibrillation
VICC	venom-induced consumption coagulopathy
VT	ventricular tachycardia
VTE	venous thromboembolism
WBC	white blood cells
WBI	whole bowel irrigation
WCC	white cell count
yr	year

Appendix

NORMAL LABORATORY VALUES

LABORATORY REFERENCE RANGES

Ranges below are the approximate 95% confidence limits for laboratory reference values in healthy adult males and females.

Test results can vary depending on measurement conditions and the laboratory methods utilized.

Therefore, always interpret results using the local testing laboratory's quoted reference ranges.

Seek senior doctor advice if in doubt.

HAEMATOLOGY

haemoglobin	females: 115–165 g/L
	males: 130–180 g/L
erythrocytes	females: $3.8-5.8 \times 3\ 10^{12}$ /L
	males: $4.5-6.5 \times 10^{12}$ /L
haematocrit (packed cell volume)	females: 0.37–0.47
	males: 0.4–0.54
mean corpuscular volume	80–100 fL
leucocytes (white cells)	$4-11 \times 10^9$ /L
neutrophils	$2-7.5 \times 10^9$ /L (40–75%)
lymphocytes	$1.5-4 \times 10^9$ /L (20–40%)
monocytes	$0.2-0.8 \times 10^9$ /L (2–10%)
eosinophils	$0.04-0.4 \times 10^9$ /L (1–6%)
basophils	$<0.1 \times 10^9$ /L (<1%)
platelets	$150-400 \times 10^9$ /L
erythrocyte sedimentation rate (Westergren method)	females:
	under 50 years: <20 mm/h
	over 50 years: <30 mm/h
	males:
	under 50 years: <15 mm/h
	over 50 years: <20 mm/h
vitamin B_{12}	120–680 picomol/L
folate	red cell: 360–1400 nanomol/L
	serum: 7–45 nanomol/L
iron	10–30 micromol/L

ferritin	females: 15–200 micrograms/L
	males: 30–300 micrograms/L
transferrin saturation	15–45%

ELECTROLYTES, GLUCOSE

sodium	135–145 mmol/L
potassium	plasma: 3.4–4.5 mmol/L
	serum: 3.8–4.9 mmol/L
chloride	95–110 mmol/L
bicarbonate	22–32 mmol/L
urea	3–8 mmol/L
creatinine	females: 50–110 micromol/L
	males: 60–120 micromol/L
glucose	fasting: 3–5.4 mmol/L
	random: 3–7.7 mmol/L
calcium	ionised: 1.16–1.3 mmol/L
	total: 2.1–2.6 mmol/L
magnesium	0.8–1 mmol/L
phosphate	0.8–1.5 mmol/L
urate	females: 0.15–0.4 mmol/L
	males: 0.2–0.45 mmol/L
osmolality	280–300 mosmol/kg

PROTEINS

albumin	32–45 g/L (age variable)
protein (total)	62–80 g/L
bilirubin (total)	<20 micromol/L
bilirubin (conj)	<4 micromol/L

ENZYMES

GGT	females: <30 units/L
	males: <50 units/L
ALP (non-pregnant)	25–100 units/L
ALT	<35 units/L
AST	<40 units/L
lactate dehydrogenase	110–230 units/L
creatine kinase	females: 30–180 units/L
	males: 60–220 units/L
lipase	<70 U/L
amylase	0–180 Somogyi U/dL

LIPIDS

triglycerides (fasting)	<1.7 mmol/L
cholesterol (total)	<5.5 mmol/L

HDL	males: 0.9–2.0 mmol/L
	females: 1–2.2 mmol/L
LDL	2–3.4 mmol/L

ARTERIAL BLOOD GASES

pH	7.35–7.45
PaO_2	80–100 mmHg (10.6–13.3 kPa)
$PaCO_2$	35–45 mmHg (4.7–6.0 kPa)
bicarbonate	22–26 mmol/L
base excess	±2 mmol/L
anion gap	8–16
A–a gradient	<10 torr

MISCELLANEOUS

lactate	<2.0 mmol/L
CRP	<10 mg/L
free T_4	10–25 picomol/L
thyroid-stimulating hormone	0.4–5 mIU/L

INDEX